a LANGE medical book

THE PATIENT HISTORY

Evidence-Based Approach

Edited by

Lawrence M. Tierney, Jr., MD
Professor of Medicine
University of California, San Francisco
Associate Chief of Medical Service
Veterans Affairs Medical Center
San Francisco, California

Mark C. Henderson, MD
Associate Professor of Clinical Medicine
Vice Chair for Education
Department of Internal Medicine
University of California, Davis School of Medicine
Sacramento, California

Lange Medical Books/McGraw-Hill
Medical Publishing Division

New York   Chicago   San Francisco   Lisbon   London   Madrid   Mexico City   Milan
New Delhi   San Juan   Seoul   Singapore   Sydney   Toronto

12/05 Majors 39.95

 # 26.40

The Patient History: Evidence-Based Approach

234567890 DOC/DOC 098765

ISBN 0-07-140260-8
ISSN 1552-1206

Notice

Medicine is an ever-changing science. As new research and clinical experience broaden our knowledge, changes in treatment and drug therapy are required. The authors and the publisher of this work have checked with sources believed to be reliable in their efforts to provide information that is complete and generally in accord with the standards accepted at the time of publication. However, in view of the possibility of human error or changes in medical sciences, neither the authors nor the publisher nor any other party who has been involved in the preparation or publication of this work warrants that the information contained herein is in every respect accurate or complete, and they disclaim all responsibility for any errors or omissions or for the results obtained from use of the information contained in this work. Readers are encouraged to confirm the information contained herein with other sources. For example and in particular, readers are advised to check the product information sheet included in the package of each drug they plan to administer to be certain that the information contained in this work is accurate and that changes have not been made in the recommended dose or in the contraindications for administration. This recommendation is of particular importance in connection with new or infrequently used drugs.

This book was set in Adobe Garamond by Pine Tree Composition.
The editors were Isabel Nogueira, Harriet Lebowitz, and Mary E. Bele.
The production supervisor was Catherine H. Saggese.
The illustration manager was Maria T. Magtoto.
The text designer was Eve Siegel.
The cover designer was Aimee Nordin.
The index was prepared by Pamela Edwards.
RR Donnelley was printer and binder.

This book is printed on acid-free paper.

For my late brother John, a fisherman,
and for my children, Jessica, Paul, and John.

MCH

Contents

SECTION XIII COMMUNICATING THE HISTORY

Contributors

Associate Editor
Gerald W. Smetana, MD
Associate Professor of Medicine, Harvard Medical
School; Division of General Medicine and Primary
Care, Beth Israel Deaconess Medical Center, Boston,
Massachusetts
gsmetana@bidmc.harvard.edu

Authors
Antonio Anzueto, MD
Professor of Medicine, Division of Pulmonary Diseases
and Critical Care Medicine, The University of Texas
Health Science Center at San Antonio
anzueto@uthscsa.edu
Cough

Kenneth A. Arndt, MD
SkinCare Physicians of Chestnut Hill, Chestnut Hill,
Massachusetts; Clinical Professor, Section of
Dermatologic Surgery and Cutaneous Oncology, Yale
University School of Medicine, New Haven,
Connecticut; Adjunct Professor of Medicine
(Dermatology), Dartmouth Medical School, Hanover,
New Hampshire; Clinical Professor of Dermatology,
Harvard Medical School, Boston, Massachusetts
karndt@skincarephysicians.net
Inflammatory Dermatoses (Rashes)

Paul Aronowitz, MD
Program Director, Internal Medicine Residency,
California Pacific Medical Center; Associate Clinical
Professor of Medicine, Univeristy of California at San
Francisco, San Francisco, California
aronowp@sutterhealth.org
Flank Pain

Jason J.S. Barton, MD, PhD, FRCPC
Associate Professor of Neurology, Harvard Medical
School; Associate Physician of Neurology and
Ophthalmology, Beth Israel Deaconess Medical
Center, Boston, Massachusetts
jbarton@caregroup.harvard.edu
Diplopia

Carol Bates, MD
Primary Care Program Director, Department of
Medicine, Internal Medicine Residency, Beth Israel
Deaconess Medical Center; Associate Professor of
Medicine, Harvard Medical School, Boston,
Massachusetts
cbates@bidmc.harvard.edu
Vaginitis

Thomas E. Baudendistel, MD, FACP
Associate Program Director, Department of Internal
Medicine, California Pacific Medical Center,
San Francisco, California
baudent@sutterhealth.org
Jaundice

John Wolfe Blotzer, MD
Program Director, Department of Medicine, Internal
Medicine Residency, York Hospital, York, Pennsylvania
jblotzer@yorkhospital.edu
Syncope; Shoulder Pain

Alexander R. Carbo, MD
Instructor in Medicine, Harvard Medical School;
Hospitalist, Division of General Medicine, Beth Israel
Deaconess Medical Center, Boston, Massachusetts
acarbo@bidmc.harvard.edu
Diarrhea

Helen K. Chew, MD
Assistant Professor of Internal Medicine; Director,
Clinical Breast Cancer Program, Division of
Hematology and Oncology, University of California,
Davis, Sacramento, California
helen.chew@ucdmc.ucdavis.edu
Breast Complaints

Virginia U. Collier, MD, FACP
Clinical Associate Professor of Medicine, Jefferson
Medical College; Vice Chair and Residency Program
Director, Department of Medicine, Christiana Care
Health System, Newark, Delaware
vcollier@christianacare.org
Hematuria

Michelle V. Conde, MD
Clinical Associate Professor of Medicine, University of
Texas Health Science Center at San Antonio; Audie
Murphy Division, South Texas Veterans Health Care
System, San Antonio, Texas
conde@uthscsa.edu
Dizziness

Michele Coviello, MD
Instructor in Medicine, Harvard Medical School; Beth
Israel Deaconess Medical Center, Boston,
Massachusetts
mcoviell@bidmc.harvard.edu
Vaginitis

Garth Davis, MD
Assistant Professor of Medicine, Division of General
Medicine, University of California, Davis Medical
Center, Sacramento, California
garth.davis@ucdmc.ucdavis.edu
*The Evidence-Based Approach to Clinical Decision
Making; Low Back Pain*

Francesca C. Dwamena, MD
Assistant Professor, Department of Medicine,
Michigan State University, East Lansing, Michigan
francesca.dwamena@ht.msu.edu
*Patient-Centered Interviewing; Doctor-Centered
Interviewing; Pelvic Pain*

Tonya Fancher, MD, MPH
Associate Program Director, Department of Internal
Medicine, University of California, Davis School of
Medicine, Sacramento, California
tonya.fancher@ucdmc.ucdavis.edu
Weight Loss; Amenorrhea

Sara B. Fazio, MD
Instructor in Medicine, Vice Chair Core I Medicine
Clerkship, Harvard Medical School; Division of
General Internal Medicine, Beth Israel Deaconess
Medical Center, Boston, Massachusetts
sfazio@bidmc.harvard.edu
Dyspepsia

David S. Fefferman, MD
Clinical Fellow, Harvard Medical School; Division of
Gastroenterology, Beth Israel Deaconess Medical
Center
Boston, Massachusetts
dfefferm@bidmc.harvard.edu
Anorectal Pain

David Feinbloom, MD
Instructor in Medicine, Harvard Medical School;
Department of Medicine, Division of General
Medicine and Primary Care, Hospital Medicine
Program, Beth Israel Deaconess Medical Center,
Boston, Massachusetts
sfeinblo@caregroup.harvard.edu
Night Sweats

Robert D. Ficalora, MD
Senior Associate Program Director and Consultant in
Internal Medicine, Mayo Clinic College of Medicine,
Rochester, Minnesota
ficalora.robert@mayo.edu
Arm and Hand Pain; Buttock, Hip, and Thigh Pain

Paul L. Fine, MD
Clinical Associate Professor of Internal Medicine,
University of Michigan Health System, Ann Arbor
pfine@umich.edu
Dysuria

Faith T. Fitzgerald, MD
Professor of Medicine and Assistant Dean of
Humanities and Bioethics, University of California,
Davis, School of Medicine, Sacramento, California
acraffetto@ucdavis.edu
History: Art and Science

Auguste H. Fortin VI, MD, MPH
Assistant Clinical Professor of Medicine, Yale
University School of Medicine, New Haven,
Connecticut
auguste.fortin@yale.edu
*Patient-Centered Interviewing; Doctor-Centered
Interviewing; Constipation*

Juan A. Garcia, MD
Assistant Professor, Division of Pulmonary Diseases
and Critical Care Medicine, Department of Medicine,
The University of Texas Health Science Center at San
Antonio
garciaja@uthscsa.edu
Hemoptysis

Estella M. Geraghty, MD, MS
Resident, Department of Internal Medicine, California
Pacific Medical Center, San Francisco
drgeraghty@aol.com
Jaundice

Kathryn A. Glatter, MD
Assistant Professor of Medicine and
Electrophysiologist, Division of Cardiology,
University of California, Davis, Medical Center,
Sacramento, California
kaglatter@ucdavis.edu
Palpitations

Mona A. Gohara, MD
Dermatology Resident, Department of Dermatology,
Yale University School of Medicine, New Haven,
Connecticut
mona.gohara@yale.edu
Inflammatory Dermatoses (Rashes)

John D. Goodson, MD
Physician, Massachusetts General Hospital; Associate
Professor of Medicine, Harvard Medical School,
Boston, Massachusetts
jgoodson1@partners.org
Neck Pain

David Gutknecht, MD
Director, Ambulatory Clinic; Associate Program
Director, Department of Internal Medicine, Geisinger
Health System, Danville, Pennsylvania
dgutknecht@geisinger.edu
Erectile Dysfunction

Linda Harpole, MD, MPH
Assistant Professor of Medicine, Duke University
Medical Center, Durham, North Carolina
linda.h.harpole@gsk.com
Depressed Mood

Mark C. Henderson, MD, FACP
Associate Professor of Clinical Medicine; Vice Chair
for Education, Department of Internal Medicine,
University of California, Davis School of Medicine
Sacramento, California
mchenderson@ucdavis.edu
*The Evidence-Based Approach to Clinical Decision
Making; Dizziness; Syncope*

Calvin H. Hirsch, MD
Professor, Division of General Medicine, University of
California, Davis Medical Center, Sacramento,
California
chhirsch@ucdavis.edu
Urinary Incontinence; Memory Loss

Craig R. Keenan, MD
Assistant Professor, Division of General Internal
Medicine, University of California, Davis School of
Medicine, Sacramento, California
craig.keenan@ucdmc.ucdavis.edu
Insomnia; Sore Throat

Ciaran P. Kelly, MD
Associate Professor of Medicine, Division of
Gastroenterology, Beth Israel Deaconess Medical
Center,
Boston, Massachusetts
Anorectal Pain

Helaina Laks Kravitz, MD, MSPH
Staff Psychiatrist, University of California at Davis,
Counseling and Psychological Services, Davis,
California
Subtleties of Medical History Taking

Richard L. Kravitz, MD, MSPH
Professor of Internal Medicine and Director, Center
for Health Services Research in Primary Care,
University of California, Davis, Sacramento, California
rlkravitz@ucdavis.edu
Subtleties of Medical History Taking

Randall E. Lee, MD
Gastroenterologist, VA Northern California Health
Care System; Associate Clinical Professor of Medicine,
University of California, Davis, Sacramento, California
randall.lee@med.va.gov
Nausea and Vomiting

Anthony Lembo, MD
Instructor in Medicine, Harvard Medical School;
Director, GI Motility Center, Beth Israel Deaconess
Medical Center, Boston, Massachusetts
alembo@bidmc.harvard.edu
Dysphagia

Joseph Ming Wah Li, MD
Instructor in Medicine, Harvard Medical School;
Director, Hospital Medicine Program, Beth Israel
Deaconess Medical Center, Boston, Massachusetts
jli2@bidmc.harvard.edu
Abdominal Pain

Timothy S. Loo, MD
Instructor, Harvard Medical School Division of
General Medicine & Primary Care, Beth Israel
Deaconess Medical Center, Boston, Massachusetts
tloo@caregroup.harvard.edu
Weight Gain

Catherine R. Lucey, MD
Associate Professor of Clinical Medicine and Vice
Chair for Education, Department of Internal
Medicine, The Ohio State University, College of
Medicine & Public Health, Columbus, Ohio
lucey-1@medctr.osu.edu
Muscle Weakness; Dyspnea

Mia W. Marcus, MD
Clinical Fellow in Medicine, Harvard Medical School;
Senior Internal Medicine Resident, Beth Israel
Deaconess Medical Center, Boston, Massachusetts
mia_marcus@vmed.org
Hearing Loss

Kenneth R. McQuaid, MD
Professor of Clinical Medicine, University of
California, San Francisco; Director of Gastrointestinal
Endoscopy, San Francisco Veterans Affairs Medicine
Center
kenneth.mcquaid@med.va.gov
Acute Gastrointestinal Bleeding

Pablo E. Molina, MD
Fellow in Pulmonary Diseases/Critical Care Medicine,
University of Texas Health Science Center at San
Antonio, San Antonio, Texas
molinamd@yahoo.com
Cough

Mary O'Keefe, MD
Internal Medicine Residency Director, Geisinger
Health System, Danville, Pennsylvania
meokeefe@geisinger.edu
Erectile Dysfunction

Jane E. O'Rorke, MD
Assistant Professor of Medicine, University of Texas
Health Science Center at San Antonio
ororke@uthscsa.edu
Knee and Calf Pain; Ankle and Foot Pain

Sonal M. Patel, MD
Clinical Fellow in Gastroenterology, Beth Israel
Deaconess Medical Center, Harvard Medical School,
Boston, Massachusetts
spatel3@bidmc.harvard.edu
Constipation; Dysphagia

Jay I. Peters, MD
Professor of Medicine, Division of Pulmonary Diseases
and Critical Care Medicine, Department of Medicine,
The University of Texas Health Science Center at San
Antonio
peters@uthscsa.edu
Hemoptysis

Laura Pham, MD
Resident Physician, Department of Internal Medicine,
University of California, Davis School of Medicine
laura.pham@ucdmc.ucdavis.edu
Amenorrhea

Sumanth D. Prabhu, MD
Associate Professor of Medicine, Physiology and
Biophysics, Division of Cardiology, University of
Louisville Health Sciences Center; Director, Coronary
Care Unit, University of Louisville Hospital,
Louisville, Kentucky
sprabhu@louisville.edu
Chest Pain

Daniel Press, MD
Instructor in Neurology, Harvard Medical School; Staff
Neurologist, Beth Israel Deaconess Medical Center,
Boston, Massachusetts
dpress@caregroup.harvard.edu
Confusion

Eileen E. Reynolds, MD
Associate Professor of Medicine, Harvard Medical
School; Program Director, Internal Medicine
Residency, Beth Israel Deaconess Medical Center,
Boston, Massachusetts
Hearing Loss

Melissa Robinson, MD
Associate Physician Diplomate, Division of Pulmonary
and Critical Care, Department of Internal Medicine,
University of California, Davis, School of Medicine,
Sacramento, California
mrobinson@ucdavis.edu
Palpitations

Michael Ronthal, MB, BCh
Associate Professor, Harvard Medical School; Staff
Neurologist, Beth Israel Deaconess Medical Center,
Boston, Massachusetts
mronthal@caregroup.harvard.edu
Confusion

Raymond Kevin Ryan, MD
Fellow, Parkinson's Disease and Movement Disorders
Center, Beth Israel Deaconess Medical Center, Boston,
Massachusetts
rryan@bidmc.harvard.edu
Tremor

Sanjay Saint, MD, MPH
Hospitalist and Research Investigator, Ann Arbor VA
Medical Center; Associate Professor of Medicine,
Division of General Medicine, University of Michigan
Medical School, Ann Arbor, Michigan
saint@umich.edu
Dysuria

Julie V. Schaffer, MD
Dermatology Chief Resident, Department of
Dermatology, Yale University, New Haven,
Connecticut
jvotava@email.med.yale.edu
Inflammatory Dermatoses (Rashes)

Amy N. Ship, MD
Instructor in Medicine, Harvard Medical School;
Assistant in Medicine, Beth Israel Deaconess Medical
Center, Boston, Massachusetts
aship@bidmc.harvard.edu
Abnormal Vaginal Bleeding

Richard J. Simons, MD
Acting Dean for Educational Affairs and Professor of
Medicine, Pennsylvania State University College of
Medicine; Staff Physician, Penn State Milton S.
Hershey Medical Center, Hershey, Pennsylvania
rsimons@psu.edu
Fatigue

Gerald W. Smetana, MD
Associate Professor of Medicine, Harvard Medical
School; Division of General Medicine and Primary
Care, Beth Israel Deaconess Medical Center, Boston,
Massachusetts
gsmetana@bidmc.harvard.edu
*The Evidence-Based Approach to Clinical Decision
Making; Headache; Night Sweats; Diarrhea*

Robert C. Smith, MD, ScM
Professor of Medicine, Michigan State University, East
Lansing, Michigan
robert.smith@ht.msu.edu
*Patient-Centered Interviewing; Doctor-Centered
Interviewing*

Malathi Srinivasan, MD
Assistant Professor of Medicine, Department of
Medicine, University of California, Davis School of
Medicine, Sacramento, California
malathi@ucdavis.edu
Tinnitus

Daniel J. Sullivan, MD, MPH
Assistant Professor of Medicine, Harvard Medical
School and Beth Israel Deaconess Medical Center,
Boston, Massachusetts
dsulliva@bidmc.harvard.edu
Ear Pain

Daniel Tarsy, MD
Associate Professor of Neurology, Harvard Medical
School; Director, Parkinson's Disease and Movement
Disorders Center, Beth Israel Deaconess Medical
Center, Boston, Massachusetts
dtarsy@bidmc.harvard.edu
Tremor

Anjala V. Tess, MD
Instructor in Medicine, Harvard Medical School;
Hospitalist and Staff Physician, Beth Israel Deaconess
Medical Center, Boston, Massachusetts
atess@caregroup.harvard.edu
Fever

Lawrence M. Tierney, Jr., MD
Professor of Medicine, University of California, San
Francisco; Associate Chief of Medical Service, San
Francisco Veterans Affairs Medical Center
vaspa@itsa.ucsf.edu
The Case Presentation

Liana Vesga, MD
Gastroenterology Fellow, Division of Gastroenterology,
University of California, San Francisco
lvesga@itsa.ucsf.edu
Acute Gastrointestinal Bleeding

Christina C. Wee, MD, MPH
Assistant Professor of Medicine, Harvard Medical
School; Associate in Medicine, Beth Israel Deaconess
Medical Center, Boston, Massachusetts
cweekuo@bidmc.harvard.edu
Weight Gain

Jeff Wiese, MD
Associate Professor of Medicine, Tulane Health
Sciences Center; Associate Chairman of Medicine and
Chief of Medicine, Charity Hospital, New Orleans
Louisiana
jwiese@tulane.edu
Edema; Gait Abnormalities

John W. Williams, Jr., MD, MHSc
Professor of Medicine and Associate Professor of
Psychiatry, Duke University and Durham Veterans
Affairs Medical Center, Durham, North Carolina
willi007@mc.duke.edu
Depressed Mood

Michael H. Zaroukian, MD, PhD
Associate Professor of Medicine and Director,
Electronic Medical Record Systems, Michigan State
University, East Lansing, Michigan
michael.zaroukian@ht.msu.edu
Lymphadenopathy; Anxiety

Preface

The health and dignity of my patients will be my first concern.

—*Yale Physician's Oath*

Give a person a fish and you will feed them for a day: Teach them to fish and you feed them for a lifetime.
—*Chinese Proverb*

Welcome to *The Patient History.* The purpose of this book is to introduce aspiring health care professionals to the timeless art of history-taking. The patient's story lies at the heart of this endeavor, is entirely unique, and defies the categorization inherent to the printed page. However, there are fundamental principles that can be articulated to start the novice on the right path.

What makes this book different? The fundamental purpose of the history is to establish a differential diagnosis for a given symptom. Therefore we have used a patient-centered approach, organizing the book by *symptoms* rather than by diseases. Symptoms, after all, bring patients to the clinician. Second, we apply principles of evidence-based medicine to the clinical history, highlighting from the medical literature the most fruitful lines of questioning for making a diagnosis.

Is there science or evidence substantiating the clinical history as a diagnostic tool? Older data (Hampton et al, *BMJ* 1975) suggest that expert clinicians can make a diagnosis in the vast majority of patients using the history alone. Throughout the book we summarize the usefulness of historical features, that is, how historical data help confirm or refute a particular diagnosis. However, many aspects of the history have not been formally studied, and in such instances we review the epidemiology, prevalence, and prognosis of the most common conditions. This type of information, integrated with clinical experience, helps guide the interviewer toward the most important diagnostic considerations for a given symptom.

We begin the book with a section covering general principles of history-taking followed by an introduction to the evidence-based method. Subsequent sections, constituting the substance of the book, cover 60 common clinical syndromes. Each symptom chapter is organized into the following sections: background, key terminology, differential diagnosis (including the prevalence of various causes), interview framework, alarm symptoms (features that alert the clinician to the most serious diagnoses), focused questions with respective likelihood ratios, prognosis, and caveats or clinical pearls. Each chapter concludes with a Diagnostic Approach algorithm. We close the book with a chapter on how to communicate the history to colleagues or consultants.

We emphasize actual questions for use in daily practice, ranging from basic queries to those an experienced clinician might employ. Communicating effectively is paramount to obtaining an accurate history, so we also include tips for effective interviewing throughout the book. We have not covered the physical examination or laboratory evaluation, lest we detract from the focus of the book, history-taking.

Learning the clinical history requires communication skills, clinical experience with patients, practice, and the observation of master historians. Faith Fitzgerald and Larry Tierney, two such masters, open and close the book covering critical but often ignored aspects of this ancient art. We hope this book gives you the fishing gear, or tools, for a successful journey to clinical excellence.

Lawrence M. Tierney, Jr., MD
Mark C. Henderson, MD

San Francisco and
Sacramento, California
December 2004

Acknowledgments

I thank my wife, Helen, and my parents, Donna and Starr Henderson, without whose inspiration and love I would never have become a physician. Second, I thank Isabel Nogueira for tirelessly shepherding the project from its conception to near completion. Third, I thank my associate editor, Dr. Jerry Smetana, and all authors for their thoughtful, practical, and scholarly contributions. Finally, I would like to recognize Dr. Maurice Kraytman for the original concept of the Complete Patient History, Bob Badgett for his wonderful search strategy for clinical symptoms (available at http://medinformatics.uthscsa.edu/symptoms), Jennifer Bernstein for her superb copy editing, and the entire editorial staff at McGraw-Hill.

I must also thank my teacher, colleague, and friend, Dr. Larry Tierney, for the honor of collaborating with him on such a wonderful project. As a third-year medical student I nervously presented some of my first ward patients to L.T. and he inspired me to become a physician teacher. I salute many other influential teachers and mentors including (in order of appearance): Drs. Jay Stein, Jay Peters, Andrew Diehl, Charles Duncan, Cynthia Mulrow, Gary Harris, George Crawford, and Thomas Cooney.

Mark C. Henderson, MD
Sacramento, California

SECTION I
Basic Concepts

History: Art *and* Science

Faith T. Fitzgerald, MD

The medical history, say venerable clinicians righteously, is the core art of patient care. They continue to cite references that maintain that the patient's history provides the diagnosis in 85% of cases. That often-quoted figure of 85% is in doubt, however, as many of the histories now given by patients and taken by doctors are in actual content a compendium of data from the laboratories and radiology suites from previous visits to their doctors and admissions to hospital. So, for example, patients bring folders of laboratory studies with them to consultant's offices; house staff and students present patients with chief complaints of "fever, leukocytosis, and mitral vegetations on echo"; and a first concern given by a patient in clinic may be "high cholesterol." It is hard to escape the implicit conviction that laboratory and technologic data are more objective, and therefore more scientific, than the subjective information gathered by listening to a patient tell his or her story. Furthermore, the wondrous advances in technologic diagnosis appear to justify the reverence in which the results they generate are held.

Developing Skill in Listening

Without a careful history, without knowing the patient's story of what happened to them and their unique circumstances and personality, the practice of medicine becomes neither art *nor* science. Consider what opinion we would have of a bench investigator who plated known microorganisms upon an unknown medium. Would we credit the observations of a geneticist who intercalated even the most intimately analyzed base pairs into an otherwise unknown genome? The study of the patient begins with the history, a history taken by a skilled listener too, for it is only the skilled listener who can hear the vocal inflections that suggest the importance of things to the patient. It is only she who can read the nonverbal clues that illuminate the meaning of the words. It is only he who can understand not only what is said but the oftentimes vitally important information gathered when things go unsaid by patients.

The ability to take a good history cannot be acquired by lecture or syllabus, standardized patient exercises, CD-ROM, or even texts such as this one. It is an experientially acquired art, learned over time, with each successive patient story and the careful observation of what follows from it. It is often frustrating for students and junior doctors who want to know what the so-called good history should include. They mistake structure for substance. The good history varies depending not on how one orders its component sections (such as present illness, review of systems, and the like), nor on mastering the current jargon and multiple acronyms that more often obscure than facilitate understanding, but on the story that the patient needs to tell and the doctor to hear, in order that they together may go further along the path of understanding what to do next. Like any art—and like science—the ability to do a patient interview builds on the practitioner's past and requires practice. Knowing what to emphasize and what to discard, what question to ask next, and how to direct the discourse (subtly and without markedly influencing or altering its content) is difficult, and the lessons are never-ending. The only way to learn it is to do it, with real patients, again and again and again.

More than the Facts

Here we are, doctors in the 21st century, equipped with truly miraculous tools of diagnosis and therapy, and patients complain about us. Even the best educated, or especially the best educated, go to quacks. They do not trust us. Why? Perhaps because the greatest afflictions of our patients—fear, despair, fatigue, and pain—may have no objective findings. No laboratory result or image can portray them. Only through the history do patients tell us how they need our help and how best that help can be given. They have told us this time and again in surveys in which the greatest discontent with physicians of our era is that they do not listen.

The history is more than the elucidation of the facts of the case, more than a construct of symptoms. It tells the tale of the reaction a unique human being has to those symptoms and their impact on the patient's mind and life, their family, and their hopes. Listening to them is more than an ingathering of indications for further studies. It is in and of itself a major therapeutic act, and the physician, himself or herself, is a potent therapeutic instrument. In conjunction with the laying on of hands that follows in the physical examination, the meeting of doctor and patient fulfills some primal need of the vulnerable to be attended to, cared for, and cared about.

The history also gives doctors the richness of their professional lives. Decades from now, a physician in reverie about his or her career in medicine will not remember the chemistry panels, the MRI results, or even the majority of the medical scientific facts of their past practice. What they will remember, and tell to their potentially bored students, are the stories of their patients about who they were and how they acted. If endurance in memory is any indication of the importance of events, it is the history, that story of how the patient responded to duress, that is existentially most important to *both* doctor and patient.

T.S. Eliot once wrote: "Where is the wisdom we have lost in knowledge? Where is the knowledge we have lost in information?" Laboratory studies are, without doubt, essential and informative; knowledge, however, comes only with their integration with the patient's story as told by history and physical examination; wisdom is what doctors acquire when they recognize this truth.

Subtleties of Medical History Taking

Helaina Laks Kravitz, MD, & Richard L. Kravitz, MD, MSPH

When first seeing patients in clinics and on the wards, the learning curve is steep. During these early encounters, it is often a struggle to ask the right questions, follow-up on the answers, and sort the information into the appropriate categories. On the other hand, when watching a seasoned clinician take a medical history, it all seems natural and effortless. The interview flows smoothly and the medical history falls seamlessly into place. Over time, clinicians develop a personal interview style, integrating the information in this book and experience with patients. The following guidelines are some "tricks of the trade" that may help the student—at whatever stage of training or practice—to dodge some of the usual obstacles to efficient medical history taking.

Even if you are in a hurry, do not show it.

In the course of everyday clinical care, there are times when you are pressed for time. There are several patients to see, laboratory results to check, and a presentation to rehearse for morning rounds. Patients are very perceptive. If you know that you have a certain amount of time with the patient, make the most of it. Sit down rather than stand. Do not bury your head in the chart. Maintain eye contact as much as possible, looking up at the patient frequently as you jot down notes. All of these things will help the patient feel better and will not require extra time.

Take a few minutes with the chart before you see the patient.

There is a wealth of information there, and it makes sense to use it. It takes much less time to extract dates of past surgeries from the medical record than to ask a typical patient to develop the list de novo. Making use of secondary sources does not release you from the obligation to confirm key points directly (eg, "I see from your chart you were hospitalized in 1966 for kidney disease. Can you tell me more about that?"). Additionally, in patients with poor cognitive function or organizational skills, it is useful to expand secondary sources and verify with friends, family, and other physicians. Finally, beware of "chart lore," eg, the patient who carries a diagnosis of "lupus" passed down from one discharge summary to the next but who has no corroborating physical or laboratory evidence of the disease. Recognizing these caveats, it is always appropriate and usually necessary to "interview the chart" as well as the patient.

It is not necessary to gather information in the same order that it will be presented.

Oral and written presentations should be delivered in a standard format, generally beginning with the reason for consultation or the chief complaint, then moving on through the history of present illness (HPI), past history (including medications and allergies), family history, personal and social history, review of systems, physical examination, and assessment and plan. Following a standard format for presentation helps organize your thoughts about the patient, reduces the likelihood of omitting critical data, and makes a presentation easier to follow. Remember, though, that just because one *presents* information in a particular order does not mean one has to *gather* it that way.

Rigid adherence to a template means missing potential opportunities: noticing the stare of Graves disease (ordinarily part of the physical examination) as the patient describes the evolution of her abdominal complaints; asking about medications, drugs, and alcohol (usually reserved for the Past Medical History) right after the patient complains of insomnia; responding to a glint of sadness elicited during the HPI by inquiring about depressed mood and recent losses (points that might otherwise be relegated to the Social History or Review of Systems). Waiting to follow-up these observations until the "correct" time is artificial and may sacrifice diagnostic efficiency (furthermore, the interviewer may overlook them).

Admit when you are confused.

Patients will not mind repetition. They want the doctor to get it right. Do not be afraid to say, "I'm sorry, I didn't quite understand that." Occasionally, a meandering and inconsistent history is a clue to cognitive dysfunction. More often, misplaced details and chronologic meanderings simply reflect the complexity of human experience. Medical knowledge can provide a framework to understand what is happening to the patient's body. But first the critical details must be clear. Was the onset of the pain or dyspnea instantaneous, acute (hours), subacute (days to weeks), or chronic (longer)? Did the nausea and anorexia precede the pain or vice versa? Is the patient who complains of frequent urination voiding relatively small volumes each time (frequency) or large volumes (polyuria)? If something does not make sense, persist until it becomes clear.

Do not leave the story out of history.

No dimension of the medical history is more important than the chronologic relation of one event to another. It can be useful to draw out a time line, indicating when symptoms started, how they have affected the patient, and what treatments have helped or been ineffective. The chronologic pattern of symptoms not only helps establish a diagnosis but also informs the urgency of response. Recurrent headaches unchanging in pattern over a period of years are unlikely to represent serious anatomic illness whereas a new-onset headache of moderate severity may be a sign of increased intracranial pressure. Chronic stable angina can be managed as an outpatient; chest pain increasing in frequency or severity may warrant urgent coronary angiography.

When the patient's story seems hopelessly confused, ask the patient about the last time they remember feeling completely well. Then ask what they first noticed as they began to feel ill. And what next ... and what next ... and what next? A solid chronology is the foundation of diagnostic accuracy.

Address the fear factor.

Most clinicians recognize that a diagnosis of cancer is frightening and will appropriately prepare themselves to deal with the patient's emotional fallout. But there are many situations that, while seemingly trivial, are in fact overwhelming to the patient. It is important to explore the patient's own ideas about the illness. For instance, an otherwise innocuous bout of upper abdominal pain might feel ominous to a 53-year-old male patient whose father died of a myocardial infarction. Failure to address the patient's worries may lead to further escalation of his or her complaints. One approach is to say, "Many patients have thoughts about what might be causing their symptoms. I was wondering if you were worried about anything in particular?" If the response is vague, you could add, "What do *you* think is going on?"

Trust, but verify.

Do not take every answer at face value. Many one-word answers (and some polysyllabic ones) demand follow-up, especially if they do not fit with other data. For instance, a 48-year-old woman with chronic cough who answers the question "Do you smoke cigarettes?" with a "no" may have "quit" yesterday after a 30-pack-year history. Sometimes definitions need to be quantified. The alcoholic might report "one or two" drinks a night, but only the persistent clinician will learn that he considers a "drink" to be eight ounces of hard liquor (or a 32-ounce beer).

Another area that often requires clarification is the patient's medication history. It is important to review the chart and ask the patient to provide a list of prescribed medications, but this list does not always match what the patient actually takes. It is often helpful to ask the patient to bring all medications to a subsequent appointment. Sometimes a medication "is not working" simply because the patient skips doses of medications that need to be taken three or four times daily. Adding yet another medication or increasing the dose is not going to solve this problem, whereas good history taking will.

Follow your instincts.

The doctor-patient interview is ultimately a conversation between two people. If something does not seem quite right, there usually is a reason. Notice whether the affect of the patient matches the content of what is said. If the patient is describing the pain in her chest, does she seem unduly worried or casually indifferent? Does the patient look away or wring her hands when she answers certain questions? She may be withholding something. There is no need to be accusatory: a simple observation, presented as a conjecture, is often all that is needed. "You seem worried about something." "I was wondering if it feels uncomfortable to talk about this." Your instincts will often be right and may yield crucial information.

Judiciously applied, silence is golden.

Eager not to miss anything, most beginning interviewers talk too much. While it is important to clarify points of confusion, try not to interrupt the patient. As William Osler is frequently quoted as saying, "Listen to the patient. He is telling you the diagnosis." This crusty aphorism often rings true! It is easier to let the patient tell the story on his or her own terms if you remember that you will have a chance to rearrange the facts into a coherent presentation—later. And do not forget to give the patient a chance to fill in any omitted details by punctuating the interview with the phrase, "Anything else?"

Good history taking serves a twofold purpose.

Incorporating these guidelines into history taking will increase the likelihood of obtaining the correct information while forming a critical connection with the patient which is, in itself, therapeutic

Patient-Centered Interviewing

3

Francesca C. Dwamena, MD, Auguste H. Fortin VI, MD, MPH, &
Robert C. Smith, MD, ScM

Effective medical interviewing is not innate but must be systematically learned and practiced. Under the biomedical model, students are trained to elicit only symptom data using isolated doctor-centered interviewing. However, isolated doctor-centered interviewing often ignores highly relevant personal data and is devoid of the emotional content necessary to establish an effective relationship with the patient. Integrating patient-centered interviewing with doctor-centered interviewing allows the interviewer to both obtain the patient's complete story and establish the optimum doctor-patient relationship.[1]

The patient-centered history typically occurs during the first 10% of an encounter, to elicit the chief complaint and initial history of present illness (HPI). It consists of mainly psychosocial data and the patient's personal description of physical symptoms. The interviewer must synthesize this with information obtained from the doctor-centered process to obtain the patient's biopsychosocial story. This chapter presents an evidence-based patient-centered interviewing method.[2]

KEY TERMS

Biopsychosocial (BPS) model	The BPS model describes the patient as an integrated mix of his or her biologic, psychological, and social components. It differs from the biomedical model, which describes the patient only in terms of disease (physical or psychiatric).
Patient-centered interviewing	The interviewer encourages the patient to express what is most important to him or her and facilitates the narration of the patient's story.
Doctor-centered interviewing	The doctor takes charge of the interaction to acquire specific details not provided already by the patient, usually to diagnose disease or to develop the database (see Chapter 4).
Integrated patient-centered and doctor-centered interviewing	The interviewer uses both patient-centered and doctor-centered interviewing to elicit personal and symptom data from the patient and then synthesizes them into the biopsychosocial story.

RATIONALE FOR PATIENT-CENTERED INTERVIEWING

Many doctors interrupt patients and prevent them from expressing their concerns.[3] This approach results in incomplete databases by failing to elicit important psychosocial data and skews data toward physical symptoms.

Integrating patient-centered methods improves patient satisfaction, compliance, knowledge and recall, and decreases doctor shopping and lawsuits.[4–7] Patient-centered approaches have been linked to improved health outcomes such as better blood pressure and diabetic control,[8] better perinatal outcomes,[9] shortened length of stay and improved mortality in critically ill patients,[10] and improved cancer outcomes.[11]

Lack of a systematic method has hindered educators from teaching patient-centered interviewing skills.

Patient-Centered Interviewing: The Required Facilitating Skills

In order to conduct an effective patient-centered interview, the interviewer must master a core set of questioning and relationship-building skills. These skills are summarized below.

Questioning skills	• *Open-ended* – *Silence* – *Nonverbal encouragement* – *Neutral utterances and continuers* – *Reflection and echoing* – *Open-ended requests* – *Summary and paraphrasing* • *Closed-ended* – *Yes and no answers* – *Brief answers*
Relationship-building skills	• *Emotion-seeking* – *Direct inquiry* – *Indirect inquiry: self-disclosure, impact, and belief about problem* • *Emotion-handling ("NURS")* – *Naming and labeling* – *Understanding and validation* – *Respect and praise* – *Support and partnership*

Open-ended questioning skills

These skills generate the patient's agenda and elicit personal descriptions of symptoms and concerns. They encourage the patient to express what is on his or her mind (eg questions, feelings, and fears) rather than responding to what is on the interviewer's mind. In contrast, closed-ended questions focus on specific issues in the interviewer's mind (eg, diagnoses) and are used in the doctor-centered process.

Nonfocusing skills	**Allow patients to talk freely without controlling the direction of the interview.**
Silence	*The interviewer says nothing while continuing to be attentive. If the silence does not prompt a response within 5–10 seconds, the interviewer should try another skill as prolonged silence may make the patient uncomfortable.*

| Nonverbal encouragement | These include hand gestures, sympathetic facial expressions and other indications by body language that the patient should continue speaking. |
| Neutral utterances | These are brief, noncommittal statements like "oh," "uh-huh," "yes," or "Mmm." |

Focusing skills	**The interviewer directs the patient to a particular topic that the patient has already mentioned. They are critical to maintaining effectiveness and efficiency of the interview.**
Reflecting or echoing	The interviewer encourages the patient to elaborate on the story behind a word or phrase by repeating it (eg, "your chest hurts...").
Open-ended requests	These are statements like "go on" or "tell me more about this chest pain" that are used to maintain focus on a particular subject.
Summarizing or paraphrasing	Similar to echoing but a little more detailed, eg, "your chest hurts and you are afraid you are having a heart attack like your brother did last year."

Relationship-building skills

These skills are used to encourage the patient to express their emotions and to nurture them once they do.

Emotion-seeking skills	
Direct inquiry	The best way to elicit the patient's emotions is by asking directly, for example, "How does that make you feel?" or "How did it make you feel emotionally?" If a patient is already expressing an emotion (eg, crying), the interviewer should develop it further, with a statement like "I can see that this is still very difficult for you. Tell me what it has been like for you." If direct inquiry fails to elicit an emotional response, it is important to continue to seek it using indirect inquiry.
Indirect inquiry	This is a way of generating emotions in patients when direct inquiry is ineffective.
• Self-disclosure	The interviewer uses previous experiences to elicit emotional expression. For example, "I had a similar experience and it made me upset" or "Most people would be unhappy about that."
• Impact on patient or his or her loved ones	The interviewer asks, "How has it affected your life?" Patients usually respond with some information about their personal life: "Well I cannot walk my dogs in the mornings like I used to do." The interviewer can then directly inquire about emotions, eg, "What is that like for you?"
• Patient's explanatory model for his or her symptoms	Patients often worry that their symptoms are the result of a serious illness (eg, cancer), so this skill may lead to emotional expression. You might ask, "What do you think is causing your headache?" The patient might respond, "Could be cancer I guess." You could follow-up with, "How do you feel about that?"

Once the interviewer elicits an emotional expression, he can address it using the emotion-handling skills: Naming, Understanding, Respecting and Supporting (which can be recalled with the mnemonic, "NURS").

Emotion–handling skills	Allow the interviewer to express empathy and help manage the patient's emotions.
Naming	The interviewer names the emotion, to show that he has heard the patient, eg, "So that scares you."
Understanding	These statements accept and validate the patient's expressed emotions, for example, "I can understand how that might upset you."
Respect	These are statements that praise the patient (eg, "You did the right thing by coming in.") or acknowledge his or her plight (eg, "You have been through a lot.").
Support	These statements indicate the interviewer's willingness to work to manage the patient's problems, eg, "I am here to help in any way I can."

Patient-centered Interviewing: The Process

Step 1: Setting the Stage for the Interview (30–60 seconds)

The interviewer begins the relationship by recognizing the identity of the patient, introducing himself, and ensuring patient's readiness to proceed with the interview.

1. Welcome the patient	Use a simple statement and a handshake to make the patient feel valued and set the proper tone for the interview.
2. Use the patient's name	It is best to use the last name unless the patient asks to be addressed by another name.
3. Introduce yourself and identify your specific role	Students can indicate that they are a part of the healthcare team, while being honest about their particular roles. For example, a medical student enters the exam room and says: "Welcome, Mrs. Green. My name is Frank Smith and I am the medical student with Dr. Brown. I am here to take your history" while shaking hands with the patient.
4. Ensure patient readiness and privacy	Sometimes patients' physical or emotional conditions preclude an effective interaction and may need to be addressed before starting the interview: "You look upset. Is everything all right?"
5. Remove barriers to communication	The interviewer may need to turn off a noisy television or make sure that a deaf patient can read his lips.
6. Ensure comfort and put the patient at ease	This may include making physical adjustments in the furniture or ambience of the room and conducting light conversation (eg, asking about the weather or hospital food) to put the patient at ease.

Step 2: Obtaining the Agenda Including the Chief Complaint (30–60 seconds)

The interviewer orients the patient to the expected duration and process of the interaction and elicits the patient's agenda.

1. Indicate time available	Many providers feel uncomfortable with this step because they fear it might be rude. However it helps patients gauge what they can hope to accomplish: "We have about 40 minutes today…"
2. Indicate interviewer's needs	The interviewer may need sufficient time to ask questions and conduct a physical examination on a new patient. Continuing from above, "…and I know I have a lot of questions to ask and that we will need to do a physical exam."
3. Obtain a list of all issues the patient wants to discuss	"Before we get started though, I would like to address all your concerns today." This minimizes the chance of important issues arising at the end of the allotted time and may preclude patient complaints about not being given a chance to discuss important issues.[12] Patients do not usually offer a complete list at the outset and often require prompting with questions like "Anything else?" or "Do you need any prescriptions or forms filled?" The interviewer must respectfully deter the patient from offering too many details about agenda items at this point with statements like "We will get back to the headache in a minute, but I need to know if there are other things we need to accomplish today."
4. Summarize and finalize the agenda	This step allows the interviewer to clarify the chief complaint if not already apparent, prioritize the list, and empower the patient to decide what will be addressed and what will be deferred to the next visit: "You mentioned several issues you wanted to cover. I do not think we will have time to address them all in the time we have together today. Please choose the 1 or 2 that are most troublesome to you today, and we will tackle those together. I will see you back soon to work on the others."

Step 3: Opening the History of Present Illness (HPI) (30–60 seconds)

Step 3 uses the nonfocusing, open-ended skills described earlier to open the HPI. It has 3 substeps:

1. Use an open-ended beginning question or statement.	After finalizing the agenda, begin the HPI with a question or statement like "Now tell me about your headaches."
2. Use nonfocusing open-ended skills.	Silence, neutral utterances ("uh-huh"), and nonverbal encouragement (nodding, leaning forward) may encourage the patient to talk. If the patient does not talk freely, the interviewer can use open-ended focusing questions (echoing, requests, summary) to encourage the patient to tell his story.
3. Obtain additional data from nonverbal sources.	Make a mental note of the patient's physical characteristics, appearance, and his environment. For example, the framed picture of a young army officer may be the key to diagnosing the anxiety of a reticent patient who is worried about her son at war.

Step 4: Continuing the Patient-Centered HPI (5–10 minutes of 40 minute visit)

The goal here is to facilitate the patient's description of her physical symptoms and their personal and emotional context.

1. *Use focusing open-ended skills to obtain a description of the patient's physical symptoms*

   The interviewer becomes much more active verbally, using focusing skills to elicit a description of the physical symptom. Patients often present a mixture of physical and personal information in the first few seconds of the interview, eg, "This headache has been bothering me so much that I cannot even concentrate at work. My husband thinks I am being lazy but the last thing I want to do when I get the headache is to cook and clean the house."

   If the interviewer remains silent, the patient can take the conversation in any direction (headache, work, husband, or cooking). A focusing statement like "Tell me more about the headache" (open-ended request) or "headache..." (echoing) will usually elicit the patient's description of the physical problem: "Yes, I have had headaches before, but this one is different..." If the patient does not elaborate, another focusing question like "How is it different?" may be effective. In this manner, the interviewer obtains a detailed description of the patient's physical symptom and its immediate personal context. The goal is to obtain a good overview of the problem. Be careful to avoid asking about details of onset, duration, etc. at this point so that the patient may continue to lead the interaction.

2. *Use focusing open-ended skills to develop the personal or psychosocial context of the patient's story.*

   After obtaining a brief overview of physical symptoms, use open-ended focusing questions to obtain the broader personal and psychological context by directing the patient to immediate or previous personal statements: (Continuing with the previous conversation) "So you cannot concentrate at work..." This allows clinicians to understand patients' often unheard but relevant personal concerns which, if not addressed, may lead to dissatisfaction. Sometimes patients revert to describing symptoms during this step – "Yes, I had to take off work because the headache started right in the middle of a very important project. It just started pounding and then I started feeling nauseated..." Although the interviewer may be more comfortable pursuing this diagnostic data, it is important at this juncture to direct the patient back to the personal data, knowing that the details of the physical symptom will be obtained in a few minutes during the doctor-centered portion of the interview (see Chapter 4): "We will come back to the headache and nausea in a minute. But before we do that, can you tell me a little more about your work?" Such persistence and focus on personal information introduced by the patient often yields highly relevant personal data: "We just got a new boss who has been making a lot of changes. Just the other day, he fired one of my coworkers." The interviewer has now laid the groundwork for the most important step—developing an emotional focus.

3. Use emotion-seeking skills to develop an emotional context.	Eliciting and addressing emotion is the key ingredient to an effective doctor-patient relationship. A direct inquiry about how the patient feels about the personal situation often elicits an emotion, "How did that make you feel?" Patient: "Well I felt sorry for her. Then I started worrying." If the patient does not respond with an emotion, then a more direct question like "How does it make you feel emotionally?" may be more fruitful. Once the patient offers an emotion, the interviewer should seek to expand his or her understanding of the patient's emotion with focusing open-ended skills, eg, "Tell me more about what was worrying you." Clinicians are often surprised by what they uncover with this inquiry: "Well, I do not want to add her responsibilities to mine. Just thinking about it makes my headache and nausea worse."
4. Use emotion-handling skills to address elicited emotions.	Once the interviewer elicits and probes the emotion enough to achieve reasonable understanding, he or she can address it with emotion-handling skills (NURS). An appropriate response to the emotion expressed above would be something like "So her being fired worried you (**naming**). That makes sense to me (**understanding**). It sounds like a lot to deal with (**respect**). I want to help in any way I can (**support**)." Emotion-handling skills may feel awkward to beginners, but this usually resolves with experience and an appreciation of the potential benefit to patients.
5. Use focused open-ended skills, emotion-seeking skills, and emotion-handling skills to further expand the story.	The interviewer usually can expand and deepen the patient's story and test hypotheses by multiple cycles of focusing on personal data offered by the patient using open-ended focusing skills, followed by emotion-seeking and emotion-handling skills as described above. For example the interviewer can begin to test the hypothesis that the patient is angry with her husband by saying, "So your husband thinks you are being lazy … How does that make you feel?"

Step 5: Transition to the Doctor-Centered Process (30 seconds)

The interviewer uses this step to close the patient-centered portion of the interview and open the doctor-centered process to obtain the details needed to complete the patient's history.

1. Summarize briefly	This summary should not be more than 2 or 3 sentences, "So you have a bad headache with nausea that is aggravated by your concerns about increased responsibility at work and at home."
2. Check accuracy	"Is that the gist of it?"
3. Indicate that both content and style of inquiry will change if the patient is ready	"Is it okay if I shift gears and ask some more specific questions about your headache?" If this is not done, the controlling style of the doctor-centered process may confuse the patient.

SUMMARY

The patient-centered interview consists of 5 steps and 21 sub-steps. The interviewer prepares the patient for the interaction with steps 1 and 2. In steps 3 and 4, he facilitates the sequential development of the patient's physical, personal, and emotional story using nonfocusing skills followed by focusing, emotion-seeking, and emotion-handling skills. The story is expanded and deepened by focusing the patient on revealed personal and emotional information and repeating the cycle of steps 3 and 4, while monitoring the patient's reaction to the interview. The interviewer finally uses step 5 to transition to the doctor-centered process to collect the details of the HPI and routine historical data. The doctor-centered process is described in Chapter 4.

REFERENCES

1. Engel GL. The need for a new medical model: a challenge for biomedicine. *Science.* 1977;196:129–136.

2. Smith RC, Lyles JS, Mettler J, et al. The effectiveness of intensive training for residents in interviewing. A randomized, controlled study. *Ann Intern Med.* 1998;128:118–126.

3. Beckman HB, Frankel RM. The effect of physician behavior on the collection of data. *Ann Intern Med.* 1984;101:692–696.

4. Ambady N, Laplante D, Nguyen T, et al. Surgeons' tone of voice: a clue to malpractice history. *Surgery.* 2002;132:5–9.

5. Hall JA, Roter DL, Katz NR. Meta-analysis of correlates of provider behavior in medical encounters. *Med Care.* 1988; 26:657–675.

6. Kasteler J, Kane RL, Olsen DM, Thetford C. Issues underlying prevalence of "doctor-shopping" behavior. *J Health Soc Behav.* 1976;17:329–339.

7. Levinson W, Roter DL, Mullooly JP, et al. Physician-patient communication. The relationship with malpractice claims among primary care physicians and surgeons. *JAMA.* 1997;277:553–539.

8. Kaplan SH, Greenfield S, Ware JE Jr. Assessing the effects of physician-patient interactions on the outcomes of chronic disease. *Med Care.* 1989;27(Suppl):S110–127.

9. Shear CL, Gipe BT, Mattheis JK, Levy MR. Provider continuity and quality of medical care. A retrospective analysis of prenatal and perinatal outcome. *Med Care.* 1983;21:1204–1210.

10. Lilly CM, Sonna LA, Haley KJ, Massaro AF. Intensive communication: four-year follow-up from a clinical practice study. *Crit Care Med.* 2003;31(5 Suppl):S394–399.

11. Spiegel D, Sephton SE, Terr AI, Stites DP. Effects of psychosocial treatment in prolonging cancer survival may be mediated by neuroimmune pathways. *Ann NY Acad Sci.* 1998;840:674–683.

12. White J, Levinson W, Roter D. "Oh, by the way...": the closing moments of the medical visit. *J Gen Intern Med.* 1994; 9:24–28.

SUGGESTED READING

Smith RC. *Patient-Centered Interviewing: An Evidence-Based Method.* 2nd ed. Philadelphia: Lippincott Williams & Wilkins, 2002.

Doctor-Centered Interviewing　　4

Auguste H. Fortin VI, MD, MPH, Francesca C. Dwamena, MD, &
Robert C. Smith, MD, ScM

The patient-centered part of the interview yields the patient's personal description of his or her symptom(s) and other, related personal experiences, that is, the patient's story of the "history of present illness" (HPI) (see Chapter 3). This patient-centered interview provides pertinent psychosocial data and, to a lesser extent, biomedical data about the patient and the disease.

Patient-centered data, however, are rarely complete. More details are needed to make diagnoses of disease and fill in the routine database (eg, the family history and social history). These details are acquired in the doctor-centered part of the interview, which produces pertinent biomedical data and, to a lesser extent, psychosocial data.[1] Unlike the patient-centered portion of the interview, here clinicians inquire about symptom information not yet mentioned by the patient in order to complete the HPI. Finally, other aspects of the patient's life and history are explored to diagnose other diseases outside the HPI, assess for disease risk, and come to know the patient better on a personal level.

In the doctor-centered interview, the patient is led through a series of open-ended and closed-ended questions. Each line of inquiry starts with an open-ended question or request and is followed with closed-ended questioning, moving from general information to specific details.

KEY TERMS

Doctor-centered interviewing	*The doctor takes charge of the interaction to acquire specific details not provided already by the patient, usually to diagnose disease or to fill in the routine database.*
Closed-ended questions	*Can be answered with "yes," "no," a number, or a short answer (eg, "When did your headache start?" "Where is it located?")*
Open-ended questions/requests	*Encourage the patients to tell a narrative, eg, "Tell me more about your headache."*

FILLING IN THE HPI

In the doctor-centered component of the HPI, the description of symptoms is expanded, and related symptoms, their details, and other data (eg, medications, hospitals, doctors) not yet introduced by the patient are obtained (Table 4–1).

Expanding Description of Symptoms

Symptoms already mentioned by the patient usually need further explanation. To fully understand a symptom, clinicians need to know its 7 "cardinal features"[1-3] (Table 4–2).

In the patient-centered interview, clinicians learn about many of a symptom's features, but even the most articulate patient is unlikely to have mentioned them all in the course of telling his or her story. Therefore, in the doctor-centered interview additional details are sought. Start with an open-ended request ("Tell me more about what your chest pain is like"), and then ask more specific closed-ended

Table 4–1. Filling in the history of present illness.

1. Define the cardinal features of the patient's chief complaint
2. Define the cardinal features of other symptoms (those already mentioned by the patient and those not yet introduced) in the organ system of the patient's chief complaint
3. Inquire about relevant symptoms outside the involved system
4. Inquire about relevant nonsymptom (secondary) data

Table 4–2. The 7 cardinal features of symptoms.

1. **Location and radiation**
   a. Precise location
   b. Deep or superficial
   c. Localized or diffuse
2. **Quality**
   a. Usual descriptors
   b. Unusual descriptors
3. **Quantification**
   a. Type of onset
   b. Intensity or severity
   c. Impairment or disability
   d. Numeric description
      i. Number of events
      ii. Size
      iii. Volume
4. **Chronology**
   a. Time of onset of symptom and intervals between recurrences
   b. Duration of symptom
   c. Periodicity and frequency of symptom
   d. Course of symptom
      i. Short-term
      ii. Long-term
5. **Setting**
6. **Modifying factors**
   a. Precipitating and aggravating factors
   b. Palliating factors
7. **Associated symptoms**

Modified from Smith RC. Patient centered interviewing. 2nd ed. Philadelphia: Lippincott Williams & Wilkins; 2002.

questions to elicit all the cardinal features ("You pointed to the left side of your chest; does the pain travel anywhere?"). For nonpain symptoms (eg, weakness, dizziness), all cardinal features may not apply (eg, location, radiation).

Precise location of symptoms should be determined. The location of a symptom and whether it radiates can be diagnostically important (eg, low back pain radiating to the buttock and down the postero-lateral thigh and lateral calf suggests L5–S1 nerve root impingement from a herniated disk).

The quality of a symptom can assist with diagnosis. For example, burning substernal chest pain is more likely to be due to esophageal reflux, while squeezing or crushing chest pain is more likely to be angina or myocardial infarction.

Patients sometimes describe their symptoms in unusual ways, eg, "It feels like someone is reaching inside me and tearing me apart." Such language may hint at psychological problems, although it can indicate serious illness as well.

When quantifying a pain symptom, use a numeric rating scale, "On a scale of 1 to 10, with 1 being no pain and 10 being the worst you can imagine, what number would you give this pain you're describing?"

Chronology provides the structure for the rest of the patient's disease story: the primary problem(s), when it began, its course to the present, and its previous treatment. All relevant details of this structure must be filled in to best understand the big picture—the interacting biologic, psychological (personal, emotional), and social dimensions of patients. The student or physician usually organizes the rest of the features to fit within the chronology.

Inquiring About Symptoms in Same Body System

After obtaining a complete picture of the patient's symptom story, including all relevant cardinal features, ask about symptoms in the same body system as the one described in the HPI. In essence we do a focused "review of systems" of that one body system. We want to know not just which other symptoms are present but also which ones are absent; for example, the absence of dyspnea in a patient with chest pain weighs against a diagnosis of pulmonary embolism.

Asking About Other Relevant Symptoms

It is important to ask about symptoms outside the involved body system if they are pertinent to a diagnosis you are considering. For example, in a patient with advanced rheumatoid arthritis who is feeling fatigued, asking about gastrointestinal bleeding symptoms ("any black stools?"), while outside the musculoskeletal system, is still warranted if bleeding caused by nonsteroidal anti-inflammatory drug therapy is suspected. In patients with more than one problem, inquiry in multiple systems will be required during the HPI.

Inquiring About Relevant Nonsymptom Data

Ask questions about the presence or absence of relevant secondary data not yet introduced by the patient. It is important to know any data concerning medications, diagnoses, treatments, doctors, and hospital stays. Also, asking relevant questions about possible etiologic explanations for the diagnoses being entertained may help narrow the differential diagnosis. For example, if pulmonary embolism is a concern, asking about recent long car rides or air travel is warranted.

Scanning Without Interpretation Versus Hypothesis Testing

Early in medical school, when interviewing is learned, students often do not know what might be causing a patient's symptom. By using the patient-centered and doctor-centered approaches, you will gather sufficient data to guide your search of texts and other resources to discover which diagnosis is most likely. Beginning interviewers must be exhaustive in their interviewing ("scanning" approach) because they are not interpreting the patient's responses in real time to guide further questioning.[4] It is often necessary to return to the patient with additional questions after reading about the problem and developing new hypotheses about what is causing the symptoms.

As medical knowledge and interviewing experience increase, however, students begin to have ideas or "hunches" about what might be causing a patient's symptoms. Interviewers can then ask specific questions to test these hypotheses.[5] For example, a patient with sudden shortness of breath and chest pain following a long car ride might prompt consideration of pulmonary embolism as the cause. To test this hypothesis, ask about hemoptysis, leg pain, whether the chest pain is pleuritic in quality, and if there is a prior history of deep venous thrombosis. The symptom-based chapters in this book will help students develop hypotheses and test them. With time and practice, knowledge and skills develop sufficiently to allow reliance upon the hypothesis-driven approach, although never completely abandoning the scanning approach. Similarly, with experience using hypothesis-testing skills, the above elements can be intermixed for efficiency rather than obtained sequentially.

Becoming Patient Centered When Necessary

Doctor-centered interviewing is only part of the interview, and the interviewer must return to the patient-centered mode if the patient expresses emotion, using the NURS skills (**n**aming, **u**nderstanding, **r**especting, and **s**upporting) (see Chapter 3). For example, if the patient becomes tearful when asked about her parents and then indicates that her father died last week, the interviewer must switch to the patient-centered approach. Using the NURS skills, one can learn more about this event, providing support and empathy: "That's very **sad,** I can **understand.** It's sure **been a hard time** for you. Is there anything **I can do to help?"**

Overview of the History After the HPI

At this point, all relevant details of the HPI have been obtained. Although you may have a reasonable idea about the diagnosis, much ancillary data are still needed. Some of it will be related directly to the HPI (eg, a prior history of myocardial infarction will be very germane in a patient with bloody stools if he requires major surgery). On the other hand, much of it will not relate directly to the HPI but will nonetheless represent important information about the patient (eg, personal exercise habits, education, and family history of tuberculosis).

The approach to the remainder of the history is similar to the doctor-centered part of the HPI. Questioning should begin in an open-ended fashion in each major area and then be followed by closed-ended questions to obtain the details, always remembering to return to the patient-centered skills and NURS when necessary.

PAST MEDICAL HISTORY

In the past medical history, inquire about medical issues and events not directly related to the HPI (Table 4–3). Start with open-ended questions (eg, "How was your health as a child?") and then focus as needed with closed-ended questions to establish details (eg, "Did you have chicken pox? Measles?").

Medications

Determine the medications the patient takes, including both dosages and routes of administration. Be sure to ask about over-the-counter medications and herbal or alternative remedies. Ask specifically about birth control pills, hormones, laxatives, and vitamins, as these are sometimes not considered medications by patients.

Allergies

Ask about environmental, food, and medication allergies. Determine exactly what reaction the patient had to a medication; this is important because many medication "allergies" are actually expected side effects (eg, itching with morphine) or nonallergic adverse reactions (eg, gastric bleeding from aspirin).

SOCIAL HISTORY

The social history describes behaviors and other personal factors that may impact disease risk, severity and outcome; it also helps the interviewer to get to know the patient (Table 4–4).

Table 4–3. Past medical history.

- Inquire about general state of health and past illnesses
  - Childhood: measles, mumps, rubella, chicken pox, scarlet fever, and rheumatic fever
  - Adult: hypertension, cerebrovascular accident, diabetes, heart disease, tuberculosis, venereal disease, cancer
- Inquire about past injuries, accidents, psychotherapy, unexplained problems
- Elicit past hospitalizations (medical, surgical, obstetric, and psychiatric)
- Review the patient's immunization history
  - Childhood: measles, mumps, rubella, polio, hepatitis B, chicken pox, tetanus/pertussis/diptheria
  - Adult: tetanus boosters, hepatitis B, hepatitis A, influenza, pneumococcal pneumonia
- Obtain the patient's obstetric history and menstrual history
  - Age of menarche, cycle length, length of menstrual flow, number of tampons/pads used per day
  - Number of pregnancies, complications; number of live births, spontaneous vaginal deliveries/cesarean sections; number of spontaneous and therapeutic abortions
  - Age of menopause
- List current medications, including dose and route
  - Ask specifically about over-the-counter medicines, alternative remedies, contraceptives, vitamins, laxatives
- Review allergies
  - Environmental, medications, foods
  - Ensure that medication "allergies" are not actually expected side effects or nonallergic adverse reactions

As students gain experience, they learn which questions are most important to ask for a particular patient encounter. Discussing the highlighted items will identify targets for risk factor modification and assist in building the doctor-patient relationship. Such issues, although rarely brought up by patients, should be discussed openly and in a nonjudgmental fashion to both garner trust and obtain accurate information. This type of information may need to be obtained over multiple patient encounters.

The psychosocial data collected in the social history complements the personal and emotional information obtained in the patient-centered portion of the interview. Hearing a patient's story and responding to his emotions is therapeutic and crucial to the doctor-patient relationship.

Some of the most important areas of the social history are detailed below; Table 4–4 lists all them all.

Habits

Ask about tobacco use, including forms of tobacco (eg, pipe, snuff, chewing tobacco) and number of pack-years for cigarette use.

Determine whether the patient consumes alcohol and whether it may be a health problem. Ask, "Do you drink beer, wine, or spirits? How much alcohol do you drink? Has alcohol ever been a problem in your life? When was your last drink?" A positive response to the last question (that is, the last drink was within 24 hours) has a positive predictive value of 68% and a negative predictive value of 98% for alcohol abuse.[6] Then, if necessary you can follow-up with the "CAGE" questions[7,8]:

- "Have you thought about **C**utting down?"
- "Have you ever gotten **A**nnoyed when people talk to you about your drinking?"
- "Have you ever felt **G**uilty about your drinking?"
- "Do you ever have a drink first thing in the morning (**E**ye opener)?"

Table 4–4. Social history.[a]

Habits

- **Caffeine use**

- **Tobacco use**
    - Forms
    - Pack-years

- **Alcohol use**
    - Type and amount consumed at 1 time/daily/weekly
    - "CAGE" questions

- **Drug use**
    - "Street" drugs
    - Illicit use of prescription drugs

Health Promotion

- **Diet**

- **Physical activity/exercise history**

- Functional status

- **Safety**
    - Seatbelt use
    - Safety helmet use
    - Smoke detectors in home
    - Safe gun storage

- **Screening**
    - Cervical cancer
    - Breast cancer
    - Colon cancer
    - Lipids
    - Hypertension
    - Diabetes
    - HIV
    - Syphilis
    - Tuberculosis
    - Glaucoma

Personal life

- **Occupation**
    - Occupational exposures

- **Home life**

- **Personal relationships and support systems**

- **Sexuality**
    - Orientation

Table 4–4. Social history.[a] (cont.)

- — Practices
- — Any difficulty
- **Domestic partner violence/abuse**
- **Stress**
- **Health beliefs**
- **Spirituality/religion**
- Important life experiences
  - — Upbringing and family relationships
  - — Schooling
  - — Military service
  - — Financial situation
  - — Aging
  - — Retirement
  - — Life satisfaction
  - — Cultural/ethnic background

[a]Items in bold should be asked about in most new patient encounters: they have high yield for risk factor modification, assist in building the doctor-patient relationship, and/or are important to patients but rarely brought up by them.

An affirmative answer to 2 or more CAGE questions has a sensitivity and specificity of > 90% for alcohol dependence.[6]

Determine whether the patient uses or abuses either "street" drugs or prescription drugs, and quantify the amount.

Personal Life

Occupation

A patient's occupation can affect health.[9] Ask, "Do you work outside the home?" "What kind of work do you do? How long have you done this work? What other jobs have you had? Have you ever been exposed to fumes, dust, radiation, or loud noise at work? Do you think your work is affecting your symptoms now?" If the patient does not work outside the home, ask what a typical day is like.

Home Life and Sexuality

A good way to inquire about home life is to ask, "Does anyone else live at home with you? Tell me about him or her." This may provide a comfortable segue into asking about sexuality.[10] Some suggested questions include the following:

- "Is there someone special in your life? Are you and this person having sex?"
- "Do you have sex with men, women, or both?"
- "Do you have sex with people who might be at risk for having sexually transmitted diseases or HIV (injection drug users, cocaine users, prostitutes, unknown partners, gay or bisexual men)?"
- "Are you using condoms to prevent disease? What percent of the time?
- "Do you have any other questions or concerns about sex?"
- "Are there any other sexual relationships that I should know about?"

To detect sexual problems, ask:
- "Have you noticed any recent changes or problems in your sexual functioning?"
- Men: "Do you have any problems having or maintaining an erection?" "Any trouble having an orgasm?"
- Women: "Do you have pain during intercourse?" "Any problems with lubrication or becoming aroused?" "Do you have difficulty having an orgasm?"
- "Has your illness affected your sexual functioning?"

Do not assume a patient's sexuality. Avoid questions such as "Are you married or single?" or (to a woman), "Do you have a boyfriend?" Gender-neutral language (eg, "partner") communicates to gay, lesbian, bisexual, and transgender patients that it is safe for them to be honest and open with the interviewer.

As with the rest of the medical interview, we must obviously tailor our questions to the particular encounter. For example, it would not be appropriate to take a detailed sexual history from a person in acute congestive heart failure in a crowded emergency department. Once the patient is stabilized and in a more private setting, you could return to these questions.

Table 4–5. Family history

1. Inquire about age and health (or cause or death) of grandparents, parents, siblings, and children
2. Ask specifically about family history of:
- Diabetes
- Tuberculosis
- Cancer
- Hypertension
- Stroke
- Heart disease
- Hyperlipidemia
- Bleeding problems
- Anemias
- Kidney disease
- Asthma
- Tobacco use
- Alcoholism
- Weight problems
- Mental illness
    — depression
    — suicide
    — schizophrenia
    — multiple somatic concerns
- Symptoms similar to those the patient is experiencing

Table 4–6. Review of systems.

General	Mouth and Throat		Male Genital

General

Usual state of health
Fever
Chills
Night sweats
Appetite
Weight change
Weakness
Fatigue
Pain
Anhedonia

Skin

Rashes
Itching
Hives
Easy bruising
Change in moles

Head

Dizziness
Headaches
Trauma

Eyes

Use of glasses
Change in vision
Double vision
Pain
Redness
Discharge
History of glaucoma
Cataracts

Ears

Hearing loss
Use of hearing aid
Discharge
Pain
Tinnitus

Nose

Nosebleeds
Discharge
Loss of smell

Mouth and Throat

Bleeding gums
Pain on swallowing
Difficulty swallowing
Hoarseness
Tongue burning
Tooth pain

Neck

Lumps
Goiter
Stiffness

Chest

Cough
Pain
Shortness of breath
Sputum production
Hemoptysis
Wheezing

Breasts

Lumps
Discharge
Pain
Self-examination

Cardiac

Chest pain
Palpitations
DOE
PND

Vascular

Pain in legs, calves, thighs, hips, buttocks when walking
Leg swelling
Thrombophlebitis
Ulcers

Gastrointestinal

Appetite
Nausea
Vomiting/hematemesis

Swallowing difficulty/pain
Heartburn
Abdominal pain
Constipation
Diarrhea
Change in stool color/caliber
Melena
Rectal bleeding
Hemorrhoids

Urinary

Frequency/nocturia
Urgency
Difficulty starting stream
Incontinence
Hematuria
Dysuria

Female Genital

Lesions/discharge/itching
Age at menarche
Interval between menses
Duration of menses
Amount of flow
Last menses
Bleeding between periods
Pregnancies
Abortions/miscarriages
Libido
Dyspareunia
Orgasm function
Age at menopause
Menopausal symptoms
Postmenopausal bleeding

Male Genital

Lesions/discharge
Erectile function
Orgasm function
Testis swelling/pain
Libido
Hernia

Neuropsychiatric

Fainting
Paralysis
Numbness
Tingling
Tremors
Loss of memory
Mood changes
Sleep
Nervousness
Speech disorders
Gait disorders
Hallucinations
Seizures

Musculoskeletal

Weakness
Pain
Stiffness

DOE, dyspnea on exertion; PND, paroxysmal nocturnal dyspnea

Domestic Partner Violence

An estimated 2 to 4 million US women are physically abused each year, with domestic violence occurring in as many as 1 of every 4 US families. Although it may feel uncomfortable, physicians must learn to sensitively inquire about domestic partner violence, since patients are unlikely to broach this important issue themselves. One suggested approach[11] is "Have you ever been hit, slapped, kicked, or otherwise physically hurt by someone? Has anyone ever forced you to have sexual activities?"

Spirituality and Religious Beliefs

Spirituality and religious beliefs are important to many patients, especially in times of illness. One suggested mnemonic for asking about these issues is FICA[12]:

F: Faith and belief: "Do you consider yourself to be a spiritual or religious person?" "What is your faith or belief?" "What gives your life meaning?"

I: Importance and influence: "What importance does faith have in your life?" "Have your beliefs influenced that way you take care of yourself and your illness?" "What role do your beliefs play in regaining your health or coping with illness?"

C: Community: "Are you a part of a spiritual or religious community?" "Does the community support you? If so, how?" "Is there a group of people you really love or who are important to you?"

A: Address in care: "Would you like me to address these issues in your health care?"

FAMILY HISTORY

The family history is a critical source of information outlined in Table 4–5. Ask about the age and health of the patient's immediate family as well as the causes of death and ages of first-degree relatives. Patients with recent losses may exhibit emotion, which should be addressed with "NURS."

Screen for genetic and environmental illnesses by asking about a family history of diseases such as cancer, heart disease, diabetes, tuberculosis, alcoholism, and asthma.

REVIEW OF SYSTEMS

The review of systems (ROS) is a head-to-toe survey to uncover symptoms not elicited earlier in the interview. Part of the ROS was already performed (see Filling in the HPI). Now, the remaining body systems are surveyed to ensure that the database is complete (Table 4–6). At this point, the interviewer should already have a reasonable idea about the major diagnostic possibilities, from data gathered in the HPI and past medical history. The ROS is not used to elucidate key features of the present illness.[1] Rather, it is used to screen for any additional symptoms *unrelated* to the HPI (eg, abnormal vaginal bleeding in a patient with suspected pneumonia). Finally, do not extensively probe for every possible symptom in the ROS; try to identify only those symptoms that cause significant problems for the patient.

As always, the interviewer should be prepared to return to patient-centered techniques if the patient shows emotion.

Doctor-centered interviewing helps uncover diagnostically important information and a routine database about the patient. Coupled with the information from the patient-centered interview, the interviewer develops the patient's biopsychosocial story, encompassing not only the patient's disease problems but also the personal and emotional context in which they occur.[12]

REFERENCES

1. Smith RC. *Patient centered interviewing.* 2nd ed. Lippincott Williams & Wilkins; 2002:1–16.

2. Bickley LS, Hoekelman RA, Bates B. *Bates' Guide to Physical Examination and History Taking.* 7th ed. Lippincott; 1999.

3. Morgan WL, Engel GL. *The Clinical Approach to the Patient.* WB Saunders; 1969.

4. Barrows HS, Pickell GC. *Developing Clinical Problem-Solving Skills: A Guide to More Effective Diagnosis and Treatment.* W.W. Norton; 1991.

5. Elstein AS. Psychological research on diagnostic reasoning. In: Lipkin M, Putnam SM, Lazare A, editors. *The Medical Interview.* Springer-Verlag; 1995:504–510.

6. Fiellin DA, Reid MC, O'Connor PG. Screening for alcohol problems in primary care: a systematic review. *Arch Intern Med.* 2000;160:1977–1989.

7. Ewing JA. Detecting alcoholism. The CAGE questionnaire. *JAMA.* 1984;252:1905–1907.

8. Clark W. Effective interviewing and intervention for alcohol problems. In: Lipkin M, Putnam SM, Lazare A, editors. *The Medical Interview.* Springer-Verlag; 1995:284–293.

9. Landrigan PJ, Barker DB. The recognition and control of occupational disease. *JAMA.* 1991;266:676–680.

10. Williams S. The sexual history. In: Lipkin M, Putnam SM, Lazare A, editors. *The Medical Interview.* Springer-Verlag; 1995:235–250.

11. MacCauley JG, Kern DE et al. The "Battering Syndrome": Prevalence and clinical characteristics of domestic violence in primary care internal medicine practices. *Ann Intern Med.* 1995;123:737–746.

12. Puchalski C, Romer AL. Taking a spiritual history allows clinicians to understand patients more fully. *J Palliat Med.* 2000;3:129–137.

SUGGESTED READING

Engel GL. The need for a new medical model: a challenge for biomedicine. *Science.* 1977;196:129–136.

Smith RC. Videotape of Evidence-Based Interviewing: (1) Patient-Centered Interviewing and (2) Doctor-Centered Interviewing. Marketing Division, Instructional Media Center, Michigan State University. P.O. Box 710, East Lansing, MI 48824.

The Evidence-Based Approach to Clinical Decision Making

5

Garth Davis, MD, Mark C. Henderson, MD, & Gerald W. Smetana, MD

Students think of history taking as an intuitive process: the patient presents a complaint, a complete history and physical examination is performed, a diagnosis is made. In reality, it is an exercise in clinical reasoning, where the historian applies principles of epidemiology, statistics, and probability to arrive at a diagnosis.

For every symptom there is a differential diagnosis including common maladies and rare diseases. Epidemiologic factors such as the patient's age and gender affect the likelihood of certain diagnoses. For instance, the likelihood of migraine as the cause of a recent onset headache in a 25-year-old woman is much higher than for a 65-year-old man with the same symptom.[1] From this starting point, we consider a list of potential diagnoses of varying likelihood and seriousness. Experienced clinicians use each piece of additional epidemiologic and clinical information to continually narrow the diagnostic possibilities. Think of this process as an inverted funnel. Initial considerations are broad, but as the history progresses, a smaller number of possible diagnoses remain.

Focused questioning further characterizes the patient's complaint; the presence or absence of various clinical findings makes certain diagnoses more or less likely. In this way, asking a question is analogous to performing a diagnostic test. Returning to our example, the presence of photophobia, nausea, and throbbing pain each increase the probability of migraine. In contrast, headache duration of greater than 3 days makes migraine less likely.

When taking the medical history, the clinician integrates information about disease **prevalence** (eg, epidemiology) with the **sensitivity** and **specificity** of historical information to determine the **likelihood** of various diagnoses.

KEY TERMS

Sensitivity	*Proportion of people with the disease that have a clinical finding (or positive test). Also known as the true positive rate.*
Specificity	*Proportion of people without the disease that do not have a clinical finding (or have a negative test). Also known as the true negative rate.*
Prevalence	*The proportion of people with the disease in question in a given population.*
Pretest probability	*The proportion of people with the disease in question prior to knowledge of a particular clinical finding or test result.*

(continued)

KEY TERMS

Posttest probability	*Proportion of patients with the specified test result (or clinical finding) who have the disease.*
Positive predictive value	*Proportion of people with a positive test or clinical finding who have the disease.*
Negative predictive value	*Proportion of people with a negative test or without a clinical finding who do not have the disease.*
Likelihood ratio	*The likelihood of a given test result or clinical finding in a patient with a disease compared with the likelihood of the same result in a patient without disease.*

PROBABILITY AND UNCERTAINTY[2]

One of the most troubling aspects of clinical decision making is uncertainty. Clinical information cannot determine the presence or absence of disease with absolute certainty. Similarly, test results may help determine the likely diagnosis but do not prove that the patient has the disorder. A more realistic approach is to think in terms of the *probability* of disease. Probability can be expressed mathematically as a spectrum from 0 to 1, where 1 represents certainty of disease and 0 represents certainty of no disease.

$$0———————————————1$$
$$\text{Probability of disease}$$

This probabilistic approach is particularly important when considering diseases for which no diagnostic "gold standard" (eg, confirmatory laboratory, pathologic, or imaging test) exists. In these cases, diagnostic confidence is based entirely on the history and physical examination. Migraine is an example of such a condition. By definition, diagnostic testing is normal in patients with migraine; it is a clinical diagnosis.

Each new piece of clinical information has the potential to alter the probability of disease. Accurately interpreting how clinical information affects the probability of disease is the basis of clinical decision making.

PREVALENCE AND PRETEST PROBABILITY

For a given complaint there are myriad potential explanations or diagnoses. Some diseases are very common, others less so. Before you perform a history and physical, the likelihood of a given diagnosis is determined by the **prevalence** of that disease in the patient population. Disease prevalence is often used interchangeably with **pretest probability.**

Unfortunately, individual estimates of disease prevalence are a common source of error. Because individual experience constitutes a relatively small sample, clinicians may overestimate the prevalence of some diseases and underestimate that of others. Integrating disease prevalence from large population studies with clinical experience helps minimize errors in estimating the pretest probability of disease.

Returning to our example, we use the literature to provide data to inform our clinical decision making. Among 25-year-old women in the general population, the prevalence (pretest probability) of migraine is 18%.[1] The prevalence of migraine among 65-year-old men is only 7%. So the likelihood of migraine, based only on age and gender, is *already* 2.5 times greater in the first patient.

SENSITIVITY AND SPECIFICITY[3,4]

The relationship between a clinical finding and a given disease can be expressed in a 2 × 2 table (see below). Using this paradigm, there are 4 diagnostic possibilities or outcomes:

1. The clinical finding is present and the patient has the disease (true positive).
2. The clinical finding is present but the patient does not have the disease (false positive).

3. The clinical finding is absent but the patient has the disease (false negative).
4. The clinical finding is absent and the patient does not have the disease (true negative).

	Disease present	*Disease absent*
Clinical finding present	*True positives (TP)*	*False positives (FP)*
Clinical finding absent	*False negatives (FN)*	*True negatives (TN)*

Clinical findings with high **sensitivity** are useful for excluding diagnoses. As the sensitivity increases, the number of false negatives decreases. With a very low number of false negatives nearly everyone with the disease has the clinical finding. If a highly sensitive test is negative, the disease is unlikely (some students use the mnemonic SnNOut or **s**ensitive tests when **n**egative tend to rule **o**ut disease).

Clinical findings with a high **specificity** are useful for confirming diagnoses. As the specificity increases, the number of false positives decreases. With a very low number of false positive results, the clinical finding is only seen in those with disease. If a highly specific test is positive, the disease is probably present (some students use the mnemonic SpPIn or **s**pecific tests when **p**ositive tend to rule **in** disease).

For example, there is evidence from the literature on the frequency of various historical features in patients with migraine and tension-type headache, the 2 most common primary headaches (headaches without pathologic cause). In a large systematic review, the presence of nausea had a sensitivity of 81% and a specificity of 96% for migraine.[5] The high specificity indicates that the presence of nausea tends to "rule in" the diagnosis of migraine. Unilateral headache, in contrast, had a sensitivity of 66% and a specificity of 78% for migraine.

PREDICTIVE VALUE[4,5]

Sensitivity and specificity are independent of disease prevalence, and remain constant across different populations. Predictive value describes the performance of a test or clinical finding in a population with a specific prevalence. **Positive predictive value** (PPV) is the proportion of people with a clinical finding that have the disease (TP divided by TP + FP). **Negative predictive value** (NPV) is the proportion of people without a clinical finding that do not have the disease (TN divided by FN + TN).

Regardless of the sensitivity of a clinical finding, as a disease becomes increasingly rare, the presence of a clinical finding is less likely to indicate the presence of disease (low PPV). Conversely, as a disease becomes more common, the absence of a clinical finding is less likely to mean the disease is not present (low NPV).

POSTTEST PROBABILITY[6]

Posttest probability is the "new" probability of disease given the presence or absence of a given clinical finding (or test result). One might assume that the presence of a clinical finding with high sensitivity and specificity would naturally lead to high posttest probability—this is *not* always the case. Figure 5–1 shows the effect of pretest probability on posttest probability for a clinical finding with a sensitivity of 90% and a specificity of 90%.

When the pretest probability (prevalence) of disease is low, it remains low despite a positive test (Figure 5–1A). When the pretest probability is intermediate, the presence of a given clinical finding (or test result) greatly affects the posttest probability (Figure 5–1B). Understanding the impact of pretest probability is crucial to accurately interpreting clinical information.

LIKELIHOOD RATIOS

Likelihood ratios (LR) are another way to express the diagnostic accuracy of a clinical finding or test. The LR of any clinical finding is:

$$\frac{\text{probability of the clinical finding in patients with disease}}{\text{probability of the clinical finding in patients \textit{without} disease}}$$

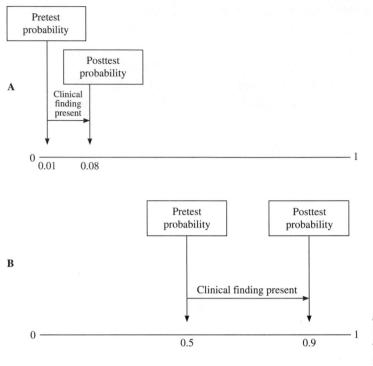

Figure 5–1. The effect of pretest probability on posttest probability for a clinical finding with a sensitivity of 90% and a specificity of 90%.

LRs are calculated from the sensitivity *and* specificity of a clinical finding. Calculation of LRs makes it possible to compare the diagnostic accuracy of 2 or more findings with different sensitivities and specificities. Because LRs are independent of disease prevalence, they can be applied to different patient populations.

For each clinical finding, there is a positive LR (LR+) and a negative LR (LR−). The LR+ is the probability of disease when the clinical finding is present; the LR− is the probability of disease when the clinical finding is absent:

$$LR+ = Sensitivity/(1\text{-specificity})$$
$$LR- = (1\text{-sensitivity})/specificity$$

LRs greater than 1 increase the probability of disease: the higher the number the greater the probability of the disease. LRs less than 1 decrease the probability of disease: the smaller the number the less likely the disease.

Likelihood ratio	Change in probability[7]	Effect on disease likelihood
10	*45%*	*Large*
5	*30%*	*Moderate*
2	*15%*	*Slight*
1	*0*	*None*
0.5	*−15%*	*Slight*
0.2	*−30%*	*Moderate*
0.1	*−45%*	*Large*

For our 2 patients with headache, the LRs for nausea as a diagnostic test for migraine are the same for each patient.

$$LR+ = \text{sensitivity}/(1-\text{specificity}) = 0.81/(1-0.96) = 20.2$$
$$LR- = (1-\text{sensitivity})/\text{specificity} = (1-0.81)/0.96 = 0.20$$

The simplest way to use LRs to calculate posttest probability is to use a nomogram (Figure 5–2).

For the 25-year-old woman with headache, the pretest probability (prevalence) of migraine is 18%. Using the nomogram, the presence of nausea (LR+ = 20.2) increases the posttest probability to 80%, essentially confirming the diagnosis of migraine. Similarly, nausea increases the probability of migraine in our 65-year-old man from 8% (pretest) to 65% (posttest).

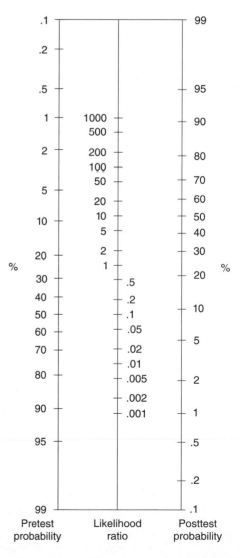

Figure 5–2. Nomogram for determining posttest probability from pretest probability and likelihood ratios. To figure the posttest probability, place a straightedge between the pretest probability and the likelihood ratio for the particular test. The posttest probability will be where the straightedge crosses the posttest probability line. (Reproduced from Tierney LM, McPhee SJ, Papadakis MA (editors). *Current Medical Diagnosis & Treatment 2004.* McGraw-Hill; 2004:1666. Adapted and reproduced, with permission, from Fagan TJ. Nomogram for Bayes theorem. (Letter.) *N Engl J Med.* 1975;293:257.)

This example illustrates the key steps in sound clinical reasoning. When considering a patient with a symptom (eg, headache), first determine the prevalence of the common diagnostic possibilities (eg, migraine) in populations similar to your patient. Then determine the impact of a clinical finding (eg, nausea) on the likelihood of disease by looking up or calculating the appropriate LRs. Finally, understand that despite a strong association between a clinical finding and a disease, the likelihood of that disease is strongly influenced by the pretest probability. Thus, a headache accompanied by nausea in a young woman is most likely a migraine. However, the presence of nausea does not clinch the diagnosis of migraine in a 65-year-old man because migraine is much less common in this population.

CAVEATS

- Clinical findings from the history and physical examination are analogous to diagnostic tests; their accuracy can be expressed in terms of sensitivity, specificity, and LRs.
- The true state of the patient is inferred (not proven) by the clinical findings.
- Using probability in clinical decision making allows you to quantify the likelihood of a suspected diagnosis.
- Disease prevalence is a good initial estimate of pretest probability.
- Clinical findings with high sensitivity are useful for excluding diagnoses and clinical findings with a high specificity are useful for confirming diagnoses.
- LRs are a convenient way to express the impact of a clinical finding on the probability of disease.
- In general, the most important determinant of posttest probability is pretest probability (unless the pretest probability is intermediate).

REFERENCES

1. Rasmussen BK, Jensen R, Schroll M, Olesen J. Epidemiology of headache in a general population—a prevalence study. *J Clin Epidemiol.* 1991;44:1147–1157.
2. Sox HC. *Medical decision making.* Boston: Butterworths; 1988.
3. Sackett DL, Straus SE, Richardson WS, Rosenberg W, Haynes RB. *Evidence Based Medicine. How to Practice and Teach EBM.* 2nd ed. Churchill Livingstone; 2000.
4. Jaeschke R, Guyatt GH, Sackett DL. Users' guides to the medical literature. III. How to use an article about a diagnostic test. B. What are the results and will they help me in caring for my patients? The Evidence-Based Medicine Working Group. *JAMA.* 1994;271:703–707.
5. Smetana GW. The diagnostic value of historical features in primary headache syndromes: a comprehensive review. *Arch Intern Med.* 2000;160:2729–2737.
6. Tierney LM, McPhee SJ, Papadakis MA, editors. *Current Medical Diagnosis & Treatment.* 43rd ed. McGraw-Hill; 2004.
7. McGee S. Simplifying likelihood ratios. *J Gen Intern Med.* 2002;17:646–649.

SECTION II
General Symptoms

Dizziness

Michelle V. Conde, MD, & Mark C. Henderson, MD

Dizziness is classically categorized into 4 subtypes: vertigo, presyncope or syncope, dysequilibrium, and lightheadedness.[1] However, it may be difficult to identify a single category in every patient, particularly in the elderly, who often manifest more than 1 subtype. Medications may also cause more than 1 subtype of dizziness.

KEY TERMS

Dysequilibrium	*Impaired walking due to difficulties with balance. It is sometimes described as dizziness "in the feet." Formally speaking, dysequilibrium does not occur in the nonambulatory patient.*
Lightheadedness	*Dizziness that is not vertigo, syncope, or dysequilibrium; this form is also called **undifferentiated dizziness**.*
Presyncope	*The feeling that one is about to faint or lose consciousness, but actual loss of consciousness is averted. **Syncope** is defined as sudden, transient loss of consciousness (see Chapter 26).*
Vertigo	*An illusion or hallucination of movement, usually rotation, either of oneself or the environment.[2]*
Benign paroxysmal positional vertigo (BPPV)	*BPPV is a common peripheral vestibular disorder that is caused by migration of inner ear otoliths (calcific particles) to the posterior semicircular canal. The otoliths amplify any movement in the plane of the canal, resulting in brief episodes of vertigo following changes in head position.*
Vertebrobasilar insufficiency (VBI)	*Reduced blood flow to the brainstem that causes the following symptoms: vertigo, cranial nerve dysfunction (eg, diplopia, hoarseness, dysarthria, dysphagia), or cerebellar dysfunction (eg, ataxia). Sensory and motor impairment may also occur. VBI may result in transient ischemic attack (TIA) or stroke.*

ETIOLOGY

The etiology of dizziness depends on the clinical setting. A systematic review including over 4500 patients from primary care offices, dizziness clinics, or emergency departments showed that dizziness was due to peripheral vestibular or psychiatric causes in roughly 60% of cases.[3] The cause was unknown in approximately 1 in 7 patients.

Differential Diagnosis	Frequency[a,3]
Peripheral vestibulopathy	**44%**
BPPV	16%
Vestibular neuronitis/labyrinthitis	9%
Meniere's disease	5%
Other (including medication-related, recurrent vestibulopathy)	14%
Nonvestibular, nonpsychiatric	**24%**
Presyncope (including volume depletion, cardiac arrhythmia, or other cardiovascular etiology)	6%
Dysequilibrium	5%
Other (including anemia, metabolic causes, parkinsonism, medication-related)	13%
Psychiatric	**16%**
Psychiatric disorder	11%
Hyperventilation	5%
Central vestibulopathy	**10%**
Cerebrovascular	6%
Tumor	< 1%
Other (including multiple sclerosis, migraine headache)	3%
Unknown	**13%**

[a]Derived from frequencies of specific causes of dizziness across 12 studies. Total percentage > 100% because dizziness was attributed to more than 1 cause in some patients.

GETTING STARTED

- Review medication list before seeing the patient and validate during the interview.
- Avoid leading questions. It may be necessary to follow up with a few close-ended questions directed at the most likely disorder.

Open-ended questions

Tell me about your symptoms. Describe the sensation you've been having without using the word dizzy.

Go over the last time you had this sensation, from start to finish.

Let's review all your medications, including over-the-counter medications, nutritional supplements, or herbal medicines.

Tips for effective interviewing

- *Let patients use their own words.*
- *Avoid interrupting.*
- *Listen to the patient's description for diagnostic clues.*

INTERVIEW FRAMEWORK

- Assess for alarm symptoms.
- Review medication list.
- Categorize into 1 or more dizziness subtypes: vertigo, presyncope/syncope, dysequilibrium, or light-headedness.
- In determining the etiology of each subtype, consider temporal pattern and duration of symptoms, accompanying symptoms, precipitating factors, risk factors, and comorbidities.

IDENTIFYING ALARM SYMPTOMS

Serious causes of dizziness are uncommon. However, most studies have oversampled persons with chronic dizziness and underrepresented persons with acute forms of dizziness who may be more likely to have life-threatening illnesses.[4] So these data may underestimate the prevalence of serious disorders in patients with acute dizziness.

Selected serious diagnoses	Frequency[a,3]
Cerebrovascular disease (stroke, TIA)	6%
Cardiac arrhythmia	1.5%
Brain tumor	< 1%

[a]Derived from frequencies of specific causes of dizziness across 12 studies.

Identification of these serious disorders requires detailed questioning aimed at eliciting cardinal symptoms of heart disease, neighborhood neurologic symptoms, and associated risk factors. Any focal neurologic symptoms should prompt immediate brain imaging to rule out serious central nervous system (CNS) causes of vertigo, eg, VBI. Other serious diagnoses, such as anemia, hypoglycemia, and carbon monoxide poisoning, are suggested by selected laboratory tests.

Alarm symptoms	Serious causes	Benign causes
Chest discomfort or presyncope/syncope	See Chapter 24 See Chapter 26	
Acute onset vertigo plus neurologic deficits (eg, diplopia, hemiparesis, dysarthria)	VBI Brainstem mass Meningoencephalitis Cranial polyneuritis Vasculitis (involving the eighth nerve) Multiple sclerosis or other demyelinating diseases Partial seizure	Basilar artery migraine
Acute vertigo (lasting > 1 day), nausea, vomiting, severe imbalance	Cerebellar stroke/mass (patient usually unable to walk without falling)	Acute vestibular neuronitis/labyrinthitis (patient tilts to one side but is still able to walk)

(continued)

Alarm symptoms	Serious causes
Sudden onset severe vertigo, facial paralysis, otalgia, external ear vesicular eruption, hearing loss	Ramsay Hunt syndrome (herpes zoster oticus)
History of diabetes (insulin and/or oral hypoglycemic use)	Hypoglycemia

FOCUSED QUESTIONS

After having the patient tell his or her own story, follow up with a few close-ended questions directed at the most likely subtype.

Questions	Think about
When you have these spells, do you just feel lightheaded or do you see the world spin around you, as if you had just gotten off a merry-go-round?	Vertigo (if answer is "spin")[2]
Do you feel these spells in your head or in your legs? Do you have trouble with your balance?	Dysequilibrium (if answer is "in the legs")
Have you ever passed out?	Syncope
Have you ever felt you might pass out but did not (like the feeling you get when you stand up too quickly)?	Presyncope
Patient responses are vague; nonspecific descriptions that do not fit into above categories (eg, "I'm just dizzy")	Lightheadedness or undifferentiated dizziness

Vertigo

Once vertigo is identified, knowing the temporal pattern and duration may help narrow the differential diagnosis. Further characterize the vertigo by assessing its quality, time course, associated symptoms, and modifying symptoms.

Questions	Think about
Quality	
Is the vertigo mild?	Central causes (vertigo less intense in central causes versus peripheral causes)
Is the vertigo intense? Does it confine you to bed or make you stop what you are doing?	Meniere's disease Vestibular neuronitis/labyrinthitis BPPV Recurrent vestibulopathy
Time course	**Think about**
Was the onset abrupt?	VBI BPPV Meniere's disease Perilymphatic fistula (versus gradual onset, as in acoustic neuroma)
Did the symptoms begin over a few hours and then peak after 1 day?	Vestibular neuronitis

Do the symptoms recur?	Meniere's disease BPPV Recurrent vestibulopathy VBI (assess for other neurologic symptoms)

Associated symptoms | **Think about**

Do you have nausea, vomiting, or sweating?	Usually peripheral disorders, eg, Meniere's disease, vestibular neuronitis/labyrinthitis, or recurrent vestibulopathy; occasionally VBI
Do you have discharge from ear?	Suppurative otitis media
Do you have double vision, weakness, or numbness on 1 side of the body?	VBI Brainstem mass Basilar artery migraine Partial seizure
Do you have headache?	Basilar artery migraine Cerebellar mass
Is there ringing in your ear?	Meniere's disease Acoustic neuroma Drug toxicity (eg, aminoglycoside antibiotics, salicylates, and loop diuretics)
Ear fullness or stuffiness before the vertigo?	Meniere's disease Middle/inner ear disease
Do you have hearing loss?	Meniere's disease (fluctuating, unilateral symptoms in 80% but may later develop bilateral disease) Acoustic neuroma Drug toxicity Labyrinthitis Labyrinthine concussion (basilar skull fracture traversing inner ear) Labyrinthine infarction (with associated neurologic signs) Perilymphatic fistula
Have you had a preceding viral illness?	Vestibular neuronitis or labyrinthitis
Do you have profound imbalance?	Cerebellar stroke/mass
Is there bleeding from your ear canal?	Temporal bone fracture

Modifying symptoms | **Think about**

Does rolling over in bed make your symptoms worse? Or bending over and straightening up or extending your neck to look up?	BPPV
Does coughing, sneezing, or straining worsen your symptoms?	Perilymphatic fistula (disruption of membranes separating the middle and inner ear with resultant perilymph leakage into middle ear, usually following barotrauma or ear surgery)
Does the vertigo occur more commonly in the morning? (matutinal vertigo)	Peripheral causes (eg, vestibular neuronitis or labyrinthitis)

Presyncope/Syncope

In a dizzy patient who has lost consciousness, syncope must be distinguished from seizure. See Chapter 26 for the diagnostic approach to presyncope/syncope.

Dysequilibrium

Visual impairment, hearing loss, peripheral neuropathy, and musculoskeletal abnormalities all contribute to the **syndrome of multiple sensory deficits,** which is a common geriatric syndrome. Ask specific questions to further delineate any sensory and/or motor impairment.

Questions	Think about
Are you having any trouble seeing?	*Visual impairment (eg, cataract)*
Are you having any trouble hearing?	*Conductive hearing impairment (eg, impacted cerumen, otitis media, otosclerosis) and/or neurosensory impairment (eg, presbycusis, the degenerative hearing loss of aging)*
Are you having any tingling or numbness in your legs or feet?	*Disorders of nerve roots, plexi, and peripheral nerves*
Do you feel weak in your legs or have incoordination in your legs?	*Musculoskeletal abnormalities (eg, cervical spondylosis, osteoarthritis, spinal stenosis); cerebellar dysfunction*

Common disorders that may cause dysequilibrium include the following:

- Diabetic peripheral neuropathy
- Parkinsonism
- Alcoholic cerebellar degeneration
- B_{12} deficiency
- Sequelae of vertebrobasilar stroke
- Bilateral vestibular hypofunction (alcohol, aminoglycoside toxicity; aminoglycoside toxicity may be accompanied by oscillopsia, which is the sensation that the eyes bounce up and down)

Lightheadedness

Frequently, underlying psychological disorders are associated with this subtype of dizziness, which is difficult for patients to describe. In addition, prescription drug toxicity and substance abuse are associated with this subtype.

Four clinical cues (S4 model) predict a subgroup of ambulatory patients likely to have underlying depressive and anxiety disorders.[5]

S4 Model[a]

Tell me what symptoms you've been experiencing.	**S**ymptom count (positive response if ≥ 6 symptoms)
During the past week have you been under stress?	**S**tress
Describe how bad your symptom is, from 10 (unbearable) to 0 (none at all).	**S**everity (positive response if ≥ 6)

| In general, would you say your health is excellent, very good, good, fair, or poor? | **S**elf-rated health (positive response for "fair" or "poor" responses) |

[a]The presence of 2 or more of these clinical cues signals the need for a more detailed psychological evaluation. The presence of all 4 predictors yields a positive likelihood ratio of 36.3 for an underlying depressive or anxiety disorder.

DIAGNOSTIC APPROACH

Keep in mind that the causes of dizziness may overlap the different subtypes. Some patients cannot describe their symptoms in a way that fits neatly into the 4 subtypes. Half of elderly patients describe 2 or more dizziness subtypes.[4] Psychiatric causes often coexist with other causes of dizziness.[6] Dysequilibrium may follow disorders that produce vertigo. Vestibular neuronitis or labyrinthitis initially presents with vertigo but may subsequently cause unsteadiness in the legs (dysequilibrium) lasting for several weeks or months. Likewise, vertebrobasilar stroke can present with vertigo followed by dysequilibrium because some patients (particularly the elderly) may also have reduced compensatory multisensory and circulatory systems.

See the algorithms for evaluating patients with dizziness and assessing those with vertigo.

CAVEATS

- A single etiology may result in more than 1 subtype of dizziness.
- Positional vertigo may be confused with postural hypotension. Both can occur on arising; however, positional vertigo occurs with a change in position that does *not* result in global cerebral hypoperfusion. For example, positional vertigo (but not postural hypotension) may occur with rolling over in bed or bending forward to put on socks or tie shoes.
- Although most central causes of vertigo produce focal neurologic symptoms, cerebellar stroke may present only with vertigo and ataxia and thus be mistaken for vestibular neuronitis.[7] The physical examination will be helpful in differentiating a central cause from a peripheral cause. For example, nystagmus due to cerebellar stroke persists for greater than 48 hours, often for weeks to months, while nystagmus associated with a peripheral lesion tends to improve after 24–48 hours.[7] The fast component of central vestibular nystagmus changes direction when the direction of gaze changes, whereas the fast component of peripheral vestibular nystagmus remains in the same direction when the direction of gaze changes.
- Vertebrobasilar TIAs may present with isolated vertigo, usually lasting minutes.[8] Atherosclerotic risk factors should heighten clinical suspicion. If recurrent, other VBI symptoms typically occur.

PROGNOSIS

In a recent community-based study, 3% of patients with persistent dizziness were severely incapacitated by their symptoms.[9] History of fainting, vertigo, or avoidance of situations that provoke dizziness predicted chronic, handicapping dizziness.

REFERENCES

1. Drachman DA, Hart CW. An approach to the dizzy patient. *Neurology.* 1972;22:323–334.

2. Hanley K, O'Dowd T, Considine N. A systematic review of vertigo in primary care. *Br J Gen Pract.* 2001;51:666–671.

3. Kroenke K, Hoffman RM, Einstadter D. How common are various causes of dizziness? A critical review. *South Med J.* 2000;93:160–167; quiz 168.

4. Sloane PD, Coeytaux RR, Beck RS, Dallara J. Dizziness: state of the science. *Ann Intern Med.* 2001;134:823–832.

5. Kroenke K, Jackson JL, Chamberlin J. Depressive and anxiety disorders in patients presenting with physical complaints: clinical predictors and outcome. *Am J Med.* 1997;103:339–347.

6. Clark MR, Sullivan MD, Fischl M, et al. Symptoms as a clue to otologic and psychiatric diagnosis in patients with dizziness. *J Psychosom Res.* 1994;38:461–470.

7. Baloh RW. Differentiating between peripheral and central causes of vertigo. *Otolaryngol Head Neck Surg.* 1998;119:55–59.

8. Grad A, Baloh RW. Vertigo of vascular origin. Clinical and electronystagmographic features in 84 cases. *Arch Neurol.* 1989;46:281–284.

9. Nazareth I, Yardley L, Owen N, Luxon L. Outcome of symptoms of dizziness in a general practice community sample. *Fam Pract.* 1999;16:616–618.

SUGGESTED READING

Baloh RW. Vestibular neuritis. *N Engl J Med.* 2003;348:1027–1032.

Drachman DA. A 69-year-old man with chronic dizziness. *JAMA.* 1998;280:2111–2119.

Hoffman RM, Einstadter D, Kroenke K. Evaluating dizziness. *Am J Med.* 1999;107:468–478.

Hotson JR, Baloh RW. Acute vestibular syndrome. *N Engl J Med.* 1998;339:680–685.

Sloane PD. Evaluation and management of dizziness in the older patient. *Clin Geriatr Med.* 1996;12:785–801.

Warner EA, Wallach PM, Adelman HM, Sahlin-Hughes K. Dizziness in primary care patients. *J Gen Intern Med.* 1992;7:454–463.

Diagnostic Approach: Dizziness

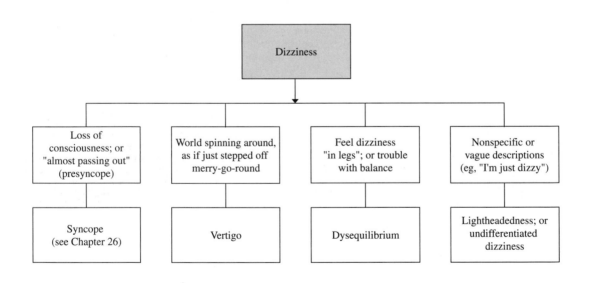

Diagnostic Approach: Vertigo

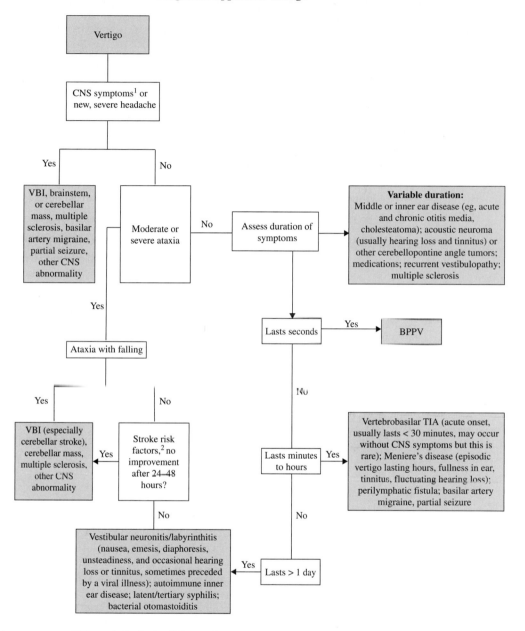

CNS, central nervous system; VBI, vertebrobasilar insufficiency; BPPV, benign paroxysmal positional vertigo.

[1]CNS symptoms: Focal sensory or motor deficits; brainstem findings, eg, dysathria, diplopia, dysphagia, hoarseness.
[2]Stroke risk factors: Advanced age, smoking, dyslipidemia, family history, diabetes mellitus, hypertension, atrial fibrillation, coronary artery disease, heart failure, peripheral vascular disease.

Fatigue

Richard J. Simons, MD

Fatigue is one of the most common symptoms encountered in primary care settings. Twenty-four percent to 32% of adult patients report significant fatigue during visits to their primary care physicians.[1,2] Fatigue is a sensation that everyone experiences from time to time; however, it is the *persistence* of fatigue that is considered abnormal. A patient with fatigue complains of lack of energy to complete tasks, exhaustion, or tiredness. Fatigue often signifies underlying medical or psychiatric disease.

The chronic fatigue syndrome (CFS) represents a very small subset of patients with chronic fatigue. CFS remains a controversial subject but probably has existed for centuries under various labels, including the Effort syndrome (soldier's heart described in 1870) and neurasthenia (1890) and more recently, the Gulf War syndrome (1991). In fact, some authorities have questioned the existence of a distinct chronic fatigue syndrome and suggest "that current definitions of chronic fatigue syndrome represent an arbitrary imposition where there may be no natural division."[3] Unfortunately, because fatigue may accompany almost any medical or psychological illness, evaluating and treating a patient with fatigue can be particularly challenging and sometimes frustrating for the clinician. A careful history with special attention to psychosocial issues, the physical examination, and a few selected laboratory tests should reveal the cause in most patients.

KEY TERMS

Chronic fatigue	*Generally implies fatigue persisting for 6 months.*
Chronic fatigue syndrome	*Unexplained, persistent, or relapsing fatigue that is of new or definite onset; is not the result of ongoing exertion; is not alleviated by rest; and results in substantial reduction in previous levels of occupational, educational, social, or personal activities **and** 4 or more of the following symptoms that persist or recur during 6 or more consecutive months of illness and that do not predate the fatigue:*

1. Self-reported impairment in short-term memory or concentration
2. Sore throat
3. Tender cervical or axillary nodes
4. Muscle pain
5. Multiple joint pain without redness or swelling
6. Headaches of a new pattern or severity
7. Unrefreshing sleep
8. Postexertional malaise lasting 24 hours.[4]

Idiopathic fatigue (IF)	*Fatigue that has not been attributed to a psychiatric or medical illness.*
Persistent fatigue	*Fatigue that generally persists for more than 1 month.*

ETIOLOGY

Approximately 70% of patients with chronic fatigue are found to have a medical or psychological explanation.[2,5] In general, psychiatric disorders (depression or anxiety) are the predominant causes of fatigue. In approximately 25% patients, a medical condition is responsible. CFS represents less than 10% of the patients with chronic fatigue.[5] More recent studies suggest that social or personal factors may be important causes of fatigue. For example, a survey of women attending a women's health symposium in Toronto, Canada attributed their fatigue to a combination of home and outside work, poor sleep, relationship problems, care of ill family members, and financial worries.[6]

Differential Diagnosis

Psychological	**Hematologic**	Antihypertensives
Depression	Anemia	Benzodiazepines
Anxiety	**Infectious**	Hypnotics
Substance abuse	Endocarditis	Narcotics
Cardiac	Mononucleosis	**Pulmonary**
Heart failure	Tuberculosis	Chronic obstructive pulmonary disease
Endocrine	HIV	Sleep apnea
Addison disease	Hepatitis	**Rheumatologic**
Diabetes mellitus	**Oncologic**	Fibromyalgia
Thyroid disease	Occult malignancy	Lyme disease
Cushing syndrome	**Pharmacologic**	Rheumatoid arthritis
Hyperparathyroidism	Antidepressants	Systemic lupus erythematosus
Gastrointestinal	Antihistamines	
Inflammatory bowel disease		
Malabsorption syndromes		

GETTING STARTED

- Ask the patient to describe his or her fatigue. Fatigue must be distinguished from excessive somnolence (excessive daytime sleepiness),[7] which suggests a primary sleep disturbance. Similarly, generalized fatigue should not be confused with exertional dyspnea or true muscle weakness. Although these symptoms may also result in a decreased ability to perform certain activities, the implications and underlying causes are much different.
- Pay attention to the chronology of the fatigue and any associated symptoms. It is essential to pinpoint the onset of fatigue. Usually the onset is insidious; however, patients with CFS often remember that the fatigue began just after a viral-type illness.
- Listen for clues to psychosocial issues. The impact of fatigue on the patient's social and occupational function should be ascertained.

Open-ended questions

Tell me about your fatigue. What do you mean when you say you are fatigued?

Tell me about your energy level. Has the fatigue changed your lifestyle?

Tips for effective interviewing

Distinguish fatigue from other symptoms such as sleepiness or shortness of breath.

Determine the impact of the patient's fatigue on the patient's lifestyle, social, and occupational function.

Tell me about any new or unusual circumstances in your life when you first noted the fatigue.	*Identify possible precipitating events.*

INTERVIEW FRAMEWORK

- Develop a clear picture and story of the patient's fatigue (including the onset).
- Probe for associated symptoms to uncover undiagnosed medical illness.
- Take a thorough medication history.
- Explore social issues.
- Screen for underlying psychiatric disorders (depression, anxiety, substance abuse).

IDENTIFYING ALARM SYMPTOMS

Significant weight loss, night sweats or fever suggests a systemic illness as a cause of the fatigue. Patients with medical illness are more likely to explain their fatigue in relation to specific activities. In contrast, patients with fatigue of psychogenic origin tend to be "tired all of the time." Patients who have a few organ-specific symptoms (eg, abdominal pain, change in bowel habits) are more likely to have an underlying medical illness whereas patients with multiple somatic complaints usually have a psychogenic cause.

Serious Diagnoses

Although most cases of fatigue result from anxiety and/or depression, a serious medical condition is sometimes the underlying cause. Serious diagnoses are often apparent at the time of presentation because of associated clinical features. Infections, heart disease, and rheumatologic disorders are suggested by the presence of fever, dyspnea or joint pain, respectively. Anemia and thyroid disease may be discovered on the basis of laboratory studies. Laboratory studies are of little diagnostic value without suggestive historical or physical examination findings.[8] Occult malignancy is a rare but often feared cause of chronic fatigue and may be suggested by the presence of weight loss, fever, or night sweats.

Alarm symptoms	Serious causes	Benign causes
Fever, night sweats	*Infection* *Lymphoma* *Occult neoplasm*	*Viral illness*
Weight loss	*Infection* *Malignancy* *Malabsorption* *Thyroid disease* *Depression* *Eating disorder*	
Sore throat	*Infectious mononucleosis* *Streptococcal pharyngitis*	*Viral illness*
Lymph node enlargement	*HIV* *Infectious mononucleosis* *Lymphoma* *Syphilis*	*Viral illness*

(continued)

Alarm symptoms	Serious causes	Benign causes
Shortness of breath	Heart failure Chronic obstructive pulmonary disease Anemia	Anxiety
Palpitations	Cardiac arrhythmia Thyrotoxicosis	Anxiety
Joint pain, stiffness	Rheumatoid arthritis Lyme disease	Viral illness
Back pain; diffuse bony pain	Metastatic carcinoma Multiple myeloma	Mechanical low back pain
Excessive thirst, urination	Diabetes mellitus Diabetes insipidus	
Abdominal pain	Peptic ulcer disease Inflammatory bowel disease Intra-abdominal malignancy Mesenteric ischemia	Irritable bowel syndrome Nonulcer dyspepsia
Jaundice	Hepatitis Pancreatic cancer Drug reaction	Gilbert syndrome
Chest pain	Coronary artery disease	Anxiety or panic disorder Gastroesophageal reflux disease
Diarrhea	Inflammatory bowel disease Malabsorption Intestinal parasite	Irritable bowel syndrome Laxative abuse
Rectal bleeding	Inflammatory bowel disease Colon cancer	Hemorrhoids
Double vision, difficulty speaking or chewing; pain with chewing	Myasthenia gravis Temporal arteritis	
Sleep disturbance	Depression Sleep apnea	Anxiety disorder

FOCUSED QUESTIONS

After characterizing the patient's fatigue and asking about alarm symptoms, the clinician should proceed to more focused, directed questions. Keep in mind that patients presenting with chronic fatigue often have undiagnosed psychiatric illness.[1,2] Patients may attribute their emotional problem to chronic fatigue. However, in a study of patients with chronic fatigue who were determined to have a psychiatric disorder, the psychiatric disorder either predated or began around the same time as the fatigue in most patients.[9] This suggests that the psychiatric disorder is likely to be primary and not merely a complication of fatigue.

Questions

Quality	*Think about*
Has your fatigue affected your ability to perform responsibilities at work or at home?	Chronic fatigue CFS
Have you stopped exercising?	Chronic fatigue CFS
Do you become more weak or tired with exertion?	Muscle or neurologic weakness
Do you become short of breath with exercise?	Cardiopulmonary disease Anemia Hyperthyroidism

Time course	*Think about*
Can you remember exactly when your fatigue started?	The patient with CFS often relates the onset after a viral-type illness.
How long have you been experiencing fatigue?	Fatigue of recent onset may be short-lived.
Do you feel more fatigued in the morning?	Depression
Do you feel tired all day?	Chronic anxiety
Do you feel more fatigued at the end of the day?	Fatigue secondary to medical illness (as opposed to psychogenic)
Did your fatigue begin following surgery?	Postoperative fatigue
Have you ever had radiation therapy?	Post-radiotherapy fatigue

Associated symptoms (see Alarm symptoms)

Modifying factors	*Think about*
Does your fatigue only appear with exertion?	Muscle weakness Cardiopulmonary disease
Is your fatigue unrelated to physical effort?	Psychogenic fatigue
Do you feel better on the weekends?	Chronic occupational stress
Does your fatigue improve after a good night's rest?	Sleep deprivation

Exploring personal or social issues	*Think about*
Have you had more stress in your life lately? Have there been any problems in your family? Have you had more pressure at work? Have you experienced a death of a close friend or relative?	Stress-related or psychogenic fatigue
When is the last time you had a vacation?	Overworked patient Lack of balance between work, family, and pleasure
Do you use alcohol? Has anyone suggested that you should reduce the amount of alcohol you drink? Do you need an alcoholic drink first thing in the morning? Have you been annoyed at anyone for suggesting that you cut back on your alcohol consumption? Do you feel guilty about the amount of alcohol you drink?	Alcoholism; the last 4 questions comprise the CAGE screening test. Two or more positive responses is associated with a relatively high sensitivity and specificity for alcoholism.[10]

(continued)

Exploring personal or social issues	*Think about*
Do you use drugs such as heroin, cocaine, or other illicit drugs?	HIV infection Hepatitis
Do you have more than 1 sexual partner?	HIV infection
Have you recently traveled to developing countries?	Parasitic infections
What medications do you take on a regular basis—both prescribed and over-the-counter? Have you recently started taking any new medications?	Medication-induced fatigue. (Common causes include antihypertensives, sedative hypnotics, antidepressants, antihistamines, narcotics)

Uncovering psychogenic illness	*Think about*
How would you describe your mood? Have you been feeling sad, blue, or down?	Depression
Have you been more irritable or angry?	Depression
Do you often feel agitated?	Depression Anxiety
Have you lost interest in or avoided social activities?	Depression
Have you lost interest in sex?	Depression
Have you had guilty feelings about anything lately?	Depression
Have you had trouble concentrating lately?	Depression
Have you lost interest in things that used to give you pleasure?	Depression
Have you experienced loss of self-esteem?	Depression
Has your appetite been disturbed?	Depression (usually decreased)
Have you had more difficulty with sleep?	Depression (often early morning awakening) Anxiety
Do you feel worse in the morning?	Depression
Do you feel hopeless?	Depression
Have you thought about suicide?	Depression
Have you been excessively nervous or anxious?	Anxiety
Are you constantly worried about something?	Anxiety
Do you experience sudden episodes of intense anxiety? If so, have you experienced chest pain, palpitations, and sweating?	Anxiety Panic attacks
Are you easily distracted?	Anxiety

DIAGNOSTIC APPROACH

In most patients with fatigue, the etiology will be determined by a careful history. If the history does not initially suggest an organic medical disorder, the physician should perform a review of systems paying attention to any alarm symptoms, and then focus the interview to uncover possible psychiatric disorders. A thorough physical examination should be performed with special attention to those organ systems suggested by the history. Laboratory studies should be directed by the history and physical examination. A complete blood cell count, serum chemistries, and thyroid-stimulating hormone measurement may be helpful. Laboratory studies rarely contribute to the diagnosis of fatigue but may help exclude potentially serious medical illness. An extensive work-up for occult medical illness is generally not warranted.[1]

PROGNOSIS

The outcome of patients with chronic fatigue is generally not favorable. In Kroenke's classic study, only 29 (28%) of 102 patients with chronic fatigue experienced some improvement in their fatigue.[1] However, Elnicki et al[11] reported that 72% of patients with fatigue (of at least 1 month duration) improved over the next 6 months. In another study, the outcome was better if the patients had fatigue for less than 3 months and no history of emotional illness.[12] Patients with CFS may have a worse prognosis in terms of improvement or recovery.[13] Even in the nondisabled elderly patient, being "tired" is associated with a greater risk of becoming disabled over the next 5 years.[14] The take home message is that a long duration of fatigue and presence of an underlying psychiatric disorder seem to predict a poor prognosis. Fortunately, IF or CFS cause neither death nor organ failure, although the associated fatigue may result in significant morbidity.

REFERENCES

1. Kroenke K, Wood DR, Mangelsdorf AD, Meier NJ, Powell JB. Chronic fatigue in primary care. Prevalence, patient characteristics and outcome. *JAMA.* 1988;260:929–934.

2. Bates DW, Schmitt W, Buchwald D, et al. Prevalence of fatigue and chronic fatigue syndrome in a primary care practice. *Arch Intern Med.* 1993;153:2759–2765.

3. Wessely S, Chalder T, Hirsch S. Psychological symptoms, somatic symptoms, and psychiatric disorder in chronic fatigue and chronic fatigue syndrome: a prospective study in the primary care setting. *Am J Psychiatry.* 1996;153:1050–1059.

4. Fukuda K, Straus SE, Hickie I, et al. The chronic fatigue syndrome: a comprehensive approach to its definition and study. International Chronic Fatigue Syndrome Study Group. *Ann Intern Med.* 1994;121:953–959.

5. Buchwald D, Umali J, Kith P, Pearlman T, Komaroff AL. Chronic fatigue and the chronic fatigue syndrome: prevalence in a Pacific Northwest health care system. *Ann Intern Med.* 1995;123:81–88.

6. Stewart D, Abbey S, Meana M, Boydell KM. What makes women tired? A community sample. *J Womens Health.* 1998;7:69–76.

7. Pigeon WR, Sateia MJ, Ferguson RJ. Distinguishing between excessive daytime sleepiness and fatigue: toward improve detection and treatment. *J Psychosom Res.* 2003;54:61–69.

8. Lane TJ, Matthews DA, Manu P. The low yield of physical examinations and laboratory investigations of patients with chronic fatigue. *Am J Med Sci.* 1990;299:313–318.

9. Lane TJ, Manu P, Matthews DA. Depression and somatization in the chronic fatigue syndrome. *Am J Med.* 1991;91:335–344.

10. Mayfield D, McLead G, Hall P. The CAGE questionnaire: validation of a new alcoholism screening instrument. *Am J Psychiatry.* 1974;131:1121–1123.

11. Elnicki DM, Shockcor WT, Brick JE, Beynon D. Evaluating the complaint of fatigue in primary care: diagnoses and outcomes. *Am J Med.* 1992;93:303–306.

12. Ridsdale L, Evans A, Jerrett W, Mandalia S, Osler K, Vora H. Patients with fatigue in general practice: a prospective study. *BMJ.* 1993;307:103–106.

13. Bombardier CH, Buchwald D. Outcome and prognosis of patients with chronic fatigue versus chronic fatigue syndrome. *Arch Intern Med.* 1995;155:2105–2110.

14. Avlund K, Damsgaard MT, Sakari-Rantala R, Laukkanen P, Schroll M. Tiredness in daily activities among non-disabled old people as determinant of onset of disability. *J Clin Epidemiol.* 2002;55:965–973.

SUGGESTED READING

Goroll AH, May LA, Mulley AG (editors). *Primary Care Medicine: Office Evaluation and Management of the Adult Patient,* 3rd ed. JB Lippincott, Philadelphia; 1995:32–38.

Kim E. A brief history of chronic fatigue syndrome. *JAMA.* 1994;272:1070.

Morrison RE, Keating HJ. Fatigue in primary care. *Obstet Gynecol Clin North Am.* 2001;28:225–240.

Stevens DL. Chronic fatigue. *West J Med.* 2001;175:315–319.

Diagnostic Approach: Fatigue

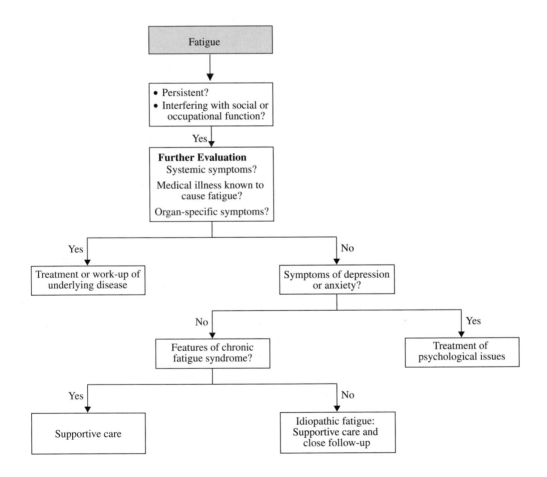

Fever

8

Anjala V. Tess, MD

Temperature regulation in the human body is controlled by hypothalamic nuclei that maintain a set point. Several mechanisms work together to achieve temperature homeostasis. For example, shivering and vasoconstriction generate heat, raising the temperature to the set point. Sweating and cutaneous vasodilation lower the temperature by increasing heat loss. **Fever** occurs when the set point itself is raised to a higher level and the body responds by raising the temperature. Macrophages and monocytes produce cytokines in response to various stimuli, which cause the hypothalamus to raise the set point.

Normal temperature is defined as 98.6 °F, although the overall mean oral temperature for healthy persons aged 18 to 40 years is actually 98.2 °F ± 0.4 °F with a diurnal variation (daily oscillations from 0.9 °F to 2.4 °F). Temperature can be measured orally or rectally: rectal temperatures measure 1 °F greater than oral values.[1]

KEY TERMS

Fever	A rise in body temperature in response to endogenous cytokines. The exact lower cutoff for fever varies from 99.4 °F to 100.4 °F. A recent study suggests that with modern thermometers, an early morning temperature of greater than 99.0 °F or an evening temperature of 100.0 °F should be considered abnormal.[1]
Fever of unknown origin (FUO)	Fever that lasts 3 weeks or longer with temperatures exceeding 100.9 °F with no clear diagnosis despite 1 week of clinical investigation.[2]
Hyperthermia	An elevation in body temperature due to loss of homeostatic mechanisms and inability to increase heat loss in response to environmental heat, as in heat stroke. Can reach levels > 105.8 °F.

ETIOLOGY

Fever is the third most common cause for visits to the emergency department and is listed in the top 20 reasons for visits to the ambulatory clinic.[3,4] Given that many conditions raise the temperature set point, the differential diagnosis of fever is broad.

Most acute febrile illnesses are readily diagnosed based on history, examination, and laboratory testing, and many resolve spontaneously. Prevalence data are unfortunately limited but a few studies have addressed the etiology of fever in specific populations, including hospitalized patients and those with FUO.[2,5]

Patient setting	Etiology	Prevalence
Hospitalized patients with fever	*Community-acquired infection*	*51%*
	Nosocomial (hospital-acquired) infection	*10%*
	Possibly infectious	*23%*
	Noninfectious	*31%*
FUO	*Infection*	*24.5%*
	Malignancy	*14.5%*
	Inflammatory disorders	*23.5%*
	Other causes	*7%*
	No diagnosis	*30%*

Differential Diagnosis for Fever	Prevalence[a]
Infection	

Bacterial *Viral* *Parasitic* *Fungal* *Rickettsial*	• Prevalence varies by season and geography. • Up to 69% of hospitalized patients may have infectious etiologies including infection of the lungs and pleura, urinary tract, blood stream, and skin.[5] • *Causes of nosocomial infections in 1 study of hospitalized patients included: bacterial infections (51%), nonbacterial infections (5%), noninfectious etiologies (25%), and unknown source (19%). Among bacterial infections, pneumonia, catheter-related sepsis, Clostridium difficile diarrhea, wound infections, and urinary tract infections were present.[6]* • *The most common infectious causes of FUO are tuberculosis and intra-abdominal abscesses.[2]* • *Patients with recent travel abroad may contract bacterial, viral, fungal, or parasitic infections. Malaria and respiratory infections are the most common infections seen, although 25% remain undiagnosed.[7]*

Malignancy

Lymphoma	• *Fever can occur in essentially any malignancy as a paraneoplastic feature.* • *The malignancies most commonly associated with FUO are Hodgkin's disease or non-Hodgkin's lymphoma.* • *10–11% of patients with Hodgkin's disease will have fever and/or night sweats (constitutional symptoms).* • *Pel-Ebstein fevers, relapsing fever for hours or days followed by days without fever, occur in 16% of cases with Hodgkin's disease.*
Leukemia	
Liver metastases	

Hepatocellular cancer	20% of patients have fever.
Renal cell cancer	33% of patients have fever.
Pancreatic cancer	

Inflammatory

Systemic lupus erythematosus (SLE)	36% of patients with SLE have fever at presentation and fever develops in up to 52% during evolution of the disease.
Rheumatic fever	
Giant cell arteritis (GCA)	42% of patients with GCA have fever at presentation
Wegener's granulomatosis	
Rheumatoid arthritis	Up to 25% of patients with rheumatoid arthritis have fever at presentation in addition to a polyarticular arthritis.
Polyarteritis nodosa	
Inflammatory bowel disease (IBD)	42% of patients with IBD will have fever, although fever tends to occur later in course of illness.
Gout	15–43% of patients with gout have fever as part of the acute attack.

Miscellaneous

Pulmonary emboli (PE)	Fever develops in 14% of patients.[8]
Drug fever	Fever can be the sole presenting symptom in up to 5% of cases of drug fever. Drug fever accounts for up to 10% of hospitalized patients with new fever.[6]
Factitious fever	Factitious fever may result from manipulation of the thermometer or self-injury, leading to infection or drug fever.
Sarcoidosis	
Adrenal insufficiency	
Hyperthyroidism	
Pancreatitis	

[a]Prevalence estimate is unavailable when not indicated.

Differential Diagnosis for Hyperthermia

	Comment
Heat stroke	May result from central nervous system (CNS) dysfunction or excessive physical exertion in a warm environment. Mortality rate is as high as 10%.

(continued)

Differential Diagnosis for Hyperthermia	Comment
Neuroleptic malignant syndrome (NMS)	*An idiosyncratic reaction to antipsychotic medications, such as butyrophenones, phenothiazines, and thioxanthenes. Cumulative data suggest incidence of 0.2% in patients treated with neuroleptic medications. Temperature exceeded 104 °F in 39% of patients.[9]*
Malignant hyperthermia	*A rare genetic abnormality in the muscle membrane that predisposes patients to severe rhabdomyolysis and temperature dysregulation. May occur with certain anesthetics although can occur with exertion in hot ambient temperatures. Fatality rate is currently 5% compared with 70% in the 1960s.*

GETTING STARTED

- Review vital signs over the preceding days to establish duration and degree of fever.
- Focus your evaluation on associated symptoms. After asking general questions, complete a full review of systems.
- Take a thorough medication history.
- Pattern of fever: Although clinicians often discuss patterns of fever, in small studies fever patterns have had limited diagnostic value. Sustained fever has been associated with gram-negative rod sepsis and CNS infections.[10] Certain malarial infections are associated with fevers that occur every 48 or 72 hours. Tertian fever is seen in certain malarial infections and occurs every 48 hours. Diurnal fever is defined as a regular rise and fall in temperature, occurring between 4 PM and midnight.

Questions	Remember
How long have you had a fever? *How and at what site did you measure your temperature?* *Describe any new symptoms you have experienced with the fever.*	• *Establish a time course for the symptom.* • *Determine the method used for measurement.* • *Listen to patient's description of the fever and associated symptoms for diagnostic clues.*

INTERVIEW FRAMEWORK

- Ask about alarm symptoms.
- Look for clues that point to the major diagnostic categories: infection, inflammatory, malignancy, or other.
- Remember to ask about recent hospitalizations, travel abroad, new medications, and sick contacts.

IDENTIFYING ALARM SYMPTOMS

Serious Diagnoses

In assessing alarm symptoms, the goal is to identify features suggesting a diagnosis that requires prompt intervention. However, certain alarm symptoms may also suggest that complications from the process causing the fever (eg, septic shock) may be developing.

Alarm symptoms	Serious causes	Benign causes
High fever (> 105.8 °F)	CNS infection NMS Heat stroke	
Rash	Meningitis Bacteremia with septic shock Rickettsial disease	Viral exanthem Drug fever
Change in mental status and level of sensorium	Meningitis Encephalitis NMS Heat stroke Bacterial infections with septic shock	
Dizziness or lightheadedness	Bacterial infection with septic shock Adrenal insufficiency PE	Viral infection with labyrinthitis
Recent chemotherapy	Nosocomial infection with neutropenia	
Shortness of breath and chest pain	PE Pneumonia Empyema	

FOCUSED QUESTIONS

Remember that the same associated symptom may occur across major diagnostic categories, eg, diarrhea may suggest a gastroenteritis or inflammatory bowel disease. Seek a constellation of symptoms that suggest a certain diagnosis. For example, diarrhea of several months duration with associated fever suggests inflammatory bowel disease rather than a viral gastroenteritis.

Questions	Think about
Have you had any sick contacts? Have you recently been in the hospital or traveled recently? Any recent procedures?	Infection
Have you lost weight? Any bony pain?	Malignancy
Do you have arthritis or a rash? Do you have a personal or family history of vasculitis or other inflammatory disease?	Inflammatory disorders

Quality	Think about
How high is your fever? • Greater than 105.8 °F	CNS infections Heat stroke NMS

Time course	Think about
How long have you had fevers? • > 3 weeks with a temperature > 100.9 °F	Establishes FUO if initial work-up is negative

(continued)

Time course	Think about
Is there a pattern to the fever?	
• Continuous or sustained (fluctuation < 0.3 °C)	Suggests CNS disease or gram-negative rod bacteremia[10]
• Diurnal (a regular rise and fall in temperature, occurring between 4 PM and midnight)	Absence of diurnal variation has been associated with, but does not establish, a noninfectious cause[10]
• Tertian fever (periodicity of 48 h)	Malaria due to Plasmodium vivax or Plasmodium ovale[7]
• Quartan fever (periodicity of 72 h)	Malaria due to Plasmodium malariae[7]

Associated symptoms	Think about
Do you have dry cough, nasal congestion, sinus pain, or a sore throat?	Acute pharyngitis (viral or bacterial) Sinusitis Upper respiratory tract infection
Any redness of your skin?	Cellulitis Phlebitis Fungal infections Drug reaction
Do you have a productive cough or shortness of breath?	Pneumonia (viral, bacterial, fungal) Bronchitis Tuberculosis
Do you have any blood in your sputum?	Pneumonia Bronchitis Tuberculosis PE Lung cancer
Do you have chest pain?	PE Pneumonia Pericarditis Bacterial endocarditis
Do you have burning with urination?	Urinary tract infection Pyelonephritis Renal cell carcinoma Urethritis Prostatitis
Do you have blood in the urine?	Urinary tract infection Pyelonephritis Renal cell carcinoma Wegener granulomatosis SLE Other vasculitic diseases of the kidney
Have you had nausea or vomiting?	Gastroenteritis (viral or bacterial) Cholecystitis Cholangitis Pyelonephritis Hepatitis Pancreatitis

Do you have diarrhea?	Gastroenteritis (viral or bacterial)
	Infectious colitis
	Parasitic infections
	IBD
Do you have any abdominal pain?	Gastroenteritis (viral or bacterial)
	Cholecystitis
	Cholangitis
	Pyelonephritis
	Hepatitis
	Pancreatic cancer
	Pancreatitis
	Liver metastasis
	Polyarteritis nodosa
	IBD
Have you noticed a yellowing of your skin (jaundice)?	Cholecystitis
	Hepatitis
	Liver abscesses
	Malignancy with involvement of the liver
Did you have associated shaking chills?	Bacteremia
	Endocarditis
Do you have night sweats, weight loss, or malaise?	Hodgkin's disease
	Non-Hodgkin's lymphoma
	Renal cell carcinoma
Have you had any stiffness or pain in your joints?	Septic arthritis
	SLE
	Rheumatic fever
	GCA
	Wegener granulomatosis
	Rheumatoid arthritis
	Polyarteritis nodosa
	IBD
Do you have a headache?	GCA
	Meningitis
	Encephalitis
	Sinusitis
Have you had jaw claudication (pain with chewing)?	GCA
Do you have easy bruising or gum bleeding?	Leukemia
	Lymphoma
Have you had difficulty with speech, double vision, arm or leg weakness, or seizure?	Meningitis
	Encephalitis
	Intracerebral hemorrhage
	Endocarditis with CNS emboli
Have you been confused?	Meningitis
	Encephalitis
	Bacterial infection with septic shock
Modifying factors (potential triggers)	**Think about**
Have you had any recent procedures, eg, dental work?	Bacterial endocarditis

(continued)

Modifying factors (potential triggers)	Think about
Have you started any new medications?	Drug fever
Have you recently started any psychiatric medications?	NMS
If you were recently in the hospital, did you have	
• *Surgery?*	Abscess Wound infection Malignant hyperthermia
• *A urinary or intravenous catheter placed?*	Catheter-associated urinary tract infection or bacteremia
• *Exposure to new antibiotics?*	C difficile colitis Drug fever
If you traveled abroad	
• *Did you consume untreated water or dairy products?*	Salmonellosis Shigellosis Hepatitis Amebiasis Brucellosis
• *Did you eat raw or undercooked meat?*	Enteric infections Cestodiasis Trichinosis
• *Were you exposed to mosquitoes?*	Malaria Dengue fever West Nile Virus infection
• *Were you exposed to ticks?*	Rickettsial disease Tularemia African trypanosomiasis Lyme disease
Have you recently had unprotected sexual intercourse or used injection drugs?	Acute HIV Hepatitis B or C infection Syphilis Gonorrhea Endocarditis
Have you ever lived in a homeless shelter or a prison?	Tuberculosis
Have you had recent exertion in the heat?	Heat stroke
Have you ever had heart valve surgery?	Endocarditis

DIAGNOSTIC APPROACH

In evaluating your patient's history look for clues that point to nosocomial infection, drug fever, or fever in the returning traveler. If these categories seem unlikely, attempt to identify the major category (infectious disease, malignancy, or inflammatory), and then use detailed questions as noted above to narrow your differential diagnosis.

CAVEATS

- In general, fever requires prompt evaluation.
- Gather as many associated symptoms and potential triggers to support a unifying diagnosis.

- Elderly and immunosuppressed patients may not mount as high a fever as younger or immunocompetent patients. These patients may present with a lower temperature or no fever at all.
- Never rely on the fever pattern alone to direct your evaluation or laboratory testing.

PROGNOSIS

- Most acute febrile illnesses either resolve or the etiology is quickly identified on the basis of history, examination, and laboratory or radiologic evaluation. The prognosis depends on the underlying diagnosis.
- In FUO cases where a cause remains elusive after several weeks, undiagnosed patients have a favorable outcome. Over 50% of patients in whom malignancies are diagnosed die within 5 years of diagnosis. Mortality is lower (22%) in patients whose fever proves due to infection.[2]
- Mortality rates can reach 10% in heat stroke patients, and 20% in those with NMS. Therefore, prompt evaluation is critical with identification of key predisposing factors. A complete list of all medications including anesthetics must be reviewed.

REFERENCES

1. Mackowiak PA, Wasserman SS, Levine MM. A critical appraisal of 98.6 °F, the upper limit of the normal body temperature, and other legacies of Carl Reinhold August Wunderlich. *JAMA*. 1992;268:578–581.
2. Mourad O, Palda V, Detsky AS. A comprehensive evidence-based approach to fever of unknown origin. *Arch Intern Med*. 2003;163:545–551.
3. McCaig L et al. National Hospital Ambulatory Medical Care Survey: 2001 Emergency Department Summary. Advance data from vital and health statistics; No. 335. Hyattsville, Maryland: National Center for Health Statistics. 2003. Available at: http://www.cdc.gov/nchs/data/ad/ad335.pdf
4. Cherry DK, Woodwell DA. National Ambulatory Medical Care Survey: 2000 summary. Advance data from vital and health statistics; No. 328. Hyattsville, Maryland: National Center for Health Statistics. 2002. Available at: http://www.cdc.gov/nchs/data/ad/ad328.pdf
5. McGowan J et al. Fever in hospitalized patients. With special reference to the medical service. *Am J Med*. 1987;82:580–586.
6. Arbo M et al. Fever of nosocomial origin: etiology, risk factors, and outcomes. *Am J Med*. 1993;95:505–515.
7. Suh KN, Kozarsky PE, Keystone JS. Evaluation of fever in the returned traveler. *Med Clin North Am*. 1999;83:997–1017.
8. Stein PD, Afzal A, Henry JW, Villareal CG. Fever in acute pulmonary embolism. *Chest*. 2000;117:39–42.
9. Caroff SN, Mann SC. Neuroleptic malignant syndrome. *Psychopharmacol Bull*. 1988;24:25–27.
10. Musher DM, Fainstein V, Young EJ, Pruett TL. Fever patterns. Their lack of clinical significance. *Arch Intern Med*. 1979;139:1225–1228.

SUGGESTED READING

Caroff S et al. Neuroleptic malignant syndrome. *Med Clinics North Am*. 1993;77:185–202.

Cervera R et al. Systemic lupus erythematosus: clinical and immunologic patterns of disease expression in a cohort of 1,000 patients. The European Working Party on Systemic Lupus Erythematosus. *Medicine (Baltimore)*. 1993;72:113–124.

Hunder GG. Giant cell arteritis and polymyalgia rheumatica. *Med Clin North Am*. 1997;81:195–219.

Mackowiak PA. Concepts of fever. *Arch Intern Med*. 1998;158:1870–1881.

Simon HB. Hyperthermia. *N Engl J Med*. 1993;329:483–487.

Weinberger A, Kesler A, Pinkhas J. Fever in various rheumatic diseases. *Clin Rheumatol*. 1985;4:258–266.

Diagnostic Approach: Fever

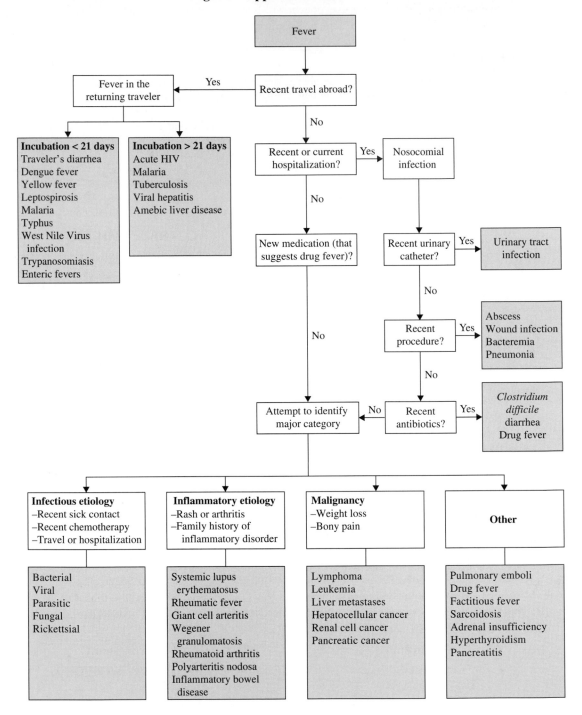

Headache

9

Gerald W. Smetana, MD

Headache is near universal and a common symptom in primary care and other practice settings. Most series place headache among the top 10 most frequent symptoms that prompt an office visit.[1] While most patients with headache will prove to have a benign cause, headache may occasionally be a symptom of a morbid or life-threatening disease. A carefully taken headache history will allow clinicians to establish a correct diagnosis with certainty in most cases, will limit the use of unnecessary and expensive diagnostic testing, and will lead to proper treatment to reduce suffering and disability. Two general approaches to history taking exist. First is to learn the alarm features that should prompt consideration of a serious pathologic cause for headache. The second is to understand the typical features of common benign headache syndromes. This approach allows clinicians to diagnose migraine, tension-type, and cluster headache with certainty based on the presence of characteristic historical features.

KEY TERMS

Aura	Complex neurologic phenomena that precede a headache. Examples include scotoma, aphasia, and hemiparesis.
Cervicogenic headache	A referred headache pain that originates from the neck. Usually due to muscle tension in neck or cervical degenerative arthritis. Also referred to as occipital neuralgia.
Negative likelihood ratio (LR−)	The decrease in the odds of a particular diagnosis if a factor is absent.
New headache	A headache of recent onset or a change in the character of a chronic headache. These are more likely to be pathologic than chronic headaches of long-standing duration.
Phonophobia	Headache is worse on exposure to loud sounds.
Photophobia	Pain or increased headache when looking into bright light.
Positive likelihood ratio (LR+)	The increase in the odds of a particular diagnosis if a factor is present.
Primary headache	A chronic, benign recurring headache without known cause such as migraine and tension-type headache.
Secondary headache	Headaches due to underlying pathology.
Thunderclap headache	The maximal intensity of headache occurs instantaneously at its onset.

ETIOLOGY

Most chronic headaches are either migraines or tension-type headaches. The etiology of headache depends on the setting. Patients who have been referred to specialized headache clinics have a disproportionately high frequency of medication-induced headache and chronic daily headache. In a study of unselected persons in the general population, the prevalence of migraine was approximately 15% among women and 6% among men.[2] The prevalence of tension-type headache was 86% among women and 63% among men. Cluster headache, the remaining primary headache syndrome, is much less common (prevalence of approximately 0.1%).[3] In a study of 872 patients with headache who sought medical attention at an emergency department (who would be expected to have a greater likelihood of new headaches due to a pathologic cause), the etiologies were infection (39.3%), tension-type headache (19.3%), posttraumatic (9.3%), hypertension-related (4.8%), migraine (4.5%), subarachnoid hemorrhage (0.9%), meningitis (0.6%), and miscellaneous or no diagnosis (20.9%).[4]

Differential Diagnosis	Prevalence[a]
Primary headaches	
Tension-type headache	12–19%[4,5]
Migraine with or without aura	3–5%[4,5]
Cluster headache	
Benign exertional, sexual, or cough headache	
Secondary headaches (common benign causes)	
Viral syndrome	39%[4]
Drug-induced headache (common offenders are caffeine, alcohol, analgesics, monosodium glutamate, birth control pills)	
Temporomandibular joint (TMJ) dysfunction	
Sinusitis	1%[5]
Cervicogenic headache	

[a]Among patients with headache seeking care at an emergency department; prevalence is unknown when not indicated.

GETTING STARTED

- Let the patient tell the headache story in his or her own words before asking more directed and focused questions.
- Remember that most headache diagnoses are based *entirely* on the history since the physical examination and laboratory testing only rarely offer diagnostic clues.
- Understand the patient's agenda. Even though most headaches are benign, patients often seek medical care due to concern for a possible brain tumor or other serious cause.

Questions	Remember
Tell me more about your headaches.	• *Listen to the story.*
When did these headaches first start?	• *Do not try to rush the interview by interrupting and*
Give me an example of your most recent	*focusing the history too soon.*
headache; tell me what you experienced	• *Reassure the patient when possible.*
from beginning to end.	

INTERVIEW FRAMEWORK

- The first goal is to determine whether this is an old or a new headache.
- The differential diagnosis completely depends on whether the headache is new or old, so failure to correctly categorize the headache at this point will lead to mistakes in diagnosis, inefficient use of time in the interview, and inappropriate diagnostic testing.
- Inquire about headache characteristics using the cardinal symptom features:

  Onset
  Aura
  Duration
  Frequency
  Pain character
  Location of pain
  Associated features
  Precipitating and alleviating factors
  Change in frequency or character over time

IDENTIFYING ALARM SYMPTOMS

- A recent progression of headache or the development of new symptoms raises concern for a pathologic cause of new headache.
- Not all secondary headaches are serious (benign examples include viral syndrome and cervicogenic headache) but headaches that worsen or become associated with new features over a period of weeks to several months are more likely to be due to a serious cause and should prompt further evaluation.

Serious Diagnoses

Serious causes for headache are rare. However, these are "can't miss" headaches due to the morbidity of overlooking these diagnoses. The estimated 1-year prevalence in the general population for selected serious causes is 0.02% for giant cell arteritis (GCA) (among patients older than 50 years),[6] 0.02% for brain tumor,[7] 0.15% for metastatic cancer,[7] 0.7% for stroke, 0.01% for subarachnoid hemorrhage, and 0.02–0.1% for arteriovenous malformation (AVM).

Diagnosis	Prevalence[a]
Miscellaneous or no diagnosis	20.9%[4]
Posttraumatic headache	9.3%[4]
Hypertensive emergency	4.8%[4]
Subarachnoid hemorrhage	0.9–1.3%[4,5,8]
Brain tumor	0.8%[8]
Meningitis	0.6%[4,8]
GCA	
Benign intracranial hypertension	
Brain abscess	
Carotid or vertebral artery dissection	
Stroke	

(continued)

Diagnosis

AVM

Carbon monoxide poisoning

[a]Among patients with headache seeking care at an emergency department; prevalence is unknown when not indicated.

After the open-ended portion of the history, specifically ask about the presence of the following alarm symptoms to assess for the possibility of a serious cause for headache and to determine the pace of subsequent evaluation or "triage." Certain symptoms *always* indicate a serious cause for headache while other symptoms increase concern for a pathologic cause but may also occur in benign headache syndromes. The absence of a particular alarm symptom generally does *not* substantially reduce the likelihood of a particular serious cause for headache. In other words, the LR– for most of these alarm symptoms approaches unity (1.0).

Alarm symptoms	Serious causes	LR+	Benign causes
Always indicates a serious cause for headache			
Visual loss	GCA Acute angle-closure glaucoma		
Dysequilibrium	Stroke Brain tumor	49[9]	
Confusion or lethargy	Meningitis Encephalitis Brain tumor Brain abscess	1.5[10]	
New onset seizure	Stroke Encephalitis Brain tumor	1.36[10]	
May indicate a serious cause for headache			
Fever	Meningitis Encephalitis Brain abscess		Viral syndrome Sinusitis
Weight loss	Brain tumor		
History of malignancy	Brain tumor	2.02[10]	
History of HIV infection	CNS lymphoma Toxoplasmosis Cryptococcal meningitis	1.80[10]	Sinusitis
History of neurosurgery or CNS shunt	Hydrocephalus Meningitis		
Eye pain	Acute angle-closure glaucoma		Cluster headache
Thunderclap headache	Subarachnoid hemorrhage	1.9[9]	Cluster headache
New onset after age 50	Brain tumor Stroke GCA		Cervicogenic headache

Progressive headache over weeks to months	Brain tumor	12[9]	
Diplopia	Brain tumor GCA Stroke AVM	3.4 (for diagnosis of GCA)[6]	Ophthalmoplegic migraine
Hemiparesis	Brain tumor Stroke Brain abscess	3.69[10]	Migraine with typical aura
Aphasia	Brain tumor Stroke Brain abscess		Migraine with typical aura
Headache causing awakening from sleep	Brain tumor	1.7–98[9]	Cluster headache
Headache worse at work	Carbon monoxide poisoning		
Headache worse with Valsalva maneuver	Brain tumor	2.3[9]	
Nausea	Brain tumor Hydrocephalus Carbon monoxide poisoning		Migraine
Neck stiffness	Meningitis		Tension-type headache Cervicogenic headache TMJ dysfunction
Onset of headache with exertion, cough, or sexual activity	Subarachnoid hemorrhage		Benign exertional, cough, or sexual headache

FOCUSED QUESTIONS

After hearing the headache story in the patient's own words and considering possible alarm symptoms, ask the following questions to begin to narrow the differential diagnosis.

Questions	Think about
Does anyone in your immediate family have migraines?	Migraine
Describe the onset of the headache.	Thunderclap headache must prompt consideration of subarachnoid hemorrhage.
How old were you when you started getting these headaches?	The longer a headache has been present, the more likely it is to be benign. Migraine and tension-type headaches usually begin in adolescence.
Is this headache the same as ones you've had before, or is it different in some way?	This question addresses the old versus new headache concept. Old headaches are usually benign.

(continued)

Questions

Why did you choose to see me for the headache today?

Do you have any awareness or warning symptoms that occur before the headache begins?

Quality

Is the headache

- *Throbbing, like a heartbeat?*

- *A bandlike tightness or pressure around your head?*

- *Piercing or sharp, as in an electric shock feeling?*

Where is the pain located in your head?

- *1 side only but can alternate between sides*

- *Always on the same side*

- *Both sides of my head*

- *Around my eye*

- *My forehead*

- *My temples*

- *The back of my head and neck*

- *Top of my head (vertex)*

Are your headaches

- *Severe and disabling?*

Think about

Determine the patient's primary agenda for the visit and most concerning feature.

The presence of a characteristic aura in a recurring headache syndrome establishes a diagnosis of migraine with certainty.

Think about

Migraine
GCA

Tension-type headache
Cervicogenic headache
TMJ dysfunction

Cluster headache
Trigeminal neuralgia

Migraine
GCA

Cluster headache
Brain tumor
AVM
GCA
Trigeminal neuralgia

Tension-type headache
GCA

Cluster headache
Trigeminal neuralgia
Acute angle-closure glaucoma
Sinusitis

Tension-type headache
Cervicogenic headache
Sinusitis

Tension-type headache
GCA
Cluster headache

Cervicogenic headache
Posterior fossa mass lesion

Sphenoid sinusitis
Cervicogenic headache

Migraine
Subarachnoid hemorrhage

- Mild?

Tension-type headache
GCA
Brain tumor (Brain tumor headaches initially are mild and nondisabling. The progression to a more severe headache over weeks to months is an important clue.)

Time course	Think about

Tell me about the onset of a typical headache.

- It occurs instantaneously and is severe in the very first second.

Subarachnoid hemorrhage

- It develops rapidly over 5–10 minutes.

Cluster headache

- It seems to get worse over the first hour or so.

Tension-type headache
Migraine

How long does each headache last?

Note that each of the common primary headache syndromes has its own characteristic duration.

- From 4 hours to 3 days

Migraine

- From 30 minutes to 1 week

Tension-type headache

- From 15 minutes to 3 hours

Cluster headache

If you have recurrent headaches, how often do they occur?

Frequencies may vary substantially from the typical frequencies below.

- Once or twice per month

Migraine

- Once or twice per week

Tension-type headache

- 1 to 4 per day

Cluster headache

What time of the day do your headaches normally occur?

- 2:00 to 3:00 AM

Cluster headache

- When I awaken in the morning

Brain tumor
Obstructive sleep apnea
TMJ dysfunction

- Afternoon

Tension-type headache

- Weekends

Migraine
Caffeine withdrawal headaches

Associated symptoms	Think about

Do you have any warning symptoms that start before your headache?

These may continue after the headache begins but should last for no more than 1 hour.

- Zigzag flashing lights on 1 side of both eyes for about 20 minutes

Classic visual aura of migraine

- Garbled speech

Aphasia occurs in 11% of all migrainous auras[3] but must consider the possibility of an acute vascular event such as carotid dissection or stroke when occurs for the first time or if symptoms last for more than 1 hour.

(continued)

Associated symptoms	Think about
• Numbness or tingling on 1 side of your face or hand?	Hemisensory symptoms occur in 20% of all migrainous auras.[3]
• Weakness on 1 side of your body	Hemiparesis accompanies 4% of migrainous auras[3] but may also represent a stroke or intracranial mass lesion and requires urgent evaluation unless it occurs as part of a stable pattern over time.
Do you have any symptoms that occur at the same time as your headache?	For cluster headache, the associated symptoms occur only on the same side as the headache
• Red eye	Acute angle-closure glaucoma Cluster headache
• Tearing	Cluster headache
• Runny nose or nasal congestion	Cluster headache
• Forehead or facial sweating	Cluster headache
• Eyelid drooping (ptosis)	Cluster headache
• Small pupil (miosis)	Cluster headache
• Nausea	Migraine Brain tumor
• Photophobia	Migraine Meningitis
• Phonophobia	Migraine

Modifying factors (headache triggers)	Think about
Have you found that anything in particular causes your headache to occur?	
• Certain foods (particularly chocolate and cheese)	Migraine
• Alcohol	Migraine Cluster headache
• Menses	Migraine (usually begins immediately before or in the first few days of menses)
• Caffeine withdrawal	Migraine
• Valsalva	Brain tumor Migraine
• Physical activity, such as walking up stairs, bending over	Migraine Brain tumor
• Turning your head and neck	Cervicogenic headache
• Touching your scalp	GCA

DIAGNOSTIC APPROACH

The first step is to distinguish between old and new headaches. In evaluation of new headaches, clinicians must pay particular attention to the alarm features. While most new headaches are due to viral syndromes and other benign diagnoses, almost all serious or pathologic headaches are new headaches.

Old headaches are usually due either to migraine or tension-type headache. The above focused questions help distinguish between these 2 diagnoses. The presence (LR+) or absence (LR−) of the following features may help distinguish migraine from tension-type headache.[3] An LR+ of 2, for example, means that the likelihood of the diagnosis increases by 2-fold if the particular feature is present. An LR− of 0.5, similarly, indicates that the likelihood of the diagnosis decreases by 2-fold if the factor is absent.

Feature	LR+[a]	LR−[a]
Nausea	19.2	0.19
Photophobia	5.8	0.25
Phonophobia	5.2	0.38
Exacerbation by physical activity	3.7	0.24
Unilateral headache	3.7	0.43
Throbbing headache	2.9	0.36
Chocolate as headache trigger	7.1	0.70
Cheese as headache trigger	4.9	0.68

[a]For the diagnosis of migraine compared with tension-type headache.
Adapted with permission from Smetana GW. The diagnostic value of historical features in primary headache syndromes. A comprehensive review. *Arch Intern Med.* 2000;160:2729-2737.

CAVEATS

- Be certain to first distinguish between old and new headaches in order to correctly move through the diagnostic algorithm.
- Migraine and tension-type headache can only be diagnosed with certainty after a pattern of similar headaches occurs over time. When faced with a patient who has an apparent first episode of migraine or tension-type headache, consider also the differential diagnosis for new headaches.
- Reconsider your working diagnosis over time if the time course appears to be too short or too long for your proposed diagnosis. Each headache diagnosis has its own characteristic natural history.
- Do not diagnose benign cough, sexual, or exertional headache until neuroimaging has confirmed that no intracranial pathology exists. It is important to exclude CNS aneurysm and Chiari malformation (tonsillar descent below the foramen magnum).
- Gender differences are important in primary headaches. Migraine headache is 3 times more common in women than in men. Cluster headache is 6 times more common in men than in women. Tension-type headache is similarly prevalent in women and men.
- Most headache diagnoses are based entirely on history taking. The more typical features that are present, the more confident the clinician can be of the diagnosis. When only a few typical features exist for a working diagnosis, expand the differential diagnosis and consider other diagnostic possibilities.
- Consider benign intracranial hypertension, dural sinus thrombosis, and new onset migraine for new headaches during pregnancy.

PROGNOSIS

Primary headache syndromes, including migraine, tension-type, and cluster headache, have an excellent prognosis, with the rare exception of stroke due to a complicated migraine. However, significant disability (lost work and school time) may result from these conditions when severe. The prognosis for new headaches depends on the ultimate diagnosis. Unrecognized and untreated, many causes for new headaches (eg, subarachnoid hemorrhage, GCA, brain tumor, meningitis) may cause significant morbidity or death.

REFERENCES

1. Cherry DK, Woodwell DA. National Ambulatory Medical Care Survey: 2000 summary. Advance data from vital and health statistics; No. 328. Hyattsville, Maryland: National Center for Health Statistics. 2002. Available at: http://www.cdc.gov/nchs/data/ad/ad328.pdf

2. Rasmussen BK, Jensen R, Schroll M, Olesen J. Epidemiology of headache in a general population. A prevalence study. *J Clin Epidemiol.* 1991;44:1147–1157.

3. Smetana GW. The diagnostic value of historical features in primary headache syndromes. A comprehensive review. *Arch Intern Med.* 2000;160:2729–2737.

4. Dhopseh V, Anwar R, Herring C. A retrospective assessment of emergency department patients with complaint of headache. *Headache.* 1979;19:37–42.

5. Morgenstern LB, Huber JC, Luna-Gonzales H, et al. Headache in the emergency department. *Headache.* 2001;41:537–541.

6. Smetana GW, Shmerling RH. Does this patient have temporal arteritis? *JAMA.* 2002;287:92–101.

7. DeAngelis LM. Brain tumors. *N Engl J Med.* 2001;344:114–123.

8. Ramirez-Lassepas M, Espinosa CE, Cicero JJ, et al. Predictors of intracranial pathologic findings in patients who seek emergency care because of headache. *Arch Neurol.* 1997;54:1506–1509.

9. Frishberg BM, Rosenberg JH, Matchar DB, et al for the US Headache Consortium. Evidence-based guidelines in the primary care setting: neuroimaging in patients with nonacute headache. 2000. Available at: http://www.aan.com/professionals/practice/index.cfm.

10. Reinus WR, Erickson KK, Wippold FJ. Unenhanced emergency cranial CT: optimizing patient selection with univariate and multivariate analysis. *Radiology.* 1993;186:763–768.

SUGGESTED READING

American College of Emergency Physicians. Clinical policy for the initial approach to adolescents and adults presenting to the emergency department with a chief complaint of headache. *Ann Emerg Med.* 1996;27:821–844.

Dalessio DJ. Diagnosing the severe headache. *Neurology.* 1994;44:S6–S12.

Frishman BM. The utility of neuroimaging in the evaluation of headache in patients with normal neurologic examinations. *Neurology.* 1994;44:1191–1197.

Diagnostic Approach: Headache

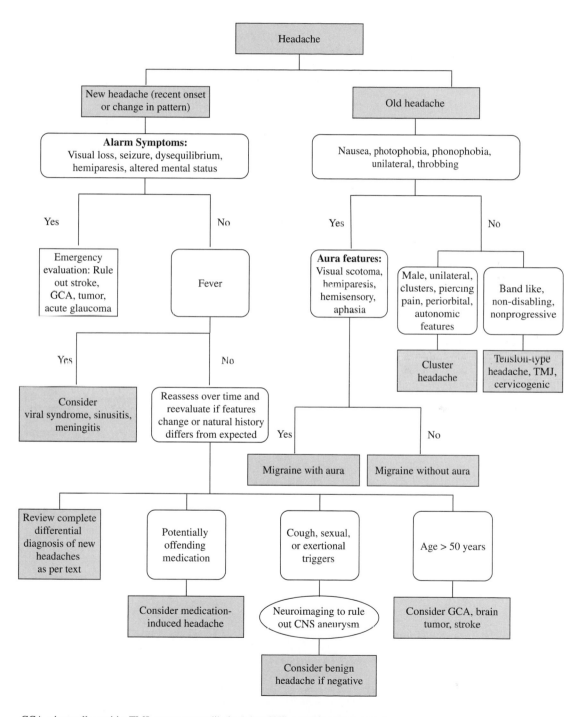

GCA, giant cell arteritis; TMJ, temporomandibular joint; CNS, central nervous system.

Insomnia

10

Craig R. Keenan, MD

Insomnia is a very common complaint. Between 30% and 50% of adults have insomnia at some time, and it is a persistent problem in about 20% of adults. The prevalence increases with age, and it is more common in women. About 10% of the population has insomnia with significant daytime consequences, including daytime sleepiness or fatigue, diminished energy, poor concentration, memory impairment, irritability, depressed or anxious mood, and interpersonal difficulties.[1]

Although definitions of insomnia vary, most patients describe problems with initiating sleep, frequent or prolonged awakenings, a feeling of nonrestorative sleep, or some combination of these symptoms. These symptoms affect daytime social and occupational functioning to varying degrees.

It is important to remember that insomnia is most often a **symptom** of an underlying problem, not a diagnosis. The history is the most important diagnostic tool in establishing the underlying diagnosis. There are few helpful physical findings, and only rarely are specialized studies (eg, polysomnography) necessary. Since eliminating or mitigating the causes of insomnia remains the cornerstone of treatment, the history is critical to successful therapy.

KEY TERMS

Adjustment sleep disorder	*Insomnia associated with acute life events (eg, medical or surgical illnesses, bereavement, divorce, stress).*
Advanced sleep phase syndrome	*A circadian rhythm disorder in which persons have difficulty with early awakenings, but no difficulty initiating sleep early at night, with normal quality and duration of sleep.[3]*
Delayed sleep phase syndrome	*A circadian rhythm disorder in which persons have difficulty falling asleep but have normal quality and duration once sleep is initiated.[3]*
Insomnia	*An experience of inadequate or poor quality sleep characterized by 1 or more of the following: difficulty falling asleep, difficulty maintaining sleep, waking up too early in the morning, or nonrefreshing sleep.[2]*
Periodic limb movement disorder (PLMD)	*An asleep phenomenon characterized by periodic episodes of repetitive and highly stereotyped limb movements. Such movements may cause insomnia via frequent awakenings. Diagnosed by polysomnography.[4]*
Primary insomnia	*Insomnia not due to medical, mental, or other disorders. Can be idiopathic, due to psychophysiologic insomnia or poor sleep hygiene.*

(continued)

KEY TERMS

Psychophysiologic insomnia	*Learned or conditioned insomnia. This subtype of primary insomnia usually arises from an episode of acute situational insomnia. The patient then associates the bed with not sleeping and so becomes hyperaroused when he or she would normally be sleeping. When the acute situation resolves, the conditioned insomnia persists.[3]*
Restless legs syndrome (RLS)	*An awake phenomenon of intense, irresistible urge to move the legs, usually associated with paresthesias or dysesthesias. The discomfort can lead to difficulty falling asleep. Diagnosed by history.[4]*
Short sleeper	*A person who has decreased total sleep time, but no significant daytime consequences. Considered a normal variant.[3]*
Sleep hygiene	*The collection of sleep habits that can either cause or ameliorate insomnia. The most important are usual rise time, usual bedtime, regularity of rise and bed times, activities around bedtime (eg, eating, drinking, exercise, sex, work), activities in sleep area (eg, computer, television, radio that are used in the bedroom), and other daytime activities (eg, daytime naps).*

ETIOLOGY

The common causes of insomnia and their prevalence are listed in the following Differential Diagnosis section.[1] Many cases are multifactorial, and nearly half are related to an underlying mental health disorder. Idiopathic insomnia is a diagnosis of exclusion and can only be diagnosed when the insomnia is not related to any of the other disorders.

The relative frequencies of the causes of insomnia have not been well studied. Studies from sleep centers vary widely, but the frequency of psychiatric causes (30–50%), psychophysiologic insomnia (15–20%), and poor sleep hygiene (15–20%) remain relatively constant.[3]

The duration of insomnia can help narrow the diagnostic possibilities. **Transient insomnia** lasts < 1 week; **short-term insomnia** lasts 1–3 weeks; and **chronic insomnia** lasts greater than 3 weeks. The causes of transient and short-term insomnia usually involve acute events, including changes in sleep environment, jet lag, changes in a work shift, environmental issues (excessive noise or extremes of temperature), stressful life events, acute medical or surgical illnesses, use of stimulant medications (eg, corticosteroids, decongestants, bronchodilators, amphetamines, or cocaine), or withdrawal from central nervous system depressant substances (eg, alcohol or benzodiazepines). Chronic insomnia often starts with an acute event such as those listed above. When it persists, however, it is generally related to a broader range of problems. The long list of potential causes can be divided into 5 main categories: medical disorders, mental disorders, neurologic disorders, medication and substance effects, and sleep disorders.

Over half of insomnia patients have recurrent, persistent, or multiple health problems that contribute to poor sleep.[1] Of the mental health conditions that cause insomnia, depressive or anxiety disorders are the most common. Nearly 80% of patients with depression have insomnia.[5] In addition, patients with persistent insomnia lasting longer than 1 year have greatly increased risk of developing major depression.[6] Medication side effects are also common causes of insomnia. The most common culprits include anticonvulsants, antidepressants, antihypertensives, antineoplastics, bronchodilators, anticholinergics, corticosteroids, decongestants, hormonal therapies, levodopa, stimulants, and nicotine. The most common primary sleep disorders that cause insomnia are RLS, PLMD, sleep apnea syndromes, and psychophysiologic insomnia. Bed partners are often very helpful in providing evidence of sleep apneas and PLMD, by reporting heavy snoring, observed apneas, and limb movements.

Lastly, some patients report chronic insomnia but have no objective evidence of a sleep disorder, a condition called sleep-state misperception. Diagnosis requires specialized studies (polysomnography or actigraphy).

Differential Diagnosis	Prevalence[a,1]
Lifestyle	
Shift-work	
Poor sleep hygiene	
Jet lag	
Stressful life events	2%
Environmental factors (eg, noise, temperature)	
Medical disorders	3.8–11.4%[1,3,4,7]
Congestive heart failure (CHF)	
Ischemic heart disease	
Chronic obstructive pulmonary disease (COPD)/asthma	
Peptic ulcer disease (PUD)	
Gastroesophageal reflux disease (GERD)	
Chronic fatigue syndrome	
Fibromyalgia	
End-stage renal disease	
Chronic pain from any cause	
Mental health disorders	**44%**
Depressive disorders	8%
Anxiety disorders (eg, posttraumatic stress disorder, generalized anxiety disorder, panic disorder)	24%
Bipolar disorder	2%
Other disorders	10%
Medications and substances	**2%**
Side effects of over-the-counter and prescription drugs	
Illicit drug use	
Alcohol abuse	
Caffeine	
Nicotine	
Withdrawal from central nervous system depressants	
Neurologic disorders	
Stroke	

(continued)

Neurologic disorders	***Prevalence**[a,1]*
Dementia	
Neurodegenerative and movement disorders	
Brain tumors	
Epilepsy	
Posttraumatic insomnia due to brain injury	
Headache syndromes	
Fatal familial insomnia	
Primary sleep disorders	**5%**
Idiopathic insomnia	
Psychophysiologic insomnia	
Sleep apnea syndromes	
Sleep-state misperception	
RLS	
PLMD	
Circadian rhythm disorders (delayed or advanced sleep phase syndromes)	
Altitude insomnia	

[a]In general population reporting insomnia and sleep dissatisfaction; prevalence is unknown when not indicated.

GETTING STARTED

- Review the patient's medical record before the visit. Potential causes of the insomnia should be identified and explored further in the interview.
- If possible, have the patient keep a sleep log for the 2 weeks before the office visit. It provides invaluable information including bed time, arising time, daytime naps, amount of time required to fall asleep, number and duration of nocturnal awakenings, total sleep time, and subjective evaluations of sleep quality (see Sample Sleep Diary).
- If possible, the patient's bed partner should attend the visit to supplement the history.

INTERVIEW FRAMEWORK

- Detail the nature and development of the sleep problem.
  - Determine the chief sleep symptom.
  - Determine the chronology of the insomnia including onset, precipitating factors, duration, and frequency.
  - Evaluate the patient's sleep hygiene.
  - Assess effects on daytime functioning and social or occupational function to gauge the severity of insomnia.
  - Review treatments that the patient has already tried and assess their efficacy.
- Expand the history to cover potentially contributing medical, psychiatric, and sleep disorders.
  - Review past medical and psychiatric history, medications, and substance use history.
  - Perform a review of symptoms that have not been covered by your other questions.

- Get collateral history from a bed partner, if possible. They can give information on the quality and quantity of sleep, daytime consequences, and nocturnal events (eg, snoring, apneas, and limb movements).
- Have the patient complete a sleep diary (if not already done). This can help determine an accurate diagnosis and may also be repeated in the future to assess response to treatment.

IDENTIFYING ALARM SYMPTOMS

The alarm symptoms associated with insomnia relate to the severity of the underlying causes.

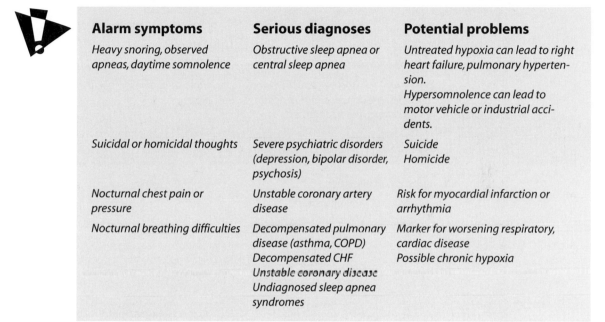

Alarm symptoms	Serious diagnoses	Potential problems
Heavy snoring, observed apneas, daytime somnolence	Obstructive sleep apnea or central sleep apnea	Untreated hypoxia can lead to right heart failure, pulmonary hypertension. Hypersomnolence can lead to motor vehicle or industrial accidents.
Suicidal or homicidal thoughts	Severe psychiatric disorders (depression, bipolar disorder, psychosis)	Suicide Homicide
Nocturnal chest pain or pressure	Unstable coronary artery disease	Risk for myocardial infarction or arrhythmia
Nocturnal breathing difficulties	Decompensated pulmonary disease (asthma, COPD) Decompensated CHF Unstable coronary disease Undiagnosed sleep apnea syndromes	Marker for worsening respiratory, cardiac disease Possible chronic hypoxia

FOCUSED QUESTIONS

After initial open-ended questions, it is usually necessary to probe more specifically to explore possible causes of insomnia.

Questions	Think about
Characterize the sleep complaint	
Describe what you mean by "insomnia."	
Is your main problem	
• Falling asleep?	Anxiety disorders Poor sleep hygiene Delayed sleep phase syndrome RLS Sleep apnea rarely causes problems falling asleep
• Early awakening?	Frequently occurs with depression Advanced sleep phase syndrome

(continued)

Questions	Think about
Characterize the sleep complaint	
• Frequent awakening?	Sleep apnea Nocturnal angina or respiratory diseases PLMD Medication effects Environmental factors
• Nonrefreshing sleep?	Sleep apnea Fibromyalgia
Determine the chronology	**Think about**
When did your problems with sleep start?	Childhood onset suggests primary insomnia
What do you think started the insomnia? Are there any life events that have affected your sleep (births, deaths, job change, move, work stress, new bedpartner, financial stress)?	The initial cause of insomnia (it may not be the ongoing cause).
How many nights per week do you have problems with sleep?	Determines severity
How long does it take you to fall asleep?	
What do you do when you cannot fall asleep?	
Do you wake up at night? If so, how many times and at what time?	
• Why do you wake up?	Specific symptoms may suggest medical conditions or medications
• How long do you remain awake?	
What do you think is causing your insomnia now?	May discover environmental factors, stressors, medical or psychiatric problems
How many hours a night do you sleep?	
Did you used to be a good sleeper?	If long-standing or began in childhood or adolescence, consider primary insomnia
Are you apprehensive in the evenings about going to sleep?	Preoccupation with insomnia suggests psychophysiologic insomnia
Assess sleep hygiene	**Think about**
Describe a usual day and night.	To determine sleep habits
What time do you get up on weekdays? On weekends? What time to you go to sleep on weekdays? On weekends?	Erratic bedtime and rise times can lead to insomnia (poor hygiene)
Describe your activities shortly before bedtime? Do you eat after 9 PM? Exercise in the late evening? Have sex? Read or watch TV in bed? Work or pay bills?	All these activities may cause insomnia
Does your bedpartner adversely affect your sleep?	Bedpartner sleep disorders (insomnia, PLMD, sleep apnea, snoring) can cause insomnia
Do you have a TV or computer in your bedroom?	Nonsleep activities can cause insomnia

Is your bedroom quiet and dark?	*Possible environmental factors (noise, light)*
Do you sleep better away from home?	*If true, suggests maladaptive conditioning (psychophysiologic insomnia)*

Evaluate effects on daytime function

The following questions may help determine the severity of insomnia.

How does your night's sleep affect your day?	
Are you fatigued or sleepy?	*Nonspecific; however, excessive daytime sleepiness or falling asleep at inappropriate times suggests sleep apnea or narcolepsy*
Do you have poor concentration?	
Are you irritable?	*Irritability may be a consequence of inadequate sleep*
Does it affect your job?	
Does it affect your personal relationships?	
Does it affect your mood during the day?	
Do you nap during the day?	*Daytime naps can cause nighttime insomnia*

Assess prior treatments

Are you or have you taken anything for your sleep? What has worked and what has not?	*Helps in devising treatment plan*
Have you tried anything else?	*Potential nonpharmacologic treatments*

Assess for substance, medical, and mental causes

Think about

What medical problems do you have? Do you have any mental health problems?	
What medications do you take? Do you take any herbal or other over-the-counter medications?	*Many herbal preparations and cold or allergy medications contain stimulants. Many prescription drugs cause insomnia.*
Do you drink caffeinated beverages or eat chocolate?	*Caffeine is a common stimulant often overlooked by patients.*
Do you smoke or use tobacco?	*Nicotine is a common stimulant*
Do you drink alcohol or use other drugs? How much?	*Alcohol and illicit drug use or withdrawal*

Review of systems

Think about

Do you feel depressed? Do you have feelings of guilt or hopelessness? How is your appetite? Do you find that you don't enjoy things that you used to enjoy? Have you lost or gained weight?	*Depressive disorders* *Bipolar disorder*
Do you feel anxious? Have panic attacks?	*Anxiety disorders*
At night do you awaken with	
• *Shortness of breath?*	*Uncontrolled asthma* *COPD*

(continued)

Review of systems	Think about
	Coronary disease
	CHF
	Sleep apnea
• Chest pain or pressure, epigastric pain?	Coronary artery disease
	GERD
	PUD
• Cough?	CHF
	Uncontrolled asthma
	COPD
	Other lung disease
Are you a heavy snorer?	Obstructive sleep apnea
Has anyone ever told you that you stop breathing or choke or that you have leg or arm jerking while you are sleeping?	Obstructive or central sleep apnea or PLMD
Do your legs sometimes twitch or can't keep still? Do you get leg pain as you try to go to sleep?	PLMD or RLS
Do you feel that you want to sleep at the wrong times?	Circadian rhythm disorders
Do you get up to urinate frequently?	Polyuria due to diuretics
	Prostate disease
	Diabetes cause frequent awakenings
Do you have headaches at night?	Headaches (due to any cause)
	Need further evaluation
Do you have pain at night that keeps you awake?	Any pain syndrome can cause insomnia

CAVEATS

- Insomnia is underrecognized in primary care practice. Less than half of primary care physicians take a sleep history, and physicians are unaware of 60% of severe cases of insomnia.[7–9]
- Insomnia frequently results from significant underlying mental health and medical disorders as well as substance abuse. Hence, identification and evaluation of insomnia can potentially lead to recognition of other important diagnoses. Targeted treatment of the underlying conditions can lead to significant improvement in patients' well being.
- Insomnia treatment addresses the underlying causes, so multiple modalities are often required. Optimizing treatment of underlying mental, medical, or sleep disorders is the primary treatment, but behavioral therapy to improve sleep hygiene is also a key component. Thus, targets for intervention are readily identified by a thorough history.

REFERENCES

1. Ohayon MM. Epidemiology of insomnia: what we know and what we still need to learn. *Sleep Med Rev.* 2002;6:97–111.
2. Insomnia: Assessment and management in primary care. NHLBI Working Group on Insomnia. *Am Fam Physician.* 1999; 59:3029–3038.
3. Sateia MJ, Doghramji K, Hauri PJ, Morin CM. Evaluation of chronic insomnia. *Sleep.* 2000;23:244–303.
4. Chesson AL, Wise M, Davila D, et al. Practice parameters for the treatment of restless legs syndrome and periodic limb movement disorder. *Sleep.* 1999;22:961–968.

5. Ohayon MM, Shapiro CM, Kennedy SH. Differentiating DSM-IV anxiety and depressive disorders in the general population: comorbidity and treatment consequences. *Can J Psychiatry.* 2000;45:166–172.

6. Ford DE, Kamerow DB. Epidemiologic study of sleep disturbances and psychiatric disorders. An opportunity for prevention? *JAMA.* 1989;262:1479–1484.

7. Hohagen F, Rink K, Kappler C, et al. Prevalence and treatment of insomnia in general practice. A longitudinal study. *Eur Arch Psychiatry Clin Neurosci.* 1993;242:329–336.

8. Schramm, E, Hohagen F, Kappler C, et al. Mental comorbidity of chronic insomnia in general practice attenders using DSM III-R. *Acta Psychiatr Scand.* 1995;91:10–17.

9. Everitt DE, Avorn J, Baker MW. Clinical decision making in the evaluation and treatment of insomnia. *Am J Med.* 1990;89:357–362.

10. Espie CA, Morin CM, editors. Insomnia: a clinical guide to assessment and treatment. New York: Kluwer Academic/Plenum Publishers; 2003:135–136.

Sample Sleep Diary [2,10]

Fill out in the Morning	Day 1	Day 2	Day 3	Day 4	Day 5	Day 6	Day 7
Rise time today							
Bedtime last night							
Estimated time to fall asleep							
Estimated number of awakenings							
Estimated total time awake during the night							
Estimated amount of sleep							
How *restful* was your sleep? 0 (not at all) 1 2 3 4 (very)							
Fill out at bedtime							
Rate how you felt today: 0 (very tired) 1 2 3 4 (wide awake)							
Number of naps (time and duration)							
Alcoholic drinks (number and time)							
Caffeinated drinks (number and time)							
Stressors from the day							
Activities this evening (eg,exercise, sex, paying bills)							
Time of evening meal and snacks							

Diagnostic Approach: Insomnia

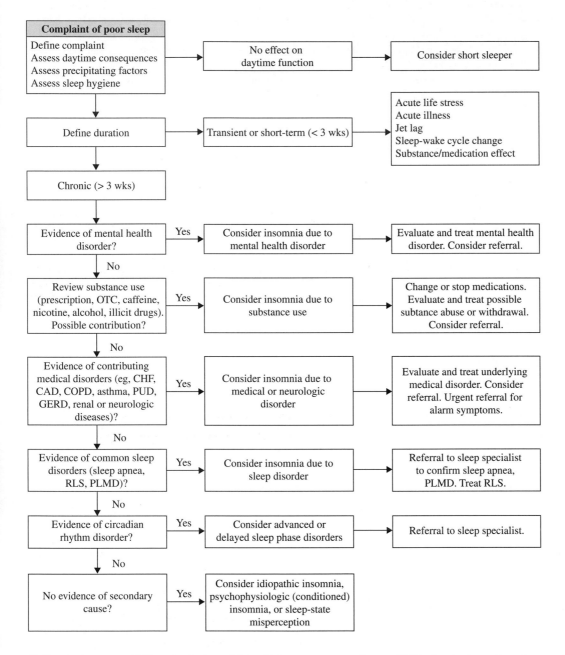

OTC, over-the-counter; CHF, congestive heart failure; CAD, coronary artery disease; COPD, chronic obstructive pulmonary disease; PUD, peptic ulcer diease; GERD, gastroesophageal reflux disease; RLS, restless legs syndrome; PLMD, periodic limb movement disorder.

Lymphadenopathy

11

Michael H. Zaroukian, MD, PhD

Lymphadenopathy is the enlargement of one or more lymph nodes. Patients may be alerted to the presence of enlarged lymph nodes by noticing visible nodular swelling, palpability, pain, or tenderness in one or more lymph node regions. It is normal to be able to palpate small lymph nodes in the neck and groin regions but generally not in the supraclavicular fossa, axilla, epitrochlear, or popliteal regions.

Lymphadenopathy generally results from infiltration of lymph nodes by inflammatory or neoplastic cells, proliferation of resident lymphocytes, or expansion due to hemorrhage or abscess formation. In primary care settings, lymphadenopathy is rarely due to malignancy; upper respiratory tract infections or nonspecific conditions account for over two thirds of cases. However, the risk of malignancy increases with age and other factors.

Careful history taking is important in determining the cause of lymphadenopathy. Patients may be concerned or even anxious that lymphadenopathy may be a manifestation of cancer. The medical interview can assist in excluding malignancy or other serious underlying disease in most patients and inform subsequent evaluation for the remainder.

KEY TERMS

Lymphadenopathy[1]	*Abnormal enlargement of one or more lymph nodes (> 1.0 cm in adults; > 1.5 cm in children and adolescents).*
Generalized lymphadenopathy[2]	*Lymph node enlargement affecting multiple body regions.*
Localized lymphadenopathy[2]	*Lymph node enlargement limited to a single body region (eg, cervical, inguinal).*

ETIOLOGY

A comprehensive discussion of the myriad agents and diseases associated with lymphadenopathy is beyond the scope of this chapter but can be found elsewhere.[3] The major causes of lymphadenopathy in the United States are listed below using the mnemonic "CINEMA DIVITT" (**c**ongenital, **i**nfectious, **n**eoplastic, **e**ndocrine, **m**etabolic, **a**llergic, **d**egenerative, **i**nflammatory/immunologic, **v**ascular, **i**diopathic or iatrogenic, **t**raumatic, **t**oxic).

Differential Diagnosis	**Prevalence[a] by Category in Primary Care[4]**
Congenital	
• Congenital syphilis	

(continued)

Differential Diagnosis	**Prevalence[a] by Category in Primary Care[4]**
Infectious[5]	*18% (upper respiratory infections)*

Infectious[5]

- *Bacteria*
  - *Atypical mycobacterial infections*
  - *Chancroid*
  - *Lyme disease*
  - *Lymphogranuloma venereum*
  - *Secondary syphilis*
  - *Skin infection (streptococci, staphylococci)*
  - *Streptococcal pharyngitis*
  - *Tuberculosis (TB)*
- *Viruses*
  - *Adenovirus*
  - *Cytomegalovirus (CMV)*
  - *Epstein-Barr virus (infectious mononucleosis)*
  - *Hepatitis B*
  - *Herpes simplex*
  - *HIV*
  - *Measles (rubeola, rubella)*
  - *Mumps*
  - *Vaccinia (smallpox vaccine)*
  - *Varicella-zoster virus (chickenpox)*
- *Fungi*
  - *Coccidioidomycosis*
  - *Cryptococcosis*
  - *Histoplasmosis*
- *Protozoa*
  - *Toxoplasmosis*
- *Mites*
  - *Scabies*

Neoplastic   *0.8–1.1% (4% if age > 40 years)*

- *Lymphoma*
- *Leukemia*
- *Metastatic solid tumors (major primary sites): breast, colon, esophagus, head and neck, kidney, lung, ovary, prostate, skin (melanoma), stomach, testes*

Endocrine

- *Adrenal insufficiency*
- *Hyperthyroidism*
- *Hypothyroidism*
- *Multiple endocrine neoplasia (see Neoplastic)*

*M*etabolic
- Lipid storage diseases
- Severe hypertriglyceridemia

*A*llergic
- Serum sickness

*D*egenerative
- Amyloidosis (secondary)

*I*nflammatory/Immunologic
- Amyloidosis (primary)
- Dermatomyositis
- Graft-versus-host disease
- Mixed connective tissue disease
- Primary biliary cirrhosis
- Rheumatoid arthritis
- Systemic lupus erythematosus
- Sarcoidosis
- Sjögren syndrome

*V*ascular
- Vasculitis
  — Churg-Strauss syndrome (adults)
  — Kawasaki disease (children)

*I*diopathic or iatrogenic   29–64%
- Nonspecific lymphadenopathy
- Prescribed medications (see Toxic)

*T*raumatic   32% (including cuts and bites, in which sec-
- Abrasions and lacerations   ondary infection causes lymphadenopathy)
- Burns
- Cat-scratch disease (Bartonella henselae)
- Operations

*T*oxic (drugs, chemicals)
- Antihypertensives
  — Atenolol
  — Captopril
  — Hydralazine
- Antimicrobials
  — Cephalosporins
  — Penicillin
  — Pyrimethamine
  — Sulfonamides

(continued)

Differential Diagnosis

Prevalence[a] by Category in Primary Care[4]

- *Antiseizure medications*
  — *Carbamazepine*
  — *Phenytoin*
  — *Primidone*
- *Antirheumatics*
  — *Allopurinol*
  — *Gold*
- *Sulindac*

[a]Prevalence estimate is unavailable when not indicated.

GETTING STARTED

- Before the visit, review the patient's problems and medications as well as his or her past, family, social, sexual, travel, and occupational history for relevant clues.
- Remember that the risk of malignancy increases with age, particularly after age 50.
- Review the anatomy of the lymphatic system and the tissues and organs that drain to each lymph node group.[6]

Open-ended questions

Tell me about the lump(s) you are feeling.

- *Where do you feel it?*
- *What does it feel like?*
- *When did you first notice it?*
- *Does it seem to be changing with time?*

Have you had any recent illnesses or other symptoms?

Tell me about your work, hobbies, pets, and travels.

Can you think of any exposures you may have had to infectious agents, chemicals, insects, or people who were ill?

Have you taken any medications lately?

Tell me about your current or past use of tobacco and alcohol.

Have you or any member of your family ever had any type of cancer?

Tell me about your sexual history.

Tips for effective interviewing

- *Establish a setting of comfort and trust*
- *Begin with open-ended questions before focusing*
- *Cover all important question areas not otherwise mentioned by the patient (see mnemonic below: **COLD RAP TAPE**)*

Character: *What is it like?*

Onset: *When did it start?*

Location: *Where do you notice it?*

Duration: *How long does it last?*

Relieving factors: *What makes it better?*

Aggravating factors: *What makes it worse?*

Precipitating factors: *What brings it on?*

Therapy: *What have you tried to make it better?*

Associated symptoms: *Do you have any other symptoms along with this?*

Past medical history: *Have you ever had anything like this before?*

Emotional impact: *What concerns do you have about this and how it may affect your life?*

INTERVIEW FRAMEWORK

- Establish the onset and course of lymph node enlargement.
- Determine the presence or absence of other symptoms and whether symptoms are localized or generalized.
- Ask about exposures related to work, home, hobbies, habits, pets, travel, sexual activity, and medications.

IDENTIFYING ALARM SYMPTOMS

Most cases of lymphadenopathy have a benign and self-limited infectious or inflammatory cause.[7,8] However, lymphadenopathy can be due to local infections, for which antimicrobial therapy can be beneficial; to potentially life-threatening diseases, such as cancer[9]; to systemic infection; and to autoimmune connective tissue disease (CTD). Remembering these conditions and the alarm symptoms associated with them facilitates earlier diagnosis and initiation of curative or palliative therapy.

Serious diagnoses	Relative prevalence in primary care settings
Cancer	1–4%
Local infections for which antimicrobial therapy may be beneficial	10–30%
Systemic infection	< 1%
Severe autoimmune disease	< 1%

Alarm symptoms	Consider
Persistence or growth over several weeks or months	Cancer Systemic inflammation/infection
Lymph node described as "hard"	Metastatic cancer
Right supraclavicular lymphadenopathy	Metastatic cancer of mediastinum, esophagus, or thorax
Left supraclavicular lymphadenopathy	Metastatic cancer originating in thorax, abdomen, or pelvis
Axillary area without local trauma or infection	Breast cancer Other metastatic cancer
Epitrochlear area without local trauma or infection	Lymphoma Sarcoidosis Secondary syphilis
Inguinal lymphadenopathy	Sexually transmitted diseases Abdominal/pelvic malignancies
Generalized lymphadenopathy	HIV infection TB Sarcoidosis Medications

(continued)

Alarm symptoms	Consider
Cervical, axillary, and inguinal lymphadenopathy associated with photosensitive rash, oral ulcers, or arthralgia	*Systemic lupus erythematosus*
Constitutional symptoms (malaise, fatigue, fever, unintentional weight loss, night sweats)	*Lymphoma* *Metastatic cancer* *Autoimmune diseases* *TB* *Systemic infection* *Medications*
Hoarseness, dysphagia, chronic cough, hemoptysis	*Metastatic cancer originating in the head and neck or lung*
Abdominal pain, hematochezia, melena, hematuria	*Cancer (gastrointestinal, genitourinary system)* *Enteric infections*

FOCUSED QUESTIONS

After listening to the patient's open-ended description of lymph node enlargement, proceed to focused questions to determine the most likely cause. It is particularly important to inquire about alarm symptoms because their presence greatly influences subsequent diagnostic decision-making.

Questions	Think about
Do you have a history of cancer?	*Metastatic cancer*
Have you traveled recently?	*Infectious causes*
Do you have a family history of head and neck cancer?	*Multiple endocrine neoplasia*
Do you drink alcohol or use tobacco? If so, how much?	*Cancer (head and neck, lung, gastrointestinal)*
Have you ever been exposed to radiation?	*Cancer*
Have you ever had a positive TB skin test? Have you been exposed to anyone with untreated TB?	*TB*
Have you been exposed to animals at work, or on a farm or ranch? Do you ever use unpasteurized milk or cheese? Do you hunt, clean, or eat the meat from wild animals? Have you been bitten or scratched by cats? Do you cut or scratch yourself often?	*Toxoplasmosis* *Cat-scratch disease* *Brucellosis* *Tularemia* *Repeated minor trauma*
Have you had a tick bite or traveled to area where Lyme disease is endemic (eg, northeast)?	*Lyme disease*
Do you engage in unprotected sexual intercourse?	*HIV infection*
Have you ever used injection drugs?	*Hepatitis B* *Syphilis*
Have you experienced fever, joint pain, or rash with recent medication use?	*Medication-associated serum sickness with lymphadenopathy*
Do you have a mole that has changed in pigmentation?	*Melanoma*

Quality

Is the swollen gland

	Think about
• *Painful or tender?*	*Infection* *Inflammatory causes*
• *Hard?*	*Metastatic cancer*
• *Draining?*	*Bacterial, mycobacterial infections*

Time course

Tell me how the lymph gland problem has changed over time. Has it

	Think about
• *Been present for over a month?*	*Malignancy*
• *Continued to increase in size?*	*Malignancy*
• *Followed use of a new medication?*	*Medication*

Associated symptoms

In addition to the lymph gland swelling, have you also had any

	Think about
• *Fevers, chills, or sweats?*	*Infections* *Lymphoma* *Hyperthyroidism*
• *Skin rash, redness, bites, insect stings, cuts or scrapes?*	*Bacterial or viral infections* *Mite infestation* *Secondary syphilis*
• *Sore throat or cold symptoms?*	*Viral or streptococcal pharyngitis*
• *Genital sores or discharge?*	*Sexually transmitted diseases*
• *Fatigue?*	*Epstein-Barr virus* *Hepatitis B infection* *CMV* *Thyroid dysfunction* *Adrenal insufficiency*
• *Unintentional weight loss?*	*Malignancy* *HIV infection* *TB*
• *Breast lumps or discharge?*	*Breast cancer*
• *Persistent cough, hoarseness, or coughing up blood?*	*Head and neck cancer* *Lung cancer* *TB* *Sarcoidosis*
• *Difficulty swallowing, abdominal pain, pencil-thin stools, blood in your stool or pitch black, tarry stool?*	*Gastrointestinal malignancy*
• *Change in a mole?*	*Melanoma*
• *Pain or nodule in a testicle?*	*Testicular cancer* *Mumps*

(continued)

Associated symptoms	Think about
• Blood in your urine?	Prostate cancer Renal malignancy
• Joint pain, mouth ulcers, rashes after sun exposure, dry mouth, dry eyes	Autoimmune CTDs Medication-associated serum sickness
Modifying symptoms	**Think about**
Does anything seem to make the lymph gland swelling better or worse, such as	
• Antibiotic use?	Better: Infection Worse: Medication-associated lymphadenopathy
• Aspirin, ibuprofen, naproxen or other nonsteroidal anti-inflammatory drugs?	Better: Inflammation Worse: Sulindac

CAVEATS

- Remember that what a patient reports as lymph node swelling may actually be another condition (eg, lipoma, sebaceous cyst, abscess, thyroid nodule).
- Lymph node swelling suggestive of a benign, self-limited condition may nevertheless prompt a strongly negative emotional response in patients or family members concerned about the possibility of malignancy.
- Nonspecific lymphadenopathy that is persistent or progressive should prompt repeat evaluation, patient education, and continued shared decision-making regarding work-up options and their relative risks, costs, and benefits.

PROGNOSIS

The prognosis of lymphadenopathy in the majority of cases seen in primary care settings is excellent, justifying reassurance and observation when the cause appears to be benign and self-limited, particularly in younger patients.[10] The prognosis of lymphadenopathy due to serious systemic infections (eg, HIV, syphilis, TB) or malignancies depends on a number of factors, including the timeliness of establishing the correct diagnosis, initiation of appropriate therapy, patient-specific immunologic and physiologic responsiveness, and the biologic characteristics of the organism or neoplasm.

REFERENCES

1. Ferrer R. Lymphadenopathy: differential diagnosis and evaluation. *Am Fam Physician.* 1998;58:1313–1320.
2. Habermann TM, Steensma DP. Lymphadenopathy. *Mayo Clin Proc.* 2000;75:723–732.
3. Henry PH, Longo DL. Enlargement of Lymph Nodes and Spleen. In: Braunwald E (editor). *Harrison's Principles of Internal Medicine,* 15th ed. The McGraw-Hill Companies, Inc; 2001.
4. Berliner N. Lymphadenopathy. In: Gotto AM, ed. *Best Practice of Medicine.* Vol. 2003. Greenwood Village, Colorado: Thomson MICROMEDEX; 2002.
5. Heitman B, Irizarry A. Infectious disease causes of lymphadenopathy: localized versus diffuse. *Lippincotts Prim Care Pract.* 1999;3:19–38.
6. Ballas ZK. Biology of the Immune System. In: Berkow R (editor). *The Merck Manual of Medical Information–Home Edition Online.* Vol. 2003. Whitehouse Station, NJ: Merck & Co., Inc.; 2000.
7. Williamson HA Jr. Lymphadenopathy in a family practice: a descriptive study of 249 cases. *J Fam Pract.* 1985;20:449–452.
8. Anthony PP, Knowles SA. Lymphadenopathy as a primary presenting sign: a clinicopathological study of 228 cases. *Br J Surg.* 1983;70:412–414.

9. Bazemore AW, Smucker DR. Lymphadenopathy and malignancy. *Am Fam Physician.* 2002;66:2103–2110.

10. Slap GB, Connor JL, Wigton RS, Schwartz JS. Validation of a model to identify young patients for lymph node biopsy. *JAMA.* 1986;255:2768–2773.

SUGGESTED READING

Fletcher RH. Evaluation of peripheral lymphadenopathy in adults. In: Rose BD, ed. *UpToDate.* 11.3 ed. Vol. 2003. Wellesley: UpToDate; 2003.

Diagnostic Approach: Lymphadenopathy

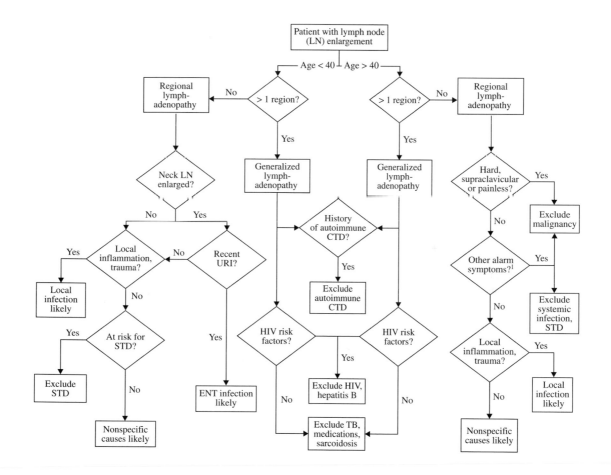

STD, sexually transmitted disease; CTD, connective tissue disease; TB, tuberculosis; URI, upper respiratory infection; ENT, ear, nose, and throat.

[1] Other alarm symptoms suggestive of malignancy include progressive lymph node enlargement over weeks and months, alcohol and tobacco use, constitutional symptoms (malaise, fatigue, fever, unintentional weight loss, night sweats), hoarseness, dysphagia, chronic cough, hemoptysis, hematuria, hematochezia, melena, abdominal pain, and axillary or epitrochlear adenopathy without local trauma or infection.

Night Sweats

12

David Feinbloom, MD, & Gerald W. Smetana, MD

Night sweats are a frequent complaint of patients who seek medical attention from primary care physicians and other health care providers. While most often benign, night sweats may be a manifestation of serious systemic disease and should prompt a thorough evaluation to determine the cause. Diagnosis requires a careful medical history, as well as an understanding of the epidemiology and differential diagnosis of this symptom.

Night sweats are drenching sweats that require the patient to change bedclothes. This definition emphasizes the need to distinguish "night sweats" from other conditions that may be associated with increased sweating but do not have the same nocturnal pattern or clinical implications. The causes of night sweats vary ranging from common, typically benign conditions to serious disorders associated with significant morbidity and mortality.

KEY TERMS

Flushing	*Acute onset of cutaneous vasodilatation with marked changes in skin color, ranging from bright red to cyanotic. While it primarily involves the face, neck and upper chest, it can extend to the whole body including the palms and soles.*
Hot flashes	*Autonomic symptoms associated with menopause. They are characterized by the sudden onset of intense warmth and redness in the face, chest, and upper back and may include palpitations, profuse sweating, and anxiety. These symptoms typically last only minutes.*
Hyperhidrosis	*Troublesome, benign increase in sweating beyond that necessary to maintain thermal homeostasis.*
Night sweats	*Drenching sweats that occur during sleep and require the patient to change bedclothes. By definition, the following features must not be present: fever, excessive bedding, or increased temperature in the sleeping quarters.*

ETIOLOGY

Although numerous causes of night sweats exist, determining a specific etiology can be challenging. Common causes include hormonal changes associated with pregnancy and menopause, gastroesophageal reflux disease (GERD), and sleep disorders. In our experience, medications commonly cause night sweats, particularly antipyretic and antidepressant medications.[1] Unfortunately, the literature on night sweats lacks scope, consistent nomenclature, or rigorous methodology, making an evidence-based approach difficult.

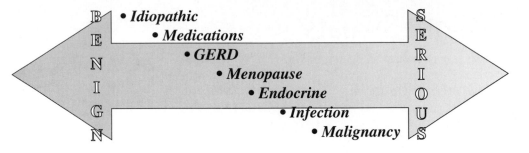

Differential Diagnosis	Prevalence[a]
Menopause	35% of women report night sweats associated with menopause[2]
Infection	
Tuberculosis	29–62% depending on series.[3] More common in reactivation tuberculosis and in younger patients.
HIV	9–70% depending on series.[4] Often seen during the acute retroviral syndrome, during coinfection with an opportunistic pathogen, or with concurrent malignancy, eg, lymphoma.
Endocarditis	17–25% depending on series[5]
Osteomyelitis	
Abscess (liver, lung, abdomen)	
Fungal	
• Histoplasmosis	
• Coccidioidomycosis	
• Blastomycosis	
Viral	
• Epstein-Barr (EBV)	
• Cytomegalovirus (CMV)	
Parasites	
• Malaria	
• Babesiosis	
Malignancy	
Hodgkin disease	Up to 25%[6]
Non-Hodgkin lymphoma	
Leukemia (chronic myelogenous leukemia [CML])	
Solid tumors	
• Renal cell carcinoma	
• Prostate cancer	

- *Medullary thyroid cancer*
- *Germ cell tumors*
- *Metastatic*

Medications[1]

Antipyretics

Nonsteroidal anti-inflammatory drugs

Clozaril	*5%*
Selective serotonin reuptake inhibitors	*5–10%*
Venlafaxine	*2%*
Donepezil	
Rituximab	*15%*
Imatinib mesylate	*10–14%*
Leuprolide acetate	*85%*
Danazol	*65%*
Bicalutamide + luteinizing hormone releasing hormone	*25%*
Anastrozole	*5%*
Raloxifene	*2–3%*
Interferon	*8%*
Saquinivir mesylate	*8%*
Triptans	*1–3%*
Cyclosporine	*Up to 4%*

Rheumatologic

Microscopic polyangiitis	*71% in 1 series[7]*

Miscellaneous

Chronic fatigue syndrome	*30–40%[8]*
Dumping syndrome	*Reported, but prevalence low*
Hyperthyroidism	*Increased sweating in 50–91%,[9] although pure night sweats are less common*

GERD[10]

[a]Prevalence is unknown when not indicated.

GETTING STARTED

- Allow the patient to describe the symptoms in his or her own words without prompting or interrupting.
- Avoid leading questions; leave time at the end to follow-up with a few close-ended questions directed at the most likely disorder.

- Patients are often uncomfortable discussing sexual behavior or illegal drug use, and clinicians must be sensitive to these concerns. At the same time, these may be important clues that increase the likelihood of particular infectious etiologies as the cause of night sweats.
- Review medication list before seeing the patient and validate them during the interview.

Questions	**Remember**
I understand that you have been having night sweats, can you tell me about them?	• *Let patients use their own words.*
Tell me what you mean by night sweats.	• *Avoid interrupting.*
	• *Listen to the patient closely, and try to identify clues that will guide your follow-up questions.*
Can you describe a typical night's sleep, from the time you go to sleep until the time you wake in the morning?	• *Reassurance that night sweats are both common and generally treatable will help the patient to provide a complete history.*
Do you have increased sweating at other times of the day?	

INTERVIEW FRAMEWORK

- The first goal is to establish that the complaint of night sweats is consistent with the working medical definition. Therefore, the clinician must first exclude fever, excessive bedding, or elevated room temperature.
- It is best to categorize night sweats into those that are benign in etiology and those that require more thorough testing in order to exclude serious illness. The following characteristics can help to make these distinctions:

  Onset: Acute, subacute, or chronic
  Duration: Daytime, nighttime, or both
  Frequency: Isolated, nightly, weekly, monthly
  Pattern: Escalating, waxing and waning
  Precipitants: Foods, medications, etc.
  Associated symptoms: Weight loss, menses, diarrhea, cough, etc.
  The presence of significant risk factors (travel to areas with endemic infections, unprotected sexual intercourse, injection drug use, etc)

IDENTIFYING ALARM SYMPTOMS

Night sweats may be the sole manifestation of a serious disease. Therefore, distinguishing between benign and serious etiologies is critical. A history of weight loss, lymphadenopathy, cough, hematuria, hemoptysis, hematochezia, rash, arthritis, back pain, diarrhea, high-risk sexual behavior, drug abuse, or disease exposure should increase clinical suspicion of a serious disease.

Serious Diagnoses

Serious causes for night sweats are uncommon. Moreover, it is unlikely that a patient will present with night sweats as the sole manifestation of serious illness. Nevertheless, serious causes of night sweats must be ruled out, since delay or failure to detect these illnesses can result in significant morbidity and mortality.

Once you have completed the open-ended portion of the medical interview, it is essential to inquire about symptoms that may suggest a serious diagnosis. While the following questions lack specificity, a positive response should prompt further questions to direct the physical examination and determine the need for diagnostic testing.

Alarm symptoms	Serious causes	Benign causes
Unintentional weight loss	Lymphoma Solid tumors Subacute endocarditis Tuberculosis HIV infection Vasculitis	Change in diet Hyperthyroidism Diabetes mellitus Malabsorption
Loss of appetite or early satiety	Lymphoma Gastrointestinal malignancy	Dyspepsia Depression Medications
Episodic diarrhea	Carcinoid tumor Medullary thyroid carcinoma Inflammatory bowel disease	Viral or bacterial Gastroenteritis Irritable bowel syndrome Medications Hyperthyroidism
Bloody or dark tarry stools	Gastric cancer Colon cancer	Gastritis Peptic ulcer disease Colonic polyps Arteriovenous malformations
Blood in urine	Uroepithelial cancer Renal cell carcinoma Vasculitis	Urinary tract infection Menses Urethritis Renal calculi
Enlarged or tender lymph nodes or glands	Lymphoma Tuberculosis Fungal infections	Viral illness (CMV, EBV, etc.) Cellulitis Drug reaction Pharyngitis
Pruritus	Lymphoma Bile duct malignancy Renal failure Polycythemia vera	Dry skin Atopic dermatitis Hypothyroidism
New back pain	Endocarditis Osteomyelitis Malignancy	Degenerative joint disease Sciatica Muscle strain
Testicular swelling or pain	Germ cell tumor Renal cell cancer	Epididymitis Trauma Orchitis Hydrocele/varicocele
Easy bruising or bleeding?	Leukemia Lymphoma	von Willebrand disease Vitamin C deficiency Steroid-induced purpura
Palpitations	Pheochromocytoma	Atrial or ventricular premature contractions Hyperthyroidism Caffeine

(continued)

Alarm symptoms	Serious causes	Benign causes
		Nicotine
		Medications
New headaches	Pheochromocytoma	Tension headache
	Central nervous system tumor	Migraine headache
	Giant cell arteritis	
Wheezing or shortness of breath	Carcinoid tumor	Asthma
	Lung cancer	Bronchospasm
	Pericardial or pleural effusion	Postnasal drip
		Medications
		Allergic reaction
New cough or a cough associated with bloody sputum	Lung cancer	Bronchitis
	Tuberculosis	Sinusitis
	Histoplasmosis	Cough variant asthma
	Coccidioidomycosis	
	Vasculitis	
High blood pressure	Pheochromocytoma	Weight gain
	Vasculitis	Essential hypertension
		Medications
Recurrent episodes of dizziness or lightheadedness	Pheochromocytoma	Hypovolemia/dehydration
	Carcinoid tumor	Benign positional vertigo
	Insulinoma	Vestibular neuronitis
Arthritis or arthralgias	HIV infection	Osteoarthritis
	Rheumatologic disease	Posttraumatic
	Endocarditis	
New or recurrent rash	HIV infection	Viral exanthems
	Vasculitis	Drug eruption
	Rickettsial disease	Dermatitis
	Syphilis	

FOCUSED QUESTIONS

After listening to the patient describe his or her night sweats, follow-up with a few close-ended questions directed at specific etiologies.

Questions	Think about
History that excludes night sweats as primary focus of inquiry	
Do these symptoms improve if you remove your blankets?	Too many coverings or overheated room
Do you have fever?	Proceed to evaluation of fever
Medications	**Think about**
What medications are you taking, and are any of them new?	Be sure to inquire about over-the-counter and herbal medications.

Do you take any medications that may suppress your immune system?

Immunosuppressant medications predispose patients to tuberculosis, fungal and viral infections, and soft-tissue abscesses.

Timing

Is this a new problem, or has it been present for many months or years?

Think about

Chronic night sweats are more likely benign, while new night sweats may suggest a more serious cause.

Do these episodes only occur at night, or are there other times as well?

Pure night sweats are most often described in patients with infections or malignancies, while continuous or episodic sweating may suggest an endocrinopathy or idiopathic hyperhidrosis.

Are these episodes associated with meals or specific foods?

Gustatory sweating
Food additive reaction

Comorbidities

Do you have diabetes?

Think about

Night sweats may occur as a result of nocturnal hypoglycemia or autonomic neuropathy. In addition, diabetes is a risk factor for infectious causes of night sweats.

Do you drink alcohol or use other drugs?

Withdrawal syndromes may be associated with night sweats. Alcoholics are predisposed to aspiration pneumonia and subsequent lung abscess formation.

Do you undergo hemodialysis?

Tuberculosis
Endocarditis

Have you had previous stomach or bowel surgery?

Tuberculosis

Have you had recent dental work or skin infection?

Endocarditis
Osteomyelitis
Soft-tissue abscess

Do you have a known history of a heart murmur, rheumatic heart disease, or a congenital valvular abnormality?

Endocarditis

Social history

Have you been homeless, institutionalized, or in prison?

Think about

Tuberculosis

Were you born in another country?

Tuberculosis is endemic in parts of Southeast Asia, Africa, and the Middle East.

Have you traveled in the United States or other countries, and if so, where?

Tuberculosis
Fungal infections
Food-borne illness
Malaria

Have you had sex with an HIV-positive individual, a prostitute, or without the use of a condom?

HIV infection
Hepatitis

(continued)

Social history	**Think about**
Do you have a history of smoking or chronic lung disease?	Lung cancer
Have you ever injected drugs?	Endocarditis HIV infection Hepatitis
Have you ever had a blood transfusion?	HIV infection Hepatitis
Focused review of systems	**Think about**
Do you have indigestion or heartburn?	GERD
Are you increasingly fatigued?	Anemia of malignancy HIV infection Infection Metastatic cancer Chronic fatigue syndrome
Do you have tremor or heat intolerance?	Hyperthyroidism
Have you had a change in your menstruation or libido?	Hyperthyroidism Premature gonadal failure Menopause Pituitary tumor
Does your sweating occur when you are anxious or emotionally upset?	Panic disorder
Do you snore or feel tired even after a good night's sleep?	Obstructive sleep apnea
Have you had a mosquito or tick bite?	Malaria Babesiosis

CAVEATS

- Night sweats that are new, accompanied by systemic symptoms, or not readily explained by benign processes *are serious until proved otherwise.*
- Be certain to exclude spurious causes of night sweats before embarking on a lengthy evaluation; likewise, fever must be excluded at the outset.
- The presence of weight loss, flushing, diarrhea, hypertension, lymphadenopathy, or cough should raise the clinical suspicion of more serious systemic disease. When unsure, err on the side of caution by ruling out more serious diagnoses.
- The clinical context is crucial in making the correct diagnosis. For example, the common causes of night sweats in a 45-year-old perimenopausal woman are quite different than in a 60-year-old man with weight loss, flank pain, and hematuria. Pay attention to demographics, comorbid illnesses, travel history, and other exposures to narrow the differential diagnosis.
- Always perform a complete review of all prescription, herbal, and over-the-counter medications.
- Reevaluate your working diagnosis over time, and pay special attention to new or contradictory information.

PROGNOSIS

The prognosis of night sweats depends on the underlying diagnosis. The majority of causes are benign and readily manageable with appropriate treatment. Serious causes of night sweats, including malignancies and infections, are less common. Failure to identify such diseases may result in unnecessary morbidity and mortality and, in the case of HIV infection and tuberculosis, pose a public health risk as well.

REFERENCES

1. *Physicians' Desk Reference,* ed. P. Staff. Vol. 57 ed. 2003, Montvale, NJ: Thompson Healthcare Press.
2. von Muhlen DG, Kritz-Silverstein D, Barrett-Connor E. A community-based study of menopause symptoms and estrogen replacement in older women. *Maturitas.* 1995;22:71–78.
3. Aktogu S et al. Clinical spectrum of pulmonary and pleural tuberculosis: a report of 5,480 cases. *Eur Respir J.* 1996; 9:2031–2035.
4. Cunningham WE et al. Constitutional symptoms and health-related quality of life in patients with symptomatic HIV disease. *Am J Med.* 1998;104:129–136.
5. Jalal S. Clinical spectrum of infective endocarditis: 15 years experience. *Indian Heart J.* 1998;50:516–519.
6. Lister TA et al. Report of a committee convened to discuss the evaluation and staging of patients with Hodgkin's disease: Cotswolds meeting. *J Clin Oncol.* 1989;7:1630–1636.
7. Kirkland GS et al. Classical polyarteritis nodosa and microscopic polyarteritis with medium vessel involvement–a comparison of the clinical and laboratory features. *Clin Nephrol.* 1997;47:176–180.
8. Komaroff AL. Clinical presentation of chronic fatigue syndrome. *Ciba Found Symp.* 1993;173:43–54, 54–61.
9. Spaulding SW, Lippes H. Hyperthyroidism. Causes, clinical features, and diagnosis. *Med Clin North Am.* 1985;69:937–951.
10. Reynolds WA. Are night sweats a sign of esophageal reflux? *J Clin Gastroenterol.* 1989;11:590–591.

SUGGESTED READING

Chambliss ML. Frequently asked questions from clinical practice. What is the appropriate diagnostic approach for patients who complain of night sweats? *Arch Fam Med.* 1999;8:168–169.

Leung AK, Chan PY, Choi MC. Hyperhidrosis. *Int J Dermatol.* 1999;38:561–567.

McWhinney IR. Significance of night sweats. *J Fam Pract.* 2002;51:457–458.

Mold JW et al. Prevalence of night sweats in primary care patients: an OKPRN and TAFP-Net collaborative study. *J Fam Pract.* 2002;51:452–456.

Ray D, Williams G. Pathophysiological causes and clinical significance of flushing. *Br J Hosp Med.* 1993;50:594–598.

Diagnostic Approach: Night Sweats

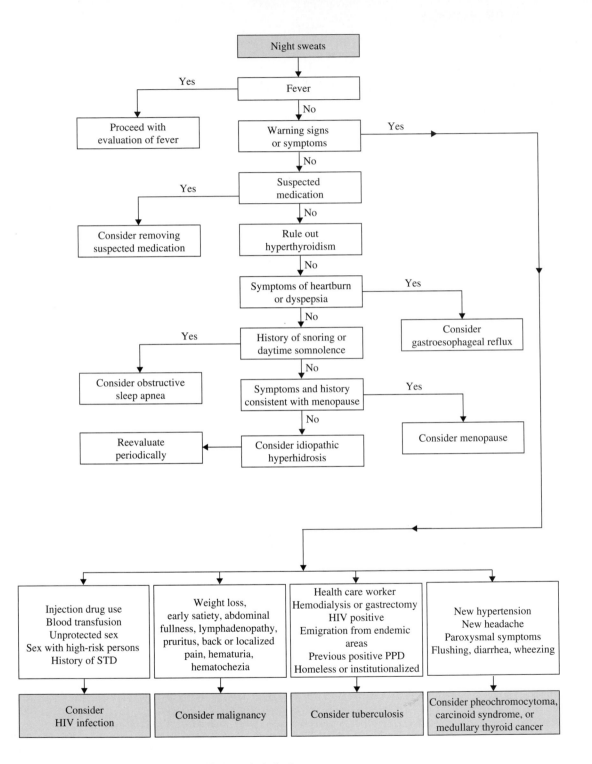

STD, sexually transmitted disease; PPD, purified protein derivative.

Muscle Weakness

13

Catherine R. Lucey, MD

In patients with weakness, the physician must first determine whether the patient merely feels weak or actually has symptoms and signs of true motor weakness. *Functional weakness* is caused by a variety of conditions including cancer, chronic infection, inflammatory diseases, depression, and fibromyalgia (see Chapter 7). In these conditions, the patient does not have objective evidence of muscle weakness but has trouble completing activities of daily living because of a lack of physical or emotional energy. In contrast, patients with true motor weakness report difficulty accomplishing specific tasks such as rising from a seated position, but their ability to perform other tasks is preserved. Furthermore, patients may also complain of weakness when pain—rather than a true loss of muscle power—prevents them from completing specific activities.

While all patients with weakness warrant a careful evaluation, this chapter focuses on patients whose history suggests true muscle weakness.

KEY TERMS[1]

Ascending paralysis	*Motor weakness that begins at the feet and progressively moves up the body.*
Bulbar symptoms	*Weakness in the muscles of the face and tongue, resulting in difficulty speaking, swallowing, and smiling.*
Descending paralysis	*Motor weakness that begins in the face and progressively moves down the body.*
Hemiparesis	*Weakness on 1 side of the body.*
Monoparesis	*Weakness of 1 limb.*
Paraparesis	*Weakness of both legs.*
Tetraparesis	*Weakness of all 4 limbs.*
Todd paralysis	*Reversible hemiplegic weakness following a partial motor seizure.*
Upper motor neuron lesions	*Abnormalities of motor pathways that descend from the brain, brainstem, or spinal column to the alpha motor neurons.*
Lower motor neuron lesions	*Abnormalities of the alpha motor neuron in the spinal gray matter or the nerves distal to the neuron.*

ETIOLOGY

Muscle weakness can be caused by primary muscle or neurologic disorders (eg, multiple sclerosis) or as a consequence of systemic disease. Since primary and secondary causes of weakness affect different aspects of the neuromuscular system, a useful categorization focuses on the anatomic localization of the lesion causing the weakness.

Category	Definition and examples
Myopathies	*Primary muscle disorders (either congenital or acquired)* *Example: Rhabdomyolysis*
Radiculopathies	*Dysfunction of the spinal nerve roots (lower motor neuron disorder)* *Example: L5 radiculopathy due to a herniated disk*
Peripheral neuropathies	*Dysfunction of a peripheral nerve (lower motor neuron disorder). Subcategories include the following:* *• Mononeuropathies: Involvement of 1 nerve* *Example: Wrist drop due to radial nerve palsy* *• Mononeuritis multiplex: Involvement of multiple peripheral nerves in an unpredictable pattern* *Example: Periarteritis nodosa with peroneal nerve weakness* *• Polyneuropathies: Simultaneous dysfunction of multiple peripheral nerves, usually causing symmetric distal symptoms* *Example: Diabetic polyneuropathy*
Central nervous system (CNS) disorders	*Dysfunction of the brain or spinal cord (myelopathy)* *Example: Multiple sclerosis, stroke*
Motor neuron disease	*Diseases affecting both upper and lower motor neurons* *Example: Amyotrophic lateral sclerosis (ALS)*
Neuromuscular junction disorders	*Conditions associated with dysfunction of the neuromuscular end plate.* *Example (acute): Botulism* *Example (chronic): Myasthenia gravis*

Differential Diagnosis

The initial differential diagnosis depends not only on the anatomic localization of the lesion but also on the duration and evolution of the symptoms. Conditions associated with a sudden, dramatic loss of muscle function or the rapid progression of muscle weakness are outlined under alarm conditions. Patients with conditions associated with insidious or episodic development of muscle weakness (outlined below) often delay seeking medical attention for weeks or months.

Condition	Associated diseases or pathophysiologic causes
Polyneuropathies[2]	*Congenital: Charcot-Marie-Tooth disease* *Toxic/metabolic: Diabetes mellitus, alcoholism, B_{12} deficiency, uremia, heavy metal poisoning* *Inflammatory: Guillain-Barré syndrome (GBS), chronic inflammatory demyelinating polyradiculopathy (CIDP), periarteritis nodosa, and other vasculitides* *Infectious: HIV and leprosy*
Polymyositis/Dermatomyositis	*Polymyositis: Idiopathic, inflammatory* *Dermatomyositis: Paraneoplastic, inflammatory*
Inclusion body myositis	*Inflammatory*
Thyroid myopathies	*Hyperthyroidism*

	Hypothyroidism (rarely)
ALS	Degenerative
Post polio syndrome	Degenerative
Multiple sclerosis	Demyelinating
Myasthenia gravis	Immunologic
Eaton-Lambert syndrome	Paraneoplastic

GETTING STARTED

The initial interview should be directed at clarifying the temporal pattern of weakness and ascertaining whether the patient's symptoms suggest true muscle weakness.

Open-ended questions	**Tips for effective interviewing**
Tell me about your weakness.	• An open-ended question will often yield significant information.
How did your weakness develop and how long has it been going on?	• The duration and evolution of the patient's symptoms is useful in determining potential etiologies.
Do you feel it is difficult to participate in all activities, or are there specific tasks that are difficult for you to do?	• Patients who describe weakness with all activities along with fatigue are likely to be suffering from functional weakness.
Do you have any pain that seems to affect or contribute to your weakness?	• The evaluation of patients with pain-associated weakness should focus on diseases that cause muscle or joint pain (eg, arthritis).

INTERVIEW FRAMEWORK

The interviewer should focus on the following elements:

- Duration of symptoms and temporal evolution of symptoms
- Distribution of symptoms
- Associated signs and symptoms
- Risk factors for conditions causing weakness from the past medical, social, and family history.

IDENTIFYING ALARM SYMPTOMS

Weakness that develops acutely over hours to a few days should be evaluated promptly, since many of the underlying conditions may cause irreversible neurologic damage or even loss of life if diagnosis and therapy are delayed.

Serious Diagnoses	**Prevalence**
Botulism	Approximately 100 cases of botulism are seen in the United States each year; 75% occur in infants, 25% are food related, and a few are related to contaminated wounds.[3]

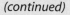

(continued)

Serious Diagnoses	Prevalence
Organophosphate poisoning	In 1999, approximately 1300 episodes of organophosphate poisoning were reported to US poison control centers.[4]
Tick paralysis	Most cases of tick paralysis occur in the Pacific Northwest and the Rocky Mountain states, although there have been sporadic cases reported in the southern United States.[5]
Stroke	There are 700,000 strokes in the United States each year; 25% occur in patients younger than 65 years.[6]
GBS	The incidence of GBS is 0.6 to 2.4 cases per 100,000, affecting men and women equally.[7]
Transverse myelitis	Transverse myelitis can occur following trauma or in association with other conditions such as multiple sclerosis or Sjögren syndrome.
Rhabdomyolysis	Hospital discharge data documents 26,000 cases of rhabdomyolysis a year.[8]
Hypokalemic periodic paralysis	Primary periodic hypokalemic paralysis is an autosomal dominant disease, whereas secondary periodic paralysis occurs sporadically.

Alarm symptoms	Serious causes	Benign causes
Rapidly progressive descending tetraparesis	Botulism Descending GBS Organophosphate poisoning Brainstem stroke	
Rapidly ascending paraparesis	GBS Transverse myelitis Spinal cord compression (neoplasm, infection, cancer, trauma, disk herniation)	
Sudden onset hemiparesis	Ischemic stroke Transient ischemic attack	Hemiplegic migraine Todd paralysis Conversion disorder
Spontaneous resolution of hemiparesis in less than 1 day	Transient ischemic attack	Hemiplegic migraine Todd paralysis Conversion disorder
Sudden onset monoparesis	Ischemic stroke Mononeuritis	Compressive neuropathy
Others have developed the same weakness	Food-related botulism Organophosphate poisoning	
Tick exposure with tetraparesis	Tick paralysis	
Diplopia or blurry vision or bulbar symptoms with developing tetraparesis	Botulism Organophosphate poisoning Descending GBS Brainstem stroke	Mononeuritis affecting cranial nerve IV, VI (diplopia) or III (blurred vision)

Localized back pain with paraparesis	GBS Transverse myelitis Spinal cord compression (neoplasm, infection, trauma)	
Radicular pain (electric pain that follows a spinal root distribution) with paraparesis	Transverse myelitis Spinal cord compression (neoplasm, infection, trauma, disk herniation)	
Headache with hemiparesis	Intracranial bleeding (subdural hematoma, subarachnoid hemorrhage, intraparenchymal bleed) CNS malignancy Brain abscess	Hemiplegic migraines
Jerking movements or seizures with hemiparesis	Ischemic stroke CNS tumor	Todd paralysis
History of heavy exercise or repetitive activities	Rhabdomyolysis	Compressive neuropathy Exertional fatigue
History of cancer	CNS malignancy Spinal cord metastases Paraneoplastic syndromes	
History of fevers or injection drug use	Epidural abscess	
Symptoms of hyperthyroidism (jitteriness, weight loss, fatigue, warmth) or known hyperthyroidism	Thyrotoxic periodic paralysis (particularly in Asian or Latino men)	

FOCUSED QUESTIONS

In the patient whose weakness has developed more insidiously, focused questions will allow the clinician to clarify the temporal pattern and identify risk factors for diseases associated with weakness. Skilled questioning may also provide the examiner with information that suggests the distribution and extent of the weakness before the physical examination is performed.

If answered in the affirmative	Think about
Personal and family history and exposures	
Do you have diabetes mellitus?	Mononeuritis Polyneuropathies Ischemic strokes
Do you have hypertension, hypercholesterolemia, vascular disease, a history of cigarette smoking or estrogen use?	Ischemic stroke

(continued)

If answered in the affirmative	Think about
Personal and family history and exposures	
Do you have hyperthyroidism or signs of hyperthyroidism?	Thyroid myopathy
	Myasthenia gravis (associated with hyperthyroidism)
Are you taking any medications?	Rhabdomyolysis due to cholesterol-lowering drugs
	Hypokalemic periodic paralysis
	Steroid-induced myopathy
	Drug-induced or exacerbated myasthenia gravis (penicillamine, aminoglycosides, quinine, procainamide, calcium channel blockers)
Do you have alcoholism or renal disease?	Alcoholic myopathy
	Alcoholic or uremic polyneuropathy
Do you have rheumatoid arthritis or a history of neck trauma?	Cervical radiculopathy or myelopathy
Do you have cancer?	Eaton-Lambert syndrome (particularly small cell lung cancer)
	Spinal cord compression
Do you have HIV or risk factors for HIV infection?	Distal symmetric polyneuropathy
	Mononeuritis multiplex
	Toxic polyneuropathies (due to nucleoside reverse transcriptase inhibitors)
	CIDP
	Myopathies (polymyositis and zidovudine-related myopathy)
Have you ever had optic neuritis?	Multiple sclerosis
Have you ever had polio?	Post polio syndrome (generally seen in the distribution affected by the primary polio infection)
Are you a vegan?	Polyneuropathy due to B_{12} deficiency
Have you been sitting, standing, or resting in one position for a long time?	Compressive peripheral neuropathy
Do you have a rash or weight loss?	Vasculitis-associated mononeuritis
	Dermatomyositis
Did anyone in your family have similar weakness?	Charcot-Marie-Tooth disease
	Familial periodic paralysis
Time course	**Think about**
Does your weakness come and go? (episodic weakness)	Myasthenia gravis
	Multiple sclerosis
	Eaton-Lambert syndrome
Has your weakness steadily gotten worse? (progressive weakness)	ALS
	Polymyositis/dermatomyositis

Chronic polyneuropathies
Post polio syndrome

Did your weakness appear dramatically and remain
constant?

Acute stroke
Compressive neuropathy or radiculopathy

Did your weakness resolve spontaneously after a few
weeks?

Compressive neuropathy
Multiple sclerosis
Mononeuritis

Distribution

Think about

Is the weakness occurring on both sides of your body at
the same time?

Spinal cord compression (neoplasm,
infection, degenerative disk disease)
Myopathies
Myasthenia gravis
Eaton-Lambert syndrome
ALS
Multiple sclerosis (transverse myelitis
variant)

Is your weakness confined to just 1 limb or part of 1 limb?

Peripheral neuropathy or radiculopa-
thy
   – Foot drop (peroneal nerve or
     L5 radiculopathy)
   – Wrist drop (radial nerve)
   – Thumb opposition weakness (me-
     dian nerve)
   – Intrinsic hand weakness (ulnar nerve)
Multiple sclerosis
Stroke

Does your weakness involve 1 side of your body or your
face?

Stroke
Transient ischemic attack
Hemiplegic migraine

Do you have difficulty lifting your head off the bed,
standing from a sitting position, or brushing your hair?
(proximal muscle weakness)

Polymyositis/dermatomyositis
Myasthenia gravis
Diabetic amyotrophy (lower extremity
proximal muscle weakness)

Is it difficult for you to stand on your toes? (distal weakness
greater than proximal weakness)

Eaton-Lambert syndrome
Inclusion body myositis
Polyneuropathy or radiculopathy

Is it difficult for you to walk on your heels?

Charcot-Marie-Tooth disease

Have you noticed a change in voice or speech or trouble
swallowing?

ALS
Polymyositis, dermatomyositis
Myasthenia gravis

Do you have trouble with double vision (diplopia)?

Mononeuritis (cranial nerve IV, VI)
Myasthenia gravis

Do you have droopy eyelids?

Myasthenia gravis
Botulism (acute)

(continued)

(continued from previous page)

Associated symptoms	**Think about**
Do you have numbness and tingling in association with your weakness?	*Multiple sclerosis* *Stroke* *Polyneuropathies* *NOT myopathies, motor neuron or neuromuscular disorders*
Can you see your muscles twitching? (fasciculations)	*ALS*
Modifying symptoms	**Think about**
Does your weakness get worse with exercise?	*Myasthenia gravis*
Does your weakness get better with exercise?	*Eaton-Lambert syndrome*

CAVEATS

- While the history can suggest the distribution of weakness and site of localization of the lesion, the physical examination is necessary to further refine the differential diagnosis. The clinical evaluation in the hands of experienced neurologists is accurate in identifying the type and cause of a given neurologic problem approximately 75% of the time.[9]
- When patients have classic symptoms and signs, it may be relatively easy to diagnose the underlying condition. However, many diseases (such as myasthenia gravis, ALS, multiple sclerosis) present variably.
- There may be more than one cause of muscle weakness. For example, the patient with Eaton-Lambert syndrome as a paraneoplastic manifestation of small cell lung cancer is also at risk for a spinal cord compression from metastatic disease.
- Specific causes of focal motor weakness, such as multiple sclerosis, may also be associated with fatigue.

PROGNOSIS

- The prognosis of acute stroke is improved if the patient receives thrombolysis within 3 hours of the onset of symptoms.[10]
- Mononeuritis due to vasculitis may respond to immunosuppressive medications.[2] Mononeuropathies due to compression/ischemia, HIV, or diabetes generally resolve spontaneously, although improved control of the underlying condition is recommended.
- Chronic progressive metabolic polyneuropathies generally do not improve.
- Eighty percent of patients with GBS will recover totally or have only minor residual neurologic dysfunction after treatment with intravenous immune globulin or plasma exchange. Death is generally due to complications of respiratory failure.[7]
- Patients with myasthenia gravis require lifelong therapy with immunosuppressants such as prednisone, azathioprine, or cyclosporine.[11]
- Recovery from an acute episode of multiple sclerosis is hastened with the administration of intravenous methylprednisolone. Interferon beta appears to decrease the likelihood of a relapse of symptoms.[12]
- ALS is a uniformly fatal disease.

REFERENCES

1. Hammerstad JP. Strength and Reflexes. In: Goetz CG. *Textbook of Clinical Neurology,* 2nd edition. Elsevier; 2003:235–278.
2. Hughes RA. Peripheral neuropathy. *BMJ.* 2002;324:466–469.

3. Shapiro RL, Hatheway C, Swerdlow DL. Botulism in the United States: a clinical and epidemiologic review. *Ann Intern Med.* 1998;129:221–228.

4. Litovitz TL, Klein-Schwatz W, White S, et al. 1999 annual report of the American Association of Poison Control Centers Toxic Exposure Surveillance System. *Am J Emerg Med.* 2000;18:517–574.

5. Spach DH, Liles WC, Campbell GL, et al. Medical progress: tick-borne diseases in the United States. *N Engl J Med.* 1993; 329:936–947.

6. American Heart Association. *Heart Disease and Stroke Statistics—2004 Update.* Dallas, Tex.: American Heart Association.

7. Chio A, Cocito D, Leone M, et al. Guillain-Barré syndrome: a prospective, population based incidence and outcome survey. *Neurology.* 2003;60:1146–1150.

8. Graves EJ, Gillum BS. Detailed diagnoses and procedures, National Hospital Discharge Survey, 1995. *Vital Health Stat.* 1997;13:1–146.

9. Chimowitz MI, Logigian EL, Caplan LR. The accuracy of bedside neurological diagnoses. *Ann Neurol.* 1990;28:78–85.

10. NINDS t-PA Stroke Study Group. Generalized efficacy of t-PA for acute stroke: subgroup analysis of the NINDS t-PA stroke trial. *Stroke.* 1997;28:2119–2125.

11. Drachman DB. Myasthenia gravis. *N Engl J Med.* 1994;330:1797–1810.

12. Noseworthy JH, Lucchinetti C, Rodriguez M, Weinshenker BG. Medical progress: multiple sclerosis. *N Engl J Med.* 2000; 343:938–952.

Diagnostic Approach: Muscle Weakness

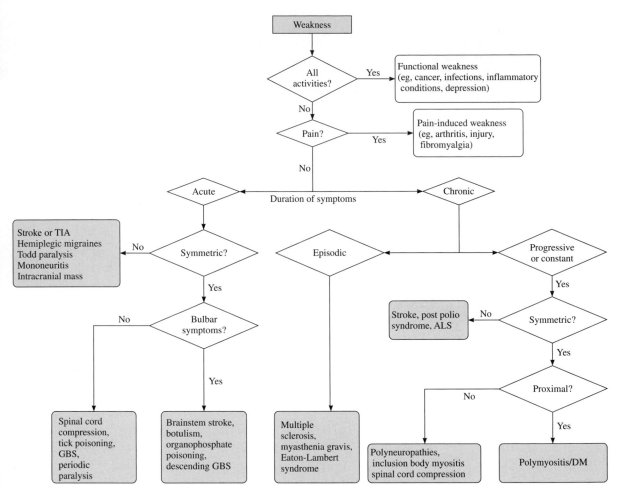

ALS, amyotrophic lateral sclerosis; DM, dermatomyositis; GBS, Guillain-Barré syndrome; TIA, transient ischemic attack.

Weight Gain

14

Timothy S. Loo, MD, & Christina C. Wee, MD, MPH

Weight gain is an absolute increase in body weight. Weight gain is usually a consequence of accumulation of excess body fat, although processes such as edema and ascites can cause substantial weight gain. Weight gain is common and a significant public health concern. Regardless of baseline weight, weight gain can lead to adverse health consequences and to the development of obesity, a major cause of morbidity and the second leading cause of preventable deaths in the United States. Over the last 2 decades, the prevalence of obesity has risen dramatically; currently, 64% of Americans are overweight and 30% are obese.

Primary weight gain is the accumulation of adipose tissue that results from an imbalance between caloric intake and energy expenditure. Less commonly, weight gain is due to secondary causes such as endocrine disorders and medication side effects. The patient history serves 3 main goals: (1) to distinguish between weight gain caused by abnormal fluid retention and weight gain caused by body fat accumulation; (2) to identify the contributing factors or secondary causes of excess fat accumulation and; (3) to screen for serious medical complications caused by weight gain or obesity.

KEY TERMS

Body mass index (BMI)	*BMI is a measure of relative weight for height. It is defined as weight in kilograms divided by the square of height in meters.[1] It correlates with other measures of body fat and is used as an inexpensive measure of weight-related health risk.*
Obesity	*A chronic disorder of excessive weight characterized by an excessive accumulation of body fat and a high health risk. It is defined as a BMI ≥ 30 kg/m^2 and further subdivided into class I (BMI 30–34.9 kg/m^2), class II (BMI 35–39.9 kg/m^2), and class III obesity (BMI ≥ 40 kg/m^2).[1]*
Overweight	*Weight above the established normal range but below the criteria for obesity. It is defined as a BMI between 25 and 29.9 kg/m^2.[1]*

ETIOLOGY

Most weight gain is primary weight gain, resulting from excess body fat accumulation due to physiologic or behavioral changes that result in an imbalance between energy intake and expenditure. The natural history of weight change depends on several factors. Weight gain is highest between the ages of 24 and 34 years; after age 55, adults tend to lose weight. Weight gain is also higher among women than men (see p. 118). African American women between 25 and 45 years have slightly higher average weight gain than whites possibly due to differences in socioeconomic status. Furthermore, weight gain can result from a change in the physiology such as during pregnancy or menopause. It can also occur when a cigarette smoker stops smoking because nicotine is a mild stimulant and appetite suppressant.

10-Year Change in BMI and Weight in the United States[2]

Age at baseline (y)	Change in BMI (kg/m²)		Change in Body Weight (lbs)[a]	
	Men	Women	Men	Women
	Mean (95% CI)	Mean (95% CI)	Mean (95% CI)	Mean (95% CI)
25–34	0.9 (0.7, 1.1)	1.3 (1.1, 1.5)	6.1 (4.7, 7.4)	7.6 (6.4, 8.7)
35–44	0.5 (0.3, 0.7)	0.9 (0.7, 1.1)	3.4 (2.0, 4.7)	5.2 (4.1, 6.4)
45–54	0.0 (−0.2, 0.2)	0.3 (0.1, 0.5)	0.0 (−1.4, 1.4)	1.7 (0.6, 2.9)
55–64	−0.3 (−0.5, −0.1)	−0.5 (−0.8, −0.2)	−2.0 (−3.4, −0.7)	−2.9 (−4.7, −1.2)
65–74	−1.1 (−1.3, −0.9)	−1.7 (−1.9, −1.5)	−7.4 (−8.8, −6.1)	−9.9 (−11.1, −8.7)

[a]Change in weight for men at an average height of 5 feet, 9 inches and change in weight for women at an average height of 5 feet, 4 inches.

Weight gain uncommonly results from secondary causes such as endocrine disorders, genetic syndromes, or medication side effects. Although the prevalence is not well established, secondary weight gain is important because it can be reversed if the underlying cause is addressed. However, secondary causes frequently coexist with primary obesity, so treatment for a specific secondary cause may not entirely reverse weight back to the normal level. Medication side effects are probably the most common secondary cause. Common offenders include glucocorticoids, anticonvulsants, antipsychotics, antidepressants, contraceptives, and diabetic medications. Endocrine disorders causing obesity include hyperinsulinemia, hypercortisolism, hypothyroidism, polycystic ovary syndrome, and hypogonadism. Obesity is also a component of several rare genetic syndromes, including Prader-Willi syndrome, Laurence-Moon syndrome, Cohen's syndrome, and Biemond syndrome.

Differential Diagnosis

Physiologic predisposition

	Comments
Primary weight gain or obesity	Most common cause of weight gain
Menopause[3]	20% of patients gain ≥ 9.9 lbs. during a 3-year period
Smoking cessation[4]	16–21% of patients who quit smoking and remain abstinent gain ≥ 33 lbs over 10 years
Increase in caloric intake	Alcohol; holiday weight gain
Decrease in physical activity level	

Medications

Glucocorticoids	Variable weight gain
Diabetic medications[5] (sulfonylurea, insulin)	Sulfonylureas: Mean weight gain of 4.0–6.8 lbs. over 3 years Insulin: Mean weight gain of 6.8 lbs. over 3 years
Anticonvulsants[6] (gabapentin, valproic acid, carbamazepine)	Valproate: 44–57% of patients affected with mean weight gain of 46.3 lbs

(continued)

Antipsychotics[7] (phenothiazines, butyrophenones, atypical agents)	Atypical antipsychotics (olanzapine, quetiapine, risperidone, ziprasidone): 9.8–29% patients affected with > 7% increase in body weight. Mean weight gain: 4.4–26.5 lbs.
Antidepressants[6,8] (tricyclic antidepressants, monoamine oxidase inhibitors, mirtazapine)	Tricyclics: 13% of patients affected with > 10% increase in body weight. Mean weight increase 1.3 to 3.1 lbs per month. SSRIs: 4–26% of patients affected with > 7% increase in body weight. Maximum weight gain 17.0–31.1 lbs. Atypical antidepressants (mirtazapine): 10–13% of patients affected with > 7% increase in body weight.
Injectable or oral contraceptives[9]	18% of patients affected with weight gain: > 4.4 lbs.

Endocrinologic disorders

Cushing syndrome

Hypothyroidism

Hyperinsulinemia

Polycystic ovary syndrome

Hypogonadism

GETTING STARTED

- Allow the patient to describe his or her weight gain.
- Try to understand the patient's concerns about weight gain. A patient may be concerned about acceleration of weight gain or the risk of obesity and its complications or may be seeking assistance to achieve weight control.
- Establish the pace and time course of weight gain and determine whether it is consistent with prior pattern of weight gain.
- Assess for any recent changes in the patient's life such as a recent stressful event, recent completion of a weight loss program, pregnancy, etc.
- Be sensitive. Patients may feel embarrassed, stigmatized, or frustrated by their weight gain.

Questions	**Remember**
Tell me about your weight gain. When did it start? How has your weight progressed over time?	• Listen to the story. • Avoid interrupting. • Listen to the course of disease and any prior attempts at weight loss for diagnostic clues.

INTERVIEW FRAMEWORK

- Assess for symptoms suggesting weight gain due to excess body fluid accumulation.
- Assess for risk factors contributing to the development of obesity including change in diet or activity level, recent menopause, or mood changes.
- Identify factors that suggest a secondary cause.
- Screen for serious medical complications associated with obesity.

IDENTIFYING ALARM SYMPTOMS

Weight gain due to the accumulation of excess body fluid can occur rapidly, resulting in serious complications. The major causes of abnormal fluid retention are congestive heart failure, renal failure, and chronic liver disease. These conditions can present acutely with pulmonary edema, peripheral edema, ascites, and metabolic derangements.

Serious diagnoses	Think
Accumulation of excess body fluid	*Congestive heart failure*
	Renal failure
	Chronic liver disease
Serious comorbid diseases and their prevalence in the obese population[10]	*Impaired glucose intolerance or diabetes (7–20%)*
	Hypertension (49–65%)
	Hyperlipidemia (34–41%)
	Coronary heart disease (10–19%)
	Sleep apnea (8–15%)

Alarm symptoms	Serious causes	Benign causes
Accumulation of excess body fluid		
Increased weight over days to weeks	*Congestive heart failure*	
	Renal failure	
	Chronic liver disease	
Difficulty breathing or coughing at night	*Congestive heart failure*	*Postnasal drip*
		Gastroesophageal reflux
		Obstructive lung disease
Inability to sleep lying flat	*Congestive heart failure*	
A recent increase in waist or pant size	*Ascites*	*Constipation*
		Flatulence
Yellowing of the skin or whites of the eyes	*Chronic liver disease*	
Tea-colored urine	*Chronic liver disease*	
Prolonged or excessive bleeding	*Chronic liver disease*	*Antiplatelet medications*
	Renal failure	*Anticoagulants*
A decrease in how much you urinate	*Renal failure*	*Benign prostatic hypertrophy*
Nausea, vomiting, or generalized itching	*Renal failure*	*Thyroid disease*
	Chronic liver disease	*Adverse drug reaction*
Swelling in the feet, ankles, or legs	*Congestive heart failure*	*Venous stasis*
	Renal failure	
	Chronic liver disease	
Development of comorbid diseases		
An increase in thirst or urination	*Diabetes*	*Diuretic use*
Blurry vision	*Diabetes*	*Refractive error*

Chest tightness or pressure brought on by exertion or emotional stress	Coronary heart disease	Anxiety or panic attack
Snoring or stop breathing during the night	Sleep apnea	
Difficulty staying awake during the day	Sleep apnea	Night shift work Jet-lag

FOCUSED QUESTIONS

After assessing for alarm symptoms, evaluate the factors contributing to the development of obesity.

Questions	**Think about**
Chronologic history When did the weight gain begin? Is this pattern consistent with previous episodes of weight gain?	Consider patient factors such as age, sex, race, and recent life events to assess whether the weight gain would be considered unusual. Weight gain often occurs with life events such as pregnancy, child rearing, smoking cessation, or a change in marital status or occupation.
Dietary practices Describe your typical diet. Have you changed your dietary habits?	**Think about** A description of dietary practices helps assess how much of the positive energy balance can be attributed to excess caloric intake.
Describe a typical breakfast, lunch, and dinner. Has this changed recently?	Fatty foods predispose to excess caloric intake because they have a higher energy density and greater palatability.
How often do you eat out or eat fast food? Has this changed?	Dining away from home facilitates overeating by providing calorically dense foods in excessively large portion sizes.
Patterns of physical activity How often do you engage in planned physical activity? Has this pattern changed?	**Think about** Sedentary patients are almost twice as likely to gain substantial weight compared with physically active patients. High fitness level has a protective effect with 1 study showing a lower mortality rate in the fit, overweight group compared with the unfit, normal weight group.[11]
Weight loss practices Are you currently trying to lose weight? When did you start? How much weight did you lose?	**Think about** Unfortunately, patients who successfully lose weight tend to regain 50% or more of the lost weight after 6 months.
Concurrent psychological conditions Have you ever been depressed? How would you describe your mood?	**Think about** Appetite disturbance can be a vegetative symptom of depression.

(continued)

Concurrent psychological conditions

*Have you been under a lot of stress lately?
Do you find yourself eating when you are
not hungry to relieve stress?*

*Do you ever go on eating binges? Have you
ever taken diuretics or laxatives to help you
lose weight? Have you ever made yourself
vomit?*

Medications

What medication(s) are you taking?

Family history

*Is there anyone else in your family who is
overweight?*

Endocrine disorders

• *Have you noticed a disproportionate
accumulation of fat in the face, trunk,
or abdomen?*

• *Have you noticed any thinning of the skin,
reddish purple streaks on the abdomen
or flank area, or easy bruising?*

• *Do you have high blood pressure?*

• *Do you have elevated blood sugar?*

• *Do you have an irregular menstrual cycle?*

• *Have you noticed increasing facial hair or
acne?*

• *Have you been more tired and fatigued?*

• *Do you have dry skin or hair loss?*

• *Have you been feeling cold?*

• *Have you been gaining weight despite a
poor appetite?*

• *Have you been constipated?*

• *Have you been experiencing episodic
confusion, headache, seizures, or visual
changes when fasting?*

• *Have you had palpitations, sweating, or
tremors when fasting?*

Think about

For some patients, eating is a coping mechanism.

*Consider eating disorders in patients (especially
young women) who admit to binge eating and show
excessive concern about body weight or shape.*

Think about

*Medications commonly associated with weight gain
are listed in the differential diagnosis section.*

Think about

*Twin, adoption, and family studies suggest that
25–40% of the variance in BMI can be attributed to
genetics.*

Think about

*Because no symptom is pathognomonic for these dis-
orders, clinical suspicion relies on the simultaneous
development and progression of a constellation of
symptoms.*

Cushing's syndrome

Hypothyroidism

Hyperinsulinemia (including insulinoma)

• Do you have irregular or infrequent menstrual periods?	Polycystic ovary syndrome
• Have you had difficulty becoming pregnant?	
• Have you noticed increasing facial hair or acne?	
In men:	
• Have you had a decrease in libido?	Hypogonadism
• Have you had difficulty obtaining erections?	
• Have you noted thinning of body and pubic hair?	
• Have you been experiencing hot flashes?	
In women:	
• Has there been a change in the pattern of your menstrual cycle?	Hypogonadism
• Have you been experiencing hot flashes?	
• Have you been experiencing insomnia?	
• Has your libido decreased?	
• Is intercourse uncomfortable or painful?	

CAVEATS

- Weight gain caused by excess body fluid accumulation can occur rapidly over days to weeks, presenting a serious condition that should be evaluated immediately. Weight gain is often not the primary presenting symptom. Since body fat accumulates more gradually, the difference in time course can help distinguish the 2 mechanisms.
- While the overwhelming majority of cases of weight gain are primary or physiologic, consider secondary causes when the degree of weight gain is inconsistent with the patient's life changes or previous weight gain pattern.
- Although a secondary cause may contribute to weight gain, it is rarely the sole cause of a patient's obesity.
- Because drug-induced weight gain is probably the most common secondary cause of obesity, always take a thorough medication history.

PROGNOSIS

- Epidemiologic studies show that mortality begins to increase modestly at a BMI above 25 kg/m^2 and that this increase accelerates significantly above a BMI of 30 kg/m^2.[1] This increase in mortality is mostly due to comorbid conditions. Weight loss, even modest amounts, does lead to improvements in the comorbid conditions; whether voluntary weight loss reduces mortality is still unknown.[1]
- Because sustained weight loss is difficult to achieve, more attention should be given to weight gain prevention.

REFERENCES

1. Expert Panel on the Identification, Evaluation, and Treatment of Overweight in Adults. Clinical Guidelines on the Identification, Evaluation, and Treatment of Overweight and Obesity in Adults. National Institutes of Health 1998. Available at: http://www.nhlbi.nih.gov/guidelines/obesity/ob_gdlns.htm

2. Williamson DF, Kahn HS, Remington PL, Anda RF. The 10-year incidence of overweight and major weight gain in US adults. *Arch Intern Med.* 1990;150:665–672.

3. Wing RR, Matthews KA, Kuller LH, Meilahn EN, Plantinga PL. Weight gain at the time of menopause. *Arch Intern Med.* 1991;151:97–102.

4. Flegal KM, Troiano RP, Pamuk ER, Kuczmarski RJ, Campbell SM. The influence of smoking cessation on the prevalence of overweight in the United States. *N Engl J Med.* 1995;333:1165–1170.

5. United Kingdom Prospective Diabetes Study (UKPDS). 13: Relative efficacy of randomly allocated diet, sulphonylurea, insulin, or metformin in patients with newly diagnosed non-insulin dependent diabetes followed for three years. *BMJ.* 1995;310:83–88.

6. Zimmermann U, Kraus T, Himmerich H, Schuld A, Pollmacher T. Epidemiology, implications and mechanisms underlying drug-induced weight gain in psychiatric patients. *J Psychiatr Res.* 2003;37:193–220.

7. Allison DB, Casey DE. Antipsychotic-induced weight gain: a review of the literature. *J Clin Psychiatry.* 2001;62(Suppl 7):22–31.

8. Fava M. Weight gain and antidepressants. *J Clin Psychiatry.* 2000;61(Suppl 11):37–41.

9. Gupta S. Weight gain on the combined pill—is it real? *Hum Reprod.* 2000;6:427–431.

10. Must A, Spadano J, Coakley EH, Field AE, Colditz G, Dietz WH. The disease burden associated with overweight and obesity. *JAMA.* 1999;282:1523–1529.

11. Lee CD, Jackson AS, Blair SN. US weight guidelines: is it also important to consider cardiorespiratory fitness? *Int J Obes Relat Metab Disord.* 1998;22(Suppl 2):S2–7.

SUGGESTED READING

Andersen RE, Blackman MR. Obesity. In: Barker RL, Burton JR, Zieve PD (editors). *Principles of Ambulatory Medicine,* 6th ed. Lippincott Williams & Wilkins. 1318–1334.

Kushner RF, Weinsier RL. Evaluation of the obese patient, practical considerations. *Med Clin North Am.* 2000;84:387–399.

Purnell JQ. Endocrinology: X Obesity, WebMD Scientific American Medicine 2003; June 2003 Update: 1–13.

Diagnostic Approach: Weight Gain

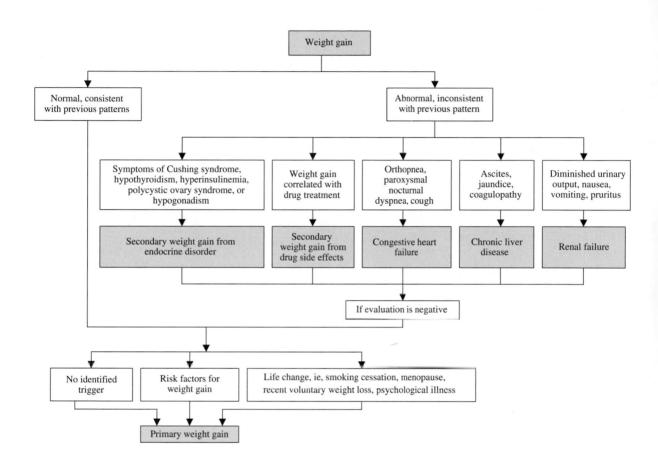

Weight Loss

15

Tonya Fancher, MD, MPH

Weight loss can be divided into 2 categories: involuntary and voluntary. Involuntary weight loss occurs in up to 13% of elderly outpatients and frequently indicates a significant medical or psychosocial condition.[1] Healthy dieting is common among both men and women; however, among young women, significant voluntary weight loss often heralds a psychiatric illness (ie, eating disorder).

KEY TERMS

Anorexia	*Loss of the desire to eat*
Bulimia	*Recurrent episodes of binge eating followed by recurrent compensatory behavior to prevent weight gain*
Involuntary weight loss	*The unintended loss of weight; sometimes not reported by the patient and only noted upon chart review*
Voluntary weight loss	*The conscious effort to lose weight; frequently not a complaint among those with eating disorders*

ETIOLOGY

The etiologies of weight loss are myriad. A recent review of involuntary weight loss found[2]:

1. Among organic causes, cancer is the most common.
2. The etiology of weight loss does not require extensive testing in most patients.
3. Psychiatric and nondiagnostic evaluations are common.

Aside from dieting, eating disorders account for the majority of voluntary weight loss. Eating disorders affect 5 to 10 million people in the United States; for women, the lifetime prevalence of anorexia nervosa ranges from 0.5% to 3.7% and from 1.1% to 4.2% for bulimia nervosa.[3] Ninety percent to 95% of anorexic patients and 80% of bulimics are female.

Differential Diagnosis: Involuntary Weight Loss[2,4]	Prevalence[a]
Cancer (gastrointestinal, hepatobiliary, hematologic, lung, breast, genitourinary, ovarian, prostate)	*16–36%*
Psychiatric illness (depression, anxiety)	*9–20%*
Gastrointestinal (peptic ulcer disease, inflammatory bowel disease, dysmotility, chronic pancreatitis, malabsorption)	*15%*

(continued)

Differential Diagnosis: Involuntary Weight Loss[2,4]   Prevalence[a]

Endocrine (diabetes, hyperthyroidism, hypothyroidism, pheochromocytoma, adrenal insufficiency)

Infection (HIV, tuberculosis, fungal disease, subacute bacterial endocarditis, parasites)

Medication (selective serotonin reuptake inhibitors, levodopa, metformin, digoxin, ephedra, other herbal and over-the-counter medication)

Cardiovascular disease (severe congestive heart failure)

Neurologic disease (stroke, dementia, Parkinson disease, multiple sclerosis)

Pulmonary disease (severe chronic obstructive pulmonary disease)

Renal disease (uremia, hemodialysis, proteinuria)

Connective tissue disease (chronic inflammatory diseases, scleroderma)

Idiopathic   *23–26%*

[a]Prevalence is unknown when not indicated.

Differential Diagnosis: Voluntary Weight Loss

Dieting

Healthy dieting[a]

- *Healthy eating plans that reduce calories but do not rule out specific food or food groups*
- *Regular exercise activity and/or exercise instruction*
- *Tips on healthy behavioral changes that also consider your cultural needs*
- *Slow and steady weight loss of about three quarters to 2 pounds per week and not more than 3 pounds per week*
- *Under medical supervision you plan to lose weight by following a special diet, such as a very-low-calorie diet*
- *A plan to keep the weight off after you have lost it*

Anorexia nervosa

Diagnostic criteria for anorexia[b]

- *15% or more below ideal body weight*
- *Fear of weight gain*
- *Body image disturbance*
- *In females, primary amenorrhea or secondary amenorrhea of 3 months duration*

Bulimia

Diagnostic criteria for bulimia[b]

- *Recurrent binge eating*
  - *Large quantity of food in discrete time period*
  - *AND*
  - *A feeling of lack of control over eating*
- *Recurrent compensatory behavior to prevent weight gain*
- *Cycle occurs at least twice weekly for 3 months*
- *Body dissatisfaction*

[a]www.nlm.nih.gov/medlineplus/weightlossdieting.html
[b]Diagnostic and Statistical Manual for Mental Disorders, Fourth Edition (DSM-IV)

GETTING STARTED

- Review the medical record to confirm weight loss. Clinically significant weight loss is 10 lb (4.5 kg) or more, or more than 5% of the baseline body weight over 6 to 12 months.[2]
- If unable to confirm weight loss, continue with thorough history and physical examination, delaying further testing until alarm signs or symptoms develop or weight loss confirmed at follow up appointment.
- Calculate the body mass index (BMI) = body weight (kg)/height (m^2)
  Calculator available at: www.cdc.gov/nccdphp/dnpa/bmi/calc-bmi.htm
- A normal BMI is 18.5–24.9 kg/m^2.
- A BMI under 18.5 kg/m^2 is considered underweight and undernourished.

Questions	Remember
Tell me about your weight loss.	• *Listen for psychosocial stressors.*
Is the weight loss voluntary or involuntary?	• *Think about the differential diagnosis.*
Is your appetite increased or decreased?	• *There are only a few causes of weight loss and increased appetite.*
How long have you been losing weight?	• *Sudden weight loss in a person with previously stable weight is worrisome.*
What did you eat yesterday?	• *Especially important for eating disorders.*
How do you feel about the way you look?	• *Most patients with eating disorders are unhappy with their appearance.*
Are your menstrual periods regular?	• *A diagnostic criterion for anorexia.*

INTERVIEW FRAMEWORK

- Involuntary weight loss is usually alarming to patients. Take time to reassure them that you will work together to find an answer.

- Assess for alarm symptoms.
- Categorize into voluntary or involuntary weight loss; increased or decreased appetite.
- A thorough review of systems will help narrow your differential diagnosis. Focus on the pulmonary and digestive system, age and gender appropriate cancers; and screen for depression (see Chapter 60).

IDENTIFYING ALARM SYMPTOMS

- With the exception of healthy dieting, significant weight loss often portends serious illness.
- Cancer accounts for nearly 33% of all patients with involuntary weight loss.[2]
- Eating disorders carry the highest premature mortality rate among all psychiatric illnesses.

Involuntary Weight Loss

Alarm signs and symptoms	If present, focus on
Dysphagia, odynophagia, early satiety, diarrhea, constipation, black tarry stools	Gastrointestinal system
Significant smoking and alcohol use	Aerodigestive and genitourinary cancer
Family history of breast or ovarian cancer	Breast or ovarian cancer
Fatigue, pallor, new lymphadenopathy	Hematologic cancer
New onset back pain or neurologic deficit	Prostate, lung, breast, renal cancer, and multiple myeloma
Excessive thirst or nervousness	Endocrinopathies
Fevers	Infections

Voluntary Weight Loss

Alarm signs and symptoms	If present, focus on
Body image disturbance or dissatisfaction	Anorexia or bulimia
Insomnia, poor concentration, irritability, tearfulness, fatigue, anhedonia	Depression
Excessive worry, restlessness, irritability, muscle tension	Anxiety

FOCUSED QUESTIONS

After having the patient tell his or her story, follow-up with a few close-ended questions to help narrow your differential diagnosis.

Questions	Think about
Time course	
Does your weight tend to fluctuate over time?	Reaction to variations in physical activity or food intake
Does the onset of weight loss correlate with starting new medications?	Drug-induced anorexia or increased metabolism

Associated symptoms

Have you lost the desire to eat?

Is your appetite increased?

Do you feel nervous, sweaty, or warm?

Do you feel thirsty or that you need to urinate more frequently?

Do you have more frequent bowel movements or diarrhea?

Do you experience facial flushing or orthostasis (and have high blood pressure)?

Have you been exercising more?

Do you have abdominal pain, early satiety, or dysphagia?

Have you ever injected drugs, had unprotected sex, or received a blood transfusion?

Are you pregnant?

Do you have congestive heart failure or chronic obstructive pulmonary disease?

Do you use cocaine, amphetamines or over-the-counter medications[a] (eg, ephedra, ephedrine, ma-huang, 5 hydroxytryptophan [5HT], teas, garcinia [hydroxycitric acid/HCA], herbal fen-phen, phenteramine, St. John's Wort, herbal laxatives or diuretics, melatonin)?

Do you take any prescribed medications?

Does fear of abdominal pain make you not want to eat?

Do you ever binge?

Have you ever used self-induced vomiting, laxatives, diuretics (water pills), or enemas to control your weight?

A positive response to any of the questions should raise concern[6]:

- *How many diets have you been on in the past year?*

- *Do you think you should be dieting?*

- *Are you dissatisfied with your body size?*

Think about

Cancer, psychiatric causes, congestive heart failure, chronic obstructive pulmonary disease, chronic infections, chronic inflammatory disease

Diabetes, hyperthyroidism, malabsorption, oropharyngeal disorders

Hyperthyroidism

Diabetes mellitus

Malabsorption

Pheochromocytoma

Increased metabolic demand

Gastrointestinal cancer

HIV infection

Hyperemesis gravidarum

Cardiac or chronic obstructive pulmonary disease cachexia

Drug-induced weight loss

Selective serotonin reuptake inhibitors, levodopa, digoxin, metformin, theophylline, opiates, methylphenidate can all contribute to weight loss

Mesenteric ischemia

Bulimia

Bulimia

Anorexia or Bulimia

(continued)

Associated symptoms	Think about
• *Does your weight affect the way you think about yourself?*	

Modifying symptoms	Think about
Do your symptoms change with different foods?	*Malabsorption*

[a]A partial list of potential medications see also: http://nccam.nih.gov/

CAVEATS

- Do not forget about Munchausen syndrome, in which patients may voluntarily lose weight to get attention.
- The elderly represent a special population. Remember the 9 D's for causes of weight loss in the elderly[7]:
  1. Dentition
  2. Dysgeusia[a]
  3. Dysphagia
  4. Diarrhea
  5. Disease (chronic)
  6. Depression
  7. Dementia
  8. Dysfunction[b]
  9. Drugs

  [a]Angiotensin-converting enzyme inhibitors are common drugs known to cause dysgeusia.
  [b]A number of factors, such as arthritis, stroke, or visual impairment, may make it increasingly difficult for elderly patients to shop or prepare food.

- If your evaluation is negative (expected in approximately 25% of cases), ensure follow-up in 3–6 months as some etiologies may emerge over time.

PROGNOSIS

- A recent review found that patients with unintentional weight loss have higher mortality rates: 9% at 24 months and 38% at 30 months.[2]
- Patients with idiopathic weight loss have a better prognosis than those with an identified etiology.
- Untreated, 18–20% of anorexia nervosa patients die within 20 years, most commonly of cardiac problems, renal failure, or suicide.
- The premature mortality rate for bulimia is 5% at 10 years.[3]
- Laxative abusers are more likely to suffer medical complications.[3]

REFERENCES

1. Wallace JI, Schwartz RS, LaCroix AZ, Uhlmann RF, Pearlman RA. Involuntary weight loss in older outpatients: incidence and clinical significance. *J Am Geriatr Soc.* 1995;43:329–337.
2. Bouras EP, Lange SM, Scolapio JS. Rational approach to patients with unintentional weight loss. *Mayo Clin Proc.* 2001;76:923–929.

3. Powers PS, Santana CA. Eating disorders: a guide for the primary care physician. *Prim Care*. 2002;29:81–98.
4. Huffman GB. Evaluating and treating unintentional weight loss in the elderly. *Am Fam Physician*. 2002;65:640–650.
5. Reife CM. Involuntary weight loss. *Med Clin North Am*. 1995;79:299–313.
6. Anstine D, Grinenko D. Rapid screening for eating disorders on college-aged females in the primary care setting. *J Adolesc Health*. 2000;26:338–342.
7. Robbins LJ. Evaluation of weight loss in the elderly. *Geriatrics*. 1989;44:31–34, 37.

SUGGESTED READING

Fairburn CG, Harrison PJ. Eating disorders. *Lancet*. 2003;361:407–416.

Pritts SD, Susman J. Diagnosis of eating disorders in primary care. *Am Fam Physician*. 2003;67:297–304.

Strasser F, Bruera ED. Update in anorexia and cachexia. *Hematol Oncol Clin North Am*. 2002;16:589–617.

Diagnostic Approach: Weight Loss

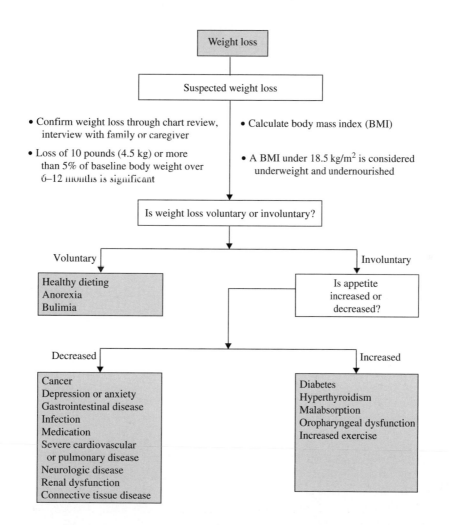

SECTION III
Otolaryngology

Ear Pain

16

Daniel J. Sullivan, MD, MPH

Ear pain is a common complaint in primary care practice, both in pediatric and adult populations. In a random sample of 411 adults in Finland, 7.5% of men and 23.4% of women had experienced ear pain that was not associated with infection in the previous 6 months.[1] The cause of ear pain may be in or near the ear, or it may be referred from a distant site. In most cases, a careful history narrows the possible causes considerably. The physical examination is also essential. Most local causes of ear pain produce specific physical findings, whereas the examination of the ear and its immediately surrounding structures are typically normal in cases of referred pain.

KEY TERMS

Acute otitis media	The presence of infected fluid in the middle ear, caused by bacterial or viral pathogens.
Negative predictive value	The likelihood, given a negative test (or the absence of a symptom), that the condition of interest is absent.
Otalgia	Ear pain.
Otitis externa	An inflammation (usually infectious) of the external auditory canal.
Pinna	The external ear, including the external acoustic meatus.
Positive predictive value	The likelihood, given a positive test (or the presence of a symptom), that the condition of interest is present.
Sensitivity	How frequently a test (or symptom) is positive (present) in those with the condition of interest.
Serous otitis	The presence of uninfected fluid in the middle ear, usually resulting from the blockage of the eustachian tube from an upper respiratory tract infection or from allergy.
Specificity	How frequently a test (or symptom) is negative (not present) in those without the condition of interest.
Tragus	The tongue-like projection of the cartilage of the ear in front of the external acoustic meatus.

ETIOLOGY

In most cases, the cause of ear pain is localized and can be divided into outer ear problems and inner ear problems. Outer ear problems are located external to the tympanic membrane and include otitis externa, ear canal foreign bodies, earwax, and mastoiditis. Occasionally, a furuncle may cause ear pain. Inner ear problems are located at the tympanic membrane or deep to it and include acute otitis media (OM)—the single most common cause of ear pain—and eustachian tube dysfunction. Injuries to the tympanic membrane, which can occur from barotrauma or from direct trauma to the ear, can also cause ear pain.

In children, acute OM is the most common cause of ear pain. The history is limited in its contribution to making a diagnosis of acute OM. In 1 study, the positive predictive value of earache for acute OM in children younger than 4 years with upper respiratory tract symptoms was 83%, with the negative predictive value being 78%.[2] Another study found that earache was the symptom that most reliably predicted acute OM in children. However, the sensitivity of earache for OM was only about 60%, with a specificity of about 85%.[3]

Ear pain may originate at a distant site. In such cases, the pain is referred to the ear via a nerve. The sensory innervation of the ear is complex, involving the vagus nerve, the glossopharyngeal nerve, the trigeminal nerve, the facial nerve, and the sensory components of the cervical (C2 and C3) nerve roots. Accordingly, a variety of conditions may cause pain to be referred to the ear including temporomandibular joint (TMJ) dysfunction; dental processes; pathology of the cranial nerves; and disease at the base of the tongue, larynx, or hypopharynx.

In 1 series of 615 patients with ear pain and a normal-appearing ear (referred pain), the following conditions were diagnosed: dental problem (38%), TMJ dysfunction (35%), cervical spine disorder (8%), neuralgia (5%), aerodigestive disorder (4%), malignancy (3%), and other (6%).[4]

Differential Diagnosis	**Frequency**
Outer ear pain	
Furuncle	Relatively uncommon
Otitis externa	Common
Foreign body	Relatively common in children
Mastoiditis	Uncommon
Inner ear pain	
OM	Common
Eustachian tube dysfunction (serous OM)	Common
Barotrauma	Uncommon
Referred pain	**Prevalence[a]**
Dental problems (especially third molar)	38.4%
TMJ dysfunction	35.4%
Cervical spine (especially arthritis)	8.4%
Neuralgias (trigeminal, geniculate, sphenopalatine, glossopharyngeal)	4.9%
Gastrointestinal etiology (including gastroesophageal reflux)	3.7%
Tumors	2.9%
Other (thyroiditis, Eagle syndrome, angina, parotid disease, angina, carotid aneurysm)	6.4%

[a]Among patients referred to a tertiary ear, nose, and throat practice.[4]

GETTING STARTED

- As always, the initial approach should be open-ended. Let the patient (or parent) tell the story.
- With a young child, the parent or caretaker may be the main source of the history. Ask the caregiver why he or she believes the child is having ear pain.

- Ascertain the time course of the ear pain as well as associated symptoms and aggravating factors because the various causes of ear pain can often be distinguished by these 3 factors.

Questions	Remember
Tell me about your ear pain.	*Resist the temptation to interrupt with specific questions before the patient has had a chance to tell you the story.*
What other symptoms do you have?	
What makes the pain worse?	

INTERVIEW FRAMEWORK

It is important to differentiate relatively acute or subacute ear pain from chronic pain. In general, patients with referred pain have had pain for months or years. An exception to this rule is referred pain from a third molar abscess, which can have an acute onset.

Since several common causes of ear pain are infectious, consider infection early in the interview. The presence of fever narrows the diagnostic possibilities. The presence of other upper respiratory tract infection symptoms (eg, sore throat, nasal congestion, or cough) suggests OM or serous otitis. Seasonal allergies may also predispose to serous otitis and OM by compromising the function of the eustachian tubes.

The patient's age is an important consideration in determining the most likely cause of ear pain. Acute OM is by far the most important cause of ear pain in children but is an infrequent cause of ear pain in adults. Referred pain is very uncommon in children, but its relative frequency in adults increases with age.

IDENTIFYING ALARM SYMPTOMS

Serious Diagnoses

Serious causes of ear pain are quite rare. Clinicians should consider and exclude the following 4 serious diagnoses in any patient with ear pain: referred pain from malignancy, necrotizing (malignant) external otitis, temporal arteritis, and mastoiditis.

Referred pain from a malignancy usually has been present for some time. In 1 series of patients with referred pain, the time between onset of ear pain and tumor diagnosis ranged from 4 to 21 months, with a mean of 7.5 months.[2] These patients are typically older; the mean age at diagnosis in this series was 55.8 years.

Necrotizing (malignant) external otitis is a rare condition in which external otitis progresses to invade the temporal bone and adjacent structures. It is almost exclusively due to infection with *Pseudomonas aeruginosa*. The condition occurs in immunocompromised patients, especially older diabetic patients, and should be considered when the patient does not respond promptly to treatment for otitis externa. In a typical case, the patient complains of persistent discharge and pain in the affected ear that is frequently severe and often worse at night.[5] Early recognition of this disease is critical because it carries a relatively high mortality (up to 46% in older case series).[6]

Temporal arteritis should be considered when a patient over the age of 50 complains of the acute or subacute onset of headache, pain in the temporal area, or scalp tenderness. A relatively specific symptom of temporal arteritis is jaw claudication, which is defined as pain in the proximal jaw near the TMJ, brought on or aggravated by a brief period of chewing and relieved by resting the jaw.[8] A patient may describe this as ear pain, but careful questioning should clarify the location of the pain. Temporal arteritis rarely presents with true ear pain. Prompt diagnosis of temporal arteritis is essential because it can cause sudden and permanent blindness if untreated.

Mastoiditis generally occurs in children when OM spreads to the mastoid air cells behind the ear. A typical presentation is fever with postauricular swelling, tenderness, and erythema, which can sometimes push the ear forward by a mass effect. Patients often report becoming ill several weeks earlier, improving, but then fever and signs of local infection develop. The condition must be promptly recognized and treated because the infection may spread to nearby critical structures such as the temporal bone, meninges, and brain.

Alarm symptoms	Serious causes	Positive likelihood ratio (LR+)	Benign causes
Weight loss	Tumors	LR data do not exist but about 25% of all patients with significant weight loss will have no cause found[7]	
Persistent ear pain with discharge, worse at night	Necrotizing (malignant) external otitis		"Ordinary" external otitis
Pain near the ear with chewing in a patient over the age of 50	Temporal arteritis	4.2[8]	TMJ dysfunction
Pain and swelling behind the ear in a child with a recent upper respiratory tract infection or ear infection	Mastoiditis		Lymphadenopathy

FOCUSED QUESTIONS

Questions	Think about
Do you grind your teeth?	TMJ dysfunction
Do you swim?	Otitis externa
Do you have a skin condition such as psoriasis or seborrheic dermatitis?	Otitis externa
Do you use Q-tips or other objects to clean your ears?	Otitis externa
Have you been struck in the ear?	Barotrauma
Have you recently been scuba diving?	Barotrauma
Are you diabetic? On chemotherapy? Otherwise immunocompromised?	Necrotizing (malignant) external otitis
Is the pain worse with chewing?	TMJ dysfunction (common) or temporal arteritis (uncommon)
(For a young child) Does the child pull on his or her ear?	Acute OM

Quality	Think about
Is the ear pain	
• Severe, deep within the ear?	OM
• Like pressure or a clogged feeling?	Eustachian tube dysfunction (serous otitis) Earwax

• Burning, knife-like, or tingling?	Neuralgia (trigeminal, geniculate, sphenopalatine, glossopharyngeal, or cervical nerve root)
• Bilateral?	Otitis externa Gastroesophageal reflux TMJ dysfunction

Time course	Think about
Was the ear pain preceded by an upper respiratory tract infection?	
• By 10 days or less?	OM, eustachian tube dysfunction (serous otitis)
• By 10 or more days?	Mastoiditis
Has the pain been present for more than a few weeks?	Referred pain
Was there severe pain at the time of air travel or diving under water?	Barotrauma

Associated symptoms	Think about
Do you have fever?	OM or mastoiditis
Do you have pain and/or swelling behind the ear?	Mastoiditis
Is there a discharge from the ear?	Otitis externa or perforated eardrum from OM
Did the pain decrease dramatically after the discharge began?	Perforated eardrum from OM
Is there a loss of hearing?	OM Eustachian tube dysfunction (serous otitis) Barotrauma
Are there crackling or gurgling sounds in the affected ear?	Eustachian tube dysfunction (serous otitis)
Do you have jaw clicking?	TMJ dysfunction
Do you have itching as well as pain?	Otitis externa Primary dermatitis (psoriasis or seborrhea)
Has there been any weight loss?	Malignancy (referred pain)
Do you have seasonal allergies or hay fever?	Eustachian tube dysfunction (serous otitis)

Modifying symptoms	Think about
Does flexing the neck aggravate the pain?	Arthritis of the neck (referred pain from C2, C3 radiculopathy)
Does pulling on the ear make the pain worse?	Otitis externa
Does the pain worsen with swallowing?	Elongated styloid process (Eagle syndrome)
Is the pain worse in the morning?	TMJ dysfunction Gastroesophageal reflux
Is the pain worse with hot or cold foods?	Infected third molar
Is the pain worse at night?	Necrotizing (malignant) external otitis
Can the pain be provoked by light touch?	Neuralgia

DIAGNOSTIC APPROACH

In approaching the patient with ear pain, the first step is to distinguish between acute or subacute ear pain, and chronic ear pain. In acute ear pain, ask about fever and concurrent symptoms of an upper respiratory tract infection. Chronic ear pain is likely to be referred pain. Dental problems, especially TMJ dysfunction, are common causes of chronic ear pain, so they should be considered in any patient with long-standing ear pain.

Pain unresponsive to simple analgesics should prompt consideration of a process affecting one of the nerves that supplies sensory fibers to the ear or immediate vicinity (eg, trigeminal nerve).

CAVEATS

- The history often only provides a starting point, since the physical examination is frequently critical to making the diagnosis. Most local causes of ear pain have characteristic physical findings, while most cases of referred pain will have a normal ear examination.
- The character and severity of pain may be a helpful feature. The pain of acute OM is generally severe, often interfering with sleep. In contrast, the pain of eustachian tube dysfunction is usually modest, often described by a patient as discomfort or fullness. Referred pain from inflammation of a nerve is frequently described by patients as burning, knife-like, or "electric." It may be provoked by light touch.
- Earwax (cerumen) uncommonly causes ear pain. If earwax is present, it must be removed to exclude the possibility that the true pathology lies behind the ear drum (as in OM).

PROGNOSIS

The prognosis of ear pain is generally favorable. In most cases, the pain resolves relatively quickly with appropriate treatment. Some of the disorders causing referred ear pain are more chronic, such as TMJ dysfunction.

REFERENCES

1. Kuttila S, Kuttila M, Le Bell Y, et al. Aural symptoms and signs of temporomandibular disorder in association with treatment need and visits to a physician. *Laryngoscope.* 1999:109;1669–1673.
2. Heikkinen T, Ruuskanen O. Signs and symptoms predicting acute otitis media. *Arch Pediatr Adolesc Med.* 1995;149:26–29.
3. Kontiokari T, Koivunen P, Neimela M, et al. Symptoms of acute otitis media. *Pediatr Infect Dis J.* 1998;17:676–679.
4. Leonetti JP, Li J, Smith PG. Otalgia. An isolated symptom of malignant infratemporal tumors. *Am J Otol.* 1998; 19:496–498.
5. Handzel O, Halperin D. Necrotizing (malignant) external otitis. *Am Fam Physician.* 2003;63:309–312.
6. Chandler JR. Malignant external otitis. *Laryngoscope.* 1968;78:1257–1294.
7. Rabinovitz M, Pitlik SD, Leifer M, Garty M, Rosenfeld JB. Unintentional weight loss: a retrospective analysis of 154 cases. *Arch Intern Med.* 1986;146:186–187.
8. Smetana GW, Shmerling RH. Does this patient have temporal arteritis? *JAMA.* 2002;287:92–101.

SUGGESTED READING

Parhiscar A, Sperling N. Ear Pain. In: Lucente F, Har-El G (editors). *Essentials of Otolaryngology,* 4th ed. Lippincott Williams & Wilkins; 1999:87–96.

Wazen JJ. Referred otalgia. *Otolaryngol Clin North Am.* 1989;22:1205–1215.

Diagnostic Approach: Ear Pain

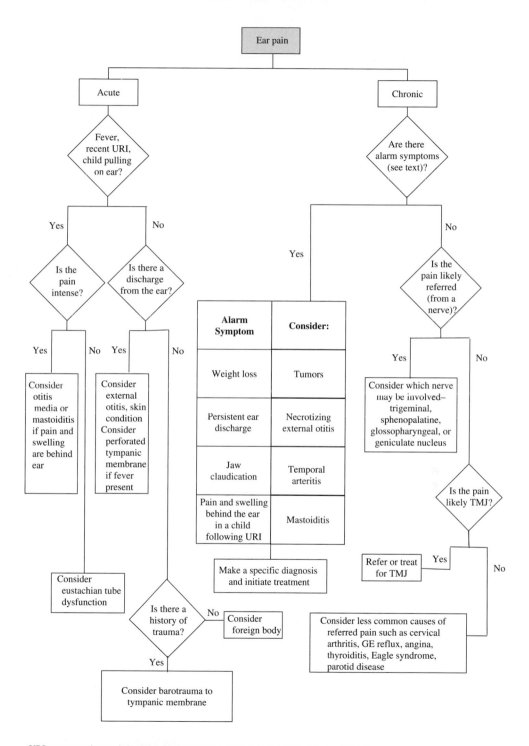

URI, upper respiratory infections; TMJ, temporomandibular joint; GE; gastroesophageal.

Hearing Loss

17

Mia W. Marcus, MD, & Eileen E. Reynolds, MD

Hearing loss is the third most common chronic condition in older Americans after hypertension and arthritis.[1] Ten percent of the US population (28 million Americans) have some degree of hearing loss.[2] The prevalence increases significantly with age; between 25% and 40% of patients over the age of 65 are affected.[1] The most common causes of hearing loss—presbycusis and noise-induced hearing loss—develop insidiously and are underreported, underdiagnosed, and undertreated. These benign causes of hearing loss, unrecognized, can lead to decreased functioning, social isolation, and depression. More dramatic but less common presentations of hearing loss, such as sudden onset hearing loss or hearing loss with associated symptoms, are more likely to be reported by patients and lead to prompt referral and treatment. A careful history allows the clinician to narrow the diagnosis and take appropriate next steps.

The approach to hearing loss involves 2 key steps. First, determine the presence of hearing loss and its severity using a screening questionnaire. Second, focus on alarm symptoms and determine the etiology through a series of specific questions.

It is important to understand the basic anatomy of the auditory system. The auditory system is divided into the **outer ear, middle ear,** and **inner ear.** The **outer ear** is composed of the pinna and external ear canal. Its functions include protection, sound localization, passive augmentation of sound and transferral of sound waves to the tympanic membrane (ear drum) causing it to vibrate. The **middle ear** includes the tympanic membrane and the ossicular chain of 3 small bones—the malleus, incus, and stapes—in the air-filled cavity behind it. The ossicular chain transmits sound vibrations from the tympanic membrane to the cochlea. The cochlea, which lies in perilymph fluid within the temporal bone, the vestibular apparatus, and the eighth cranial nerve (vestibulocochlear) comprise the **inner ear.** This is where mechanical sound is transduced into an electrical impulse via hair cells as sound travels through endolymph fluid within the cochlea to the auditory nerve.

KEY TERMS

Conductive hearing loss	Caused by disorders of the outer and middle ear whereby mechanical transmission of sound to the inner ear is blocked.
Hearing loss	Audiogram showing pure tone threshold of 40 dB or higher at 1 and 2 kHz in one ear, or at 1 or 2 kHz in both ears.[3] Normal conversation is 45–60 dB.[4]
Noise-induced hearing loss	Gradual irreversible sensorineural hearing loss due to cochlear hair cell damage as a result of exposure to continuous or intermittent loud noise. Exposure to > an average of 85 dB over 8 hours can cause noise-induced hearing loss.[4]
Ototoxic medications	Medications that cause sensorineural hearing loss from injury to the cochlear hair cells.

(continued)

KEY TERMS

Presbycusis	*Age-related sensorineural hearing loss due to both genetic and environmental factors. Usually, it is gradual and bilateral; loss of high frequency sounds occurs first.[6]*
Sensorineural hearing loss	*Caused by disorders of the inner ear (cochlea or auditory nerve) usually from damage to the cochlear hair cells.*
Sudden sensorineural hearing loss (SSNHL)	*Uncommon condition with unclear etiology. Hearing loss of at least 30 dB in 3 contiguous frequencies over a period not exceeding 3 days.[5] Most cases are unilateral. Possible causes include viral infection, vascular, autoimmune, or migraine.*
Tinnitus	*An intrinsic noise heard in the ears, described as ringing (or roaring, crickets, or bells). Usually sensorineural in origin but can also be caused by disorders of the outer and middle ears.*

ETIOLOGY

Hearing loss is categorized into 2 major types: **conductive** and **sensorineural.** Most adults with hearing loss in the United States have sensorineural hearing loss (greater than 90% of cases). Presbycusis is by far the most common cause of sensorineural hearing loss, followed by noise-induced hearing loss. Conductive hearing loss represents < 10% of hearing loss. The most common causes of conductive hearing loss in adults are cerumen impaction, otosclerosis, cholesteatoma, and tympanic membrane perforation secondary to chronic otitis media.

Differential Diagnosis[2,4,5,7–9]	Prevalence or incidence[a]
Conductive hearing loss	**< 10% of hearing loss**
Outer ear	
• *Cerumen impaction*	*Up to 30% of older patients with hearing loss[7]*
• *Otitis externa, trauma, squamous cell carcinoma, psoriasis*	
Middle ear	
• *Chronic otitis media*	*18/100,000 per year[8]*
• *Otosclerosis*	*1.0%[2]*
• *Cholesteatoma, barotrauma, tympanic membrane perforation, temporal bone trauma*	
Sensorineural	**> 90% of hearing loss (17 million)[2]**
Presbycusis	*37% of adults older than 75 years[2]*
Noise-induced	*10 million people[2,4]*
Acoustic neuroma	*1/ 60,000 adults per year[9]*
Meniere's disease	*3–5 million people[2] with 300,000 new cases per year[2]*
Genetic	
SSNHL	*4000 new cases[2] or 1/10,000 per year[5]*

Meningitis, ototoxic medications, viral cochleitis, autoimmune disease, multiple sclerosis, perilymphatic fistula, syphilis, cerebrovascular ischemia, penetrating trauma, meningioma, thyrotoxicosis, migrainous, congenital malformations, viral

Mixed

Otosclerosis, chronic otitis media, trauma, neoplasm

Meningitis, ototoxic medications, viral cochleitis, autoimmune disease, multiple sclerosis, perilymphatic fistula, syphilis, cerebrovascular ischemia, penetrating trauma, meningioma, thyrotoxicosis, migrainous, congenital malformations, viral

[a]Prevalence is unknown when not indicated.

GETTING STARTED

- First, ask the patient to describe the hearing loss in his or her own words.
- During the annual visit for either an older patient or a patient with significant noise exposure, ask about hearing loss even if he or she does not report it.
- If hearing loss is reported, determine whether the patient indeed has hearing loss and the severity. Next, focus on determining the etiology.
- The Hearing Handicap Inventory for the Elderly Screening (HHIE-S) questionnaire is the standard tool to confirm and quantify hearing loss. It takes 2–5 minutes to complete and has been validated against audiometry.[6] Using this questionnaire, the total score determines the severity of hearing loss.
- A recent preliminary study showed that the global question: "Do you have a hearing problem now?" may be more effective than the HHIE-S in identifying handicapping hearing loss in older adults.[9]

Hearing Handicap in the Elderly Screening Questionnaire (HHIE-S)[3]

Symptom	Yes	No	Sometimes
1) Does a hearing problem cause you to feel embarrassed when meeting new people?	4	0	2
2) Does a hearing problem cause you to feel frustrated when talking to members of your family?	4	0	2
3) Do you have difficulty hearing when someone whispers?	4	0	2
4) Do you feel handicapped by a hearing problem?	4	0	2

(continued)

Symptom	Yes	No	Sometimes
5) Does a hearing problem cause you difficulty when visiting friends, relatives, or neighbors?	4	0	2
6) Does a hearing problem cause you to attend religious services less often than you would like?	4	0	2
7) Does a hearing problem cause you to have arguments with family members?	4	0	2
8) Does a hearing problem cause you difficulty when listening to TV or radio?	4	0	2
9) Do you feel that your hearing limits or hampers your personal or social life?	4	0	2
10) Does a hearing problem cause you difficulty when in a restaurant with relatives or friends?	4	0	2

Scores: 0–8 = no handicap; 10–24 = mild to moderate handicap; 26–40 = severe handicap.

INTERVIEW FRAMEWORK

Before asking specific questions, review background historical data, which may suggest predisposing factors for certain types of hearing loss:

Factor	Think
Age[2,5]	
• 30–60 years old	Otosclerosis
	Meniere's disease
	Acoustic neuroma
	Autoimmune disease
	SSNHL
• > 65 years	Presbycusis
• Any age	Noise-induced
Sex[1,2,5]	
• M = F	Meniere's disease
	SSNHL
• M > F	Presbycusis
• F > M	Otosclerosis
	Vertiginous migraine
	Autoimmune disease
Other factors	
Past medical history	Autoimmune disease (systemic lupus erythematosus [SLE], rheumatoid arthritis, Wegener's granulomatosis, Sjögren syndrome, antiphospholipid syndrome, polyarteritis nodosa, giant cell arteritis, Behçet disease, Cogan syndrome)
	Diabetes
	Cardiovascular disease

	Stroke
	Renal insufficiency
	Hyperlipidemia
	Recurrent ear infections
	Multiple sclerosis
	Syphilis
	Recent head trauma
	Migraines
	Thyrotoxicosis
Medications	Loop diuretics, antibiotics (aminoglycosides, eg, gentamicin), nonsteroidal anti-inflammatory drugs (NSAIDs), aspirin, chemotherapy (cisplatin), antimalarials
Family history	Genetic: Alport, Usher, and Waardenburg syndromes; other multifactorial causes.
	Genetically predisposing conditions: presbycusis, otosclerosis (50–70% of cases have a positive family history[2]), Paget's disease, neurofibromatosis II, migraine.
Social history	Occupational noise exposure: construction, manufacturing, agriculture.
	Loud hobbies: loud music, hunting, motorcycles.
	Smoking
	Barotrauma: scuba diving, flying
Risk factors for presbycusis	Smoking
	Noise exposure
	Diabetes
	Cardiovascular disease
	Ototoxic medications
	History of recurrent ear infections
	Family history of presbycusis

IDENTIFYING ALARM SYMPTOMS

- Since most benign causes of hearing loss present gradually and bilaterally, any symptoms that differ from these are alarming.
- Sudden or rapid onset of hearing loss is the most concerning symptom for a serious cause of hearing loss.
- Other concerning symptoms include rapidly progressive, unilateral, or asymmetric hearing loss, and association with other neurologic symptoms such as tinnitus or vertigo.
- After determining the severity of hearing loss and any predisposing factors, ask specifically about the presence of alarm symptoms. Keep in mind that some benign causes of hearing loss can also present with alarm symptoms.

Serious Diagnoses

Certain uncommon causes of hearing loss require immediate recognition and prompt referral to an otolaryngologist since early management may prevent progression, complications, and irreversible damage[5]:

- Trauma
- Tumor (eg, acoustic neuroma)
- Autoimmune disease

- Cerebrovascular disease
- Meningitis
- Multiple sclerosis
- Syphilis
- Meniere's disease
- SSNHL

Alarm symptoms	Serious causes	Benign causes
Sudden or rapid onset	SSNHL Vascular embolism or insufficiency Autoimmune disease Trauma (barotrauma, tympanic membrane perforation, perilymphatic fistula, cochlear concussion) Meningitis	Viral cochleitis Migraine Otitis media Ototoxic medications
Rapidly progressive	Autoimmune disease Syphilis	Ototoxic medications
Unilateral or asymmetric	Vascular embolism or insufficiency Acoustic neuroma Meniere's disease SSNHL Autoimmune disease	Cerumen impaction Viral cochleitis
Tinnitus	Meniere's disease Acoustic neuroma Trauma (perilymphatic fistula, barotrauma) SSNHL	Noise-induced Presbycusis Otosclerosis Viral cochleitis Ototoxic medications
Vertigo	Meniere's disease Autoimmune disease Acoustic neuroma Trauma (barotrauma, perilymphatic fistula) Multiple sclerosis Syphilis Meningitis SSNHL	Thyrotoxicosis Genetic Migraine Aminoglycosides

FOCUSED QUESTIONS

Quality	Think about
Is your hearing loss	
• Mild to moderate?	Presbycusis Aminoglycosides
• Severe to profound?	Autoimmune Meningitis Syphilis

Where is your hearing loss?

- Unilateral

Viral cochleitis
SSNHL
Acoustic neuroma
Vascular
Cerumen
Meniere's disease
Migraine

- Bilateral symmetric

Presbycusis
Noise-induced
Ototoxicity
Genetic
Otosclerosis
Meningitis
Syphilis

- Bilateral asymmetric

Autoimmune
Multiple sclerosis

Time course

Think about

Was the onset of your hearing loss

- Sudden or rapid?

Viral cochleitis
Vascular embolism or insufficiency
SSNHL
Perilymphatic fistula
Barotrauma
Otitis media
Tympanic membrane perforation
Autoimmune
Migraine
Meningitis

- Gradual?

Presbycusis
Noise-induced
Ototoxicity
Acoustic neuroma

Does your hearing loss fluctuate?

Meniere's disease
Autoimmune disease
Syphilis
Genetic
Migraine
Perilymphatic fistula

Is your hearing loss getting worse over time

- Slowly?

Presbycusis
Noise-induced
Otosclerosis
Meniere's disease
Acoustic neuroma

(continued)

Time course	*Think about*
	Ototoxicity
	Multiple sclerosis
	Trauma
	Genetic
• *Rapidly?*	*Autoimmune*
	Syphilis
	Ototoxicity

Associated symptoms	*Think about*
Do you have other symptoms that have occurred with your hearing loss?	
• *Ringing in the ear(s)*	*Meniere's disease*
	Acoustic neuroma
	Noise-induced
	Presbycusis
	Ototoxicity
	SSNHL
	Migraine
	Autoimmune
	Otosclerosis
	Perilymphatic fistula
	Viral labyrinthitis
• *Ear pain or drainage*	*Infection (otitis externa, otitis media), tumor, trauma, cerumen impaction*
• *Itchy ear(s)*	*Otitis externa*
• *Fullness or pressure in your ear(s)*	*Otitis media*
	Meniere's disease
	Autoimmune
	Barotrauma
	Acoustic neuroma
	Vertiginous migraine
	Cerumen impaction
• *Fever*	*Otitis media*
	Meningitis
• *Dizziness*	*Meniere's disease*
	Autoimmune
	Acoustic neuroma
	Multiple sclerosis
	Syphilis
	Meningitis
	Aminoglycosides
	Perilymphatic fistula
	SSNHL
	Genetic
	Thyrotoxicosis
	Migraine
	Viral labyrinthitis

• *Facial numbness or weakness*	*Acoustic neuroma*
• *Double vision*	*Acoustic neuroma*
• *Headache*	*Acoustic neuroma* *Migraine* *Meningitis*
Modifying symptoms	***Think about***
Is it more difficult for you to hear	
• *High-pitched sounds?*	*Presbycusis* *Noise-induced* *Ototoxicity* *Genetic*
• *Low-pitched sounds?*	*Meniere's disease* *Migraine*
• *When there is background noise, like in a restaurant?*	*Presbycusis* *Noise-induced*
• *The TV or radio compared to others?*	*Presbycusis* *Noise-induced*
• *A conversation in a group of people rather than one-on-one?*	*Presbycusis* *Noise-induced*
Do loud noises bother you?	*Presbycusis* *Noise-induced* *Migraine*
Is it difficult to tell where sound is coming from?	*Multiple sclerosis* *Noise-induced* *Presbycusis*
Do you ever hear speech but cannot understand it?	*Presbycusis* *Acoustic neuroma* *Noise-induced*
At work, do you need to shout at someone 3 feet or less (an arm's length) away to be heard?	*Noise-induced hearing loss*

CAVEATS

- Most hearing loss results from presbycusis. However, prompt evaluation is warranted if the diagnosis is uncertain or if any alarm symptoms are present.
- Because patients with gradual hearing loss often do not report this complaint, health care providers should take the initiative to ask about it. Patients often ignore or accept hearing loss; alternatively, they may not be as aware of their problem as those around them. Therefore, always include the patient's family and friends in history taking.
- Because the HHIE-S measures a patient's perceived handicap from hearing loss, it is more likely to detect hearing loss in motivated patients who have already sought medical attention about their hearing loss.
- Many patients will not wear hearing aids. Reasons include embarrassment about cosmetic appearance, the stigma associated with using them, cost, and technical difficulty. However, technologic and cosmetic advances in the hearing aid industry may improve patient compliance.

PROGNOSIS

- Causes of reversible hearing loss include SSNHL (70–90% experience full recovery, either spontaneously or with prompt initiation of corticosteroid therapy),[5] syphilis, barotrauma, viral labyrinthitis, otitis media, tympanic membrane perforation, cochlear concussion, temporal bone fracture, ototoxicity from medications such as aspirin, antimalarials, loop diuretics, and NSAIDs.
- Causes of irreversible hearing loss include presbycusis, chronic otitis media, Meniere's disease (after repeated attacks), ototoxicity from antibiotics or chemotherapy, noise-induced, and autoimmune hearing loss.
- Since most causes of hearing loss are treatable, screening and early detection are important. Any patient with subjective hearing loss should be referred for further evaluation by an audiologist or otolaryngologist.

REFERENCES

1. Cruickshanks KJ, Wiley TL, Tweed TS, et al. Prevalence of hearing loss in older adults in Beaver Dam, Wisconsin. The Epidemiology of Hearing Loss Study. *Am J Epidemiol.* 1998;148:879–886.

2. Castrogiovanni A. Incidence and prevalence of hearing loss and hearing aid use in the United States. *ASHA.* 2002.

3. Ventry IM, Weinstein BE. Identification of elderly people with hearing problems. *ASHA.* 1983;25:37–42.

4. Rabinowitz PM. Noise-induced hearing loss. *Am Fam Physician.* 2000;61:2749–2756, 2759–2760.

5. Zadeh MH, Storper IS, Spitzer JB. Diagnosis and treatment of sudden-onset sensorineural hearing loss: a study of 51 patients. *Otolaryngol Head Neck Surg.* 2003;128:92–98.

6. Lichtenstein MJ, Bess FH, Logan SA. Validation of screening tools for identifying hearing impaired elderly in Primary Care. *JAMA.* 1988;259:2875–2878.

7. Lewis-Culinan C, Janken J. Effect of cerumen removal on the hearing ability of geriatric patients. *J Adv Nurs.* 1990; 15:594–600.

8. Ruben RJ. The disease in society: evaluation of chronic otitis media in general and cholesteatoma in particular. In: Sade J (editor). *Cholesteatoma and mastoid surgery.* Amsterdam: Kugler, 1982:111-116.

9. Harcourt JP, Vijaya-Sekaran S, Loney E, Lennox P. The incidence of symptoms consistent with cerebellopontine angle lesions in a general ENT out-patient clinic. *J Laryngol Otol.* 1999;113:518–522.

10. Gates GA, Murphy M, Rees T, Fraher A. Screening for handicapping hearing loss in the elderly. *J Fam Pract.* 2003;52:56–62.

SUGGESTED READING

Bogardus ST, Yueh B, Shekelle PG. Screening and management of adult hearing loss in primary care: clinical applications. *JAMA.* 2003;289:1986–1990.

Nadol JB. Hearing Loss. *N Engl J Med.* 1993;329:1092–1102.

Yueh B, Shapiro N, MacLean CH, Shekelle PG. Screening and management of adult hearing loss in primary care: scientific review. *JAMA.* 2003;289:1976–1985.

Diagnostic Approach: Hearing Loss

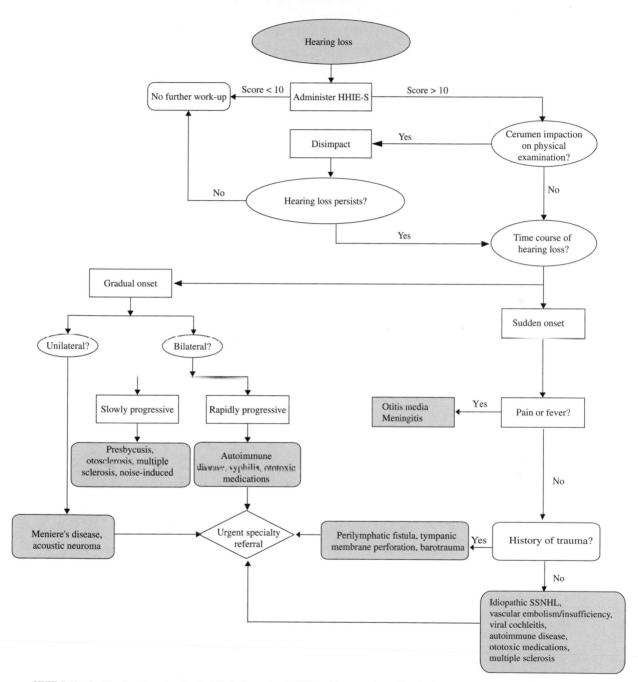

HHIE-S, Hearing Handicap Inventory for the Elderly Screening; SSNHL, sudden sensorineural hearing loss.

Tinnitus

18

Malathi Srinivasan, MD

Tinnitus is a common symptom in primary care, with great heterogeneity in presentation, severity, and etiology. The term "tinnitus" originates from the Latin word *tinnire,* which means "to ring." Although commonly defined as **ringing in the ears,** a better definition is that "tinnitus is the conscious expression of a sound that originates in an involuntary manner ...".[1] Tinnitus is reported by patients as a ringing, hissing, buzzing, pulsing, humming, or whistling.[2] Tinnitus may cause insomnia; difficulty hearing in social situations; anxiety; annoyance; frustration; and feelings of inadequacy, social anxiety, or loss of control. Only 4–8% of patients with tinnitus report moderate to severe tinnitus that interferes with their daily life.[3]

A truly evidence-based approach to tinnitus is handicapped by lack of epidemiologic and observational data. Thus, likelihood ratios for associated tinnitus symptoms cannot be generated. Most studies include very small numbers of patients.

KEY TERMS

Tinnitus	Person's perception of a simple involuntary sound that is usually not audible to the observer. The monotonous sound may range in pitch, tone, and amplitude. Often described as hissing, buzzing, ringing, pulsing, "steam escaping."
Auditory hallucination	Person's perception of an involuntary sound that is of complex structure. The sounds may be musical or voices. Not tinnitus, and indicates psychiatric disturbance.
Bilateral tinnitus	Tinnitus perceived in both ears. May be of central origin, in the central auditory pathways, or represent systemic damage (noise, medications, toxins, infection).
Objective tinnitus	Tinnitus that the physician and the patient can hear; 4% of all tinnitus patients have this form. Clonic muscular contractures and vascular bruits are common causes.
Pulsatile tinnitus	Tinnitus that pulses in time with the cardiac cycle. Almost always a vascular source, and mandates a close evaluation of the vasculature and potential vascular tumors.[4]
Subjective tinnitus	Tinnitus that only the patient can hear; 96% of all tinnitus patients have this form.
Unilateral tinnitus	Tinnitus localized to 1 ear. Typically of peripheral origin (middle ear, cochlea, acoustic nerve).

ETIOLOGY

The perception of tinnitus is extremely common in all age groups. Overall, 9% of the US population reports tinnitus, with prevalence increasing with age.[5] With age, men are 1.4–1.8 times more likely to be affected than women. With age, whites are 2.2 times more likely to be affected than blacks, while individuals from poorer families are 1.3–2.3 times more likely to report tinnitus. In children, the prevalence of tinnitus ranges from 1% to 13%.[5,6] Tinnitus and hearing loss are highly associated; although hearing loss is 2–3 times more common than tinnitus.[5] Tinnitus is highly associated with depression, anxiety, and other personality disorders. However, it is unclear whether the depression is a reaction to tinnitus-related handicap, or if existing depression makes the perception of tinnitus worse. Perception of tinnitus is altered by patient's attention to the sounds, level of stress, and ambient noise level.

A lesion anywhere along the auditory pathway can cause tinnitus (see Chapters 16 and 17). A few key points on tinnitus generation can help guide appropriate history-taking and diagnosis.[7]

Conductive system (outer ear, tympanic membrane, ossicles)

Damage to the conductive hearing system may cause bilateral tinnitus if the agent was environmental (prolonged noise exposure) or systemic (medications that damage the cochlear hairs). Usually, these causes are associated with hearing loss. Unilateral tinnitus with conductive hearing loss results from tympanic membrane damage, recurrent unilateral ear infections, ossicle damage, or trauma. A patulous eustachian tube causes blowing tinnitus, as the tympanic membrane moves in time with the respiratory cycle.

Medications That Commonly Cause Tinnitus

Class	Drug
Analgesics	Aspirin and nonsteroidal anti-inflammatory drugs (NSAIDs)
Antibiotics	Gentamicin
	Vancomycin
	Amphotericin B
	Neomycin
	Other aminoglycosides
Diuretics	Furosemide
	Chlorthalidone
Chemotherapeutic agents	Cisplatin
	Bleomycin
	Vincristine
	Methotrexate
	Nitrogen mustard
Cardiac medications	Lidocaine
	Metoprolol
	Quinine
	Flecainide
Gastrointestinal medications	Misoprostol
Psychopharmacologic medications	Benzodiazepines
	Tricyclic antidepressants
	Lithium
Vapor solvents	Cyclohexane
	Styrene

Sensorineural transduction (cochlea)

Many cochlear disorders are associated with tinnitus, such as Meniere disease and postinfectious cochlear labyrinthitis. In addition, many common medications can damage cochlear stereocilia. Damage to the cochlear stereocilia may not be reversible. Spontaneous otoacoustic emissions (SOAEs) from the cochlea can be heard by placing a small microphone in the patient's ear canal.

Central auditory pathways alteration (8th nerve and brain)

The closer the focal pathology is to the ear, the more likely that tinnitus will be unilateral. For instance, a tumor that grows out of the myelin sheath of the 8th cranial nerve (called an acoustic neuroma or schwannoma) produces unilateral tinnitus and progressive neurosensory hearing loss. Myelin or axonal brain lesions can produce bilateral tinnitus, once the auditory pathways have combined in the auditory cortex; they also often present with other neurologic deficits.

After head trauma or central nervous system (CNS) infections, tinnitus may be caused by nerve sensitivity after cortical reorganization. Normally, people habituate to background noises through a negative central feedback mechanism; thus, auditory disinhibition may cause central bilateral tinnitus. Tinnitus after sound exposure may cause "negative emotional reinforcement" (fear, anxiety, tension), triggering the limbic and autonomic nervous systems, producing fear of recurrent episodes. Finally, low serotonin levels may contribute to tinnitus and to depression.

Referred sounds

Vascular structures near the ear can cause pulsatile tinnitus. High cardiac output states may result in pulsatile tinnitus. If no obvious etiology is found, then a careful evaluation of the head and neck circulation is indicated (eg, computed tomography angiography or magnetic resonance angiography). Tonic contractions of muscles around the ear may result in "clicking," such as with palatal myoclonus or stapedius muscle myoclonus, with 175–200 contractions per minute.

Differential Diagnosis	Prevalence[a]
Subjective tinnitus	*Study of 200 patients[8]*
Cochlear origin	75%
CNS	18%
Conductive causes	4%
Vascular causes	3%
Objective tinnitus	
Pulsatile tinnitus (intracranial/extracranial)	*Study of 84 patients[9]*
• Unknown causes	32%
• Vascular structures	
– Dural arteriovenous malformations	20%
– Carotid narrowing (eg, stenosis, dissection, or fibromuscular dysplasia)	20%
– Carotid-cavernous sinus fistula	7%
– Other vascular sources	2%
– Internal carotid artery aneurysm	1%
• Nonvascular structures	
– Glomus tumor, other tumors, intracranial hypertension, etc	13%

(continued)

Objective tinnitus

Nonpulsatile tinnitus

- *Impacted cerumen*
- *Clonic muscular contractions*
- *Palatal myoclonus*
- *Stapedius spasm*
- *Tensor tympani spasm*
- *Patulous eustachian tube (persistently open)*

[a]Prevalence is unknown when not indicated.

GETTING STARTED

- The initial questions should be open-ended.
- Let the patient (or parent) tell the story.
- The degree of functional impairment should be assessed with a validated tinnitus instrument.[10]

Open-ended questions

Tell me about your tinnitus.

When did it start? How has it changed? What makes it better or worse? What else have you noticed with your tinnitus?

How does the tinnitus affect your life?

What do you think is causing this symptom?

Tips for effective interviewing

- *Create a comfortable setting.*
- *Give the patient enough time to finish his or her story.*
- *Whenever possible, do not interrupt the patient.*

INTERVIEW FRAMEWORK

During the interview, determine whether the tinnitus is unilateral or bilateral, pulsatile or nonpulsatile. Determine whether the patient has hearing loss. In past medical history, remember that both anxiety and depression have been associated with tinnitus perception. Ask about childhood or recent ear infections. Assess other comorbid conditions, such as atherosclerosis. Could the patient be pregnant? Whenever possible, have the patient bring in all of their medications, including over-the-counter and herbal medications. During social history, determine the patient's hobbies, musical interests, and occupation. Quantify the degree, loudness, and chronicity of noise exposure and whether the patient wore protective ear-wear. In the occupational history, assess if the patient was exposed to ototoxic chemicals. Occasionally, the family history may point to otosclerosis or neurofibromatosis syndromes. From both history and physical examination, assess the presence of functional deficits.

IDENTIFYING ALARM SYMPTOMS

- The most frequently occurring causes of tinnitus are benign, such as those resulting from cochlear damage or repeated sound exposure.
- Often, no clear etiology of tinnitus is found.
- It is critical to diagnose any disorder that may result in deafness or life-threatening diseases.

Alarm symptoms	Serious causes	Benign causes
Episodic tinnitus, vertigo, nausea, and hearing loss	Meniere disease	Labyrinthitis (self-limited)
Pulsatile tinnitus	Vascular tumor Arterial or venous stenosis, aneurysm, or shunt	Pseudotumor cerebri High cardiac output states (pregnancy, hyperthyroidism) Flow murmur
Bilateral progressive conductive hearing loss and tinnitus	Otosclerosis	Tympanic membrane scarring Recurrent infection Chronic noise exposure
Unilateral progressive hearing loss	Acoustic neuroma (8th nerve tumor)	Conductive hearing loss (eg, recurrent middle ear infection or trauma to ear structures) Sensorineural hearing loss (eg, ototoxic medications)
Bilateral sensorineural hearing loss	Toxin-associated tinnitus	Chronic noise exposure SOAEs
Headaches	Intracranial tumors Glomus tumors Pseudotumor cerebri	Migraine
Focal neurologic symptoms	Multiple sclerosis Strokes or transient ischemic attack Intracranial tumor	
New seizures	Intracranial tumor Intracranial cavitary lesion	Unrelated causes of seizure (alcohol withdrawal, primary seizure disorder)
Weight loss, fevers, fatigue	Intracranial tumor Giant cell arteritis	

FOCUSED QUESTIONS

Questions	Think about
Quality	
Does the tinnitus sound like it is blowing, in time with your breathing?	Patulous eustachian tube
Does the tinnitus sound like it is clicking?	Myoclonic muscular contractions (stapedius, palatal muscles, etc)
Does the tinnitus pulse in time with your heartbeat?	Vascular causes of tinnitus High cardiac output states
Is the tinnitus low-pitched, with intermittent sound muffling?	Incomplete cerumen impaction

(continued)

(continued from previous page)

Associated symptoms and exposures	Think about
Do you play an instrument or in a band? Have you attended loud concerts?	*Sound-associated sensorineural damage*
Are you a boxer?	*Stereocilia damage or cortical reorganization problems*
Have you been exposed to solvents?	*Cochlear stereocilia damage*
Have you had a recent viral infection (especially mumps, rubella, cytomegalovirus)?	*Labyrinthitis*
Do you use Q-tips to clean your ears? Is sound muffled?	*Cerumen impaction* *Tympanic membrane scarring*
Does aspirin make the tinnitus better?	*SOAEs (a small percentage improve with aspirin)*
Have you been taking large amounts of aspirin or NSAIDs?	*NSAID-associated cochlear and neuronal damage*
Does anyone in your family have early deafness?	*Otosclerosis (autosomal dominant)*
Do you feel like you become significantly dizzy or can't keep your balance intermittently?	*Meniere disease* *Labyrinthitis*
Have you recently had heavy or chronic blood loss?	*Anemia-associated high cardiac output states*

DIAGNOSTIC APPROACH

After taking the tinnitus history, a focused physical examination should be performed to look for objective tinnitus diagnoses. It includes careful examination of the head, the neck, the external auditory meatus, and the tympanic membrane. Testing the acoustic reflex and tympanic membrane mobility (office procedures); screening tests for conductive or sensorineural hearing loss (Weber, Renee, and office screening tools for hearing loss); and a full neurologic screening examination are also important.

Patients with mild to moderate tinnitus, no hearing loss, and no signs of neurologic, cardiac, or otologic dysfunction can be monitored at regular intervals. However, patients with subjective or objective hearing loss require a full audiologic examination.

PROGNOSIS

Tinnitus is difficult to control. To date, no cure exists for this symptom complex. Multiple clinical trials of tinnitus therapy show no significant, reproducible benefit of medication.[11] Medications (antidepressants, benzodiazepines, pain modulators) and complementary medicines (*Ginkgo biloba,* ginseng, etc) have only modest success. The placebo effect in most tinnitus studies ranges from 5% to 30%. Other therapies for benign causes include tinnitus retraining therapy, somatic modulation, cognitive retraining therapy, amplification devices, cochlear implantation, and tinnitus maskers. At best, these have only mild to moderate benefits.

REFERENCES

1. McFadden D. Tinnitus: Facts, Theories and Treatments. Report of Working Group 89. Committee on Hearing, Bioacoustics and Biomechanics. National Research Council. National Academy Press; 1982.
2. Stouffer JL, Tyler RS. Characterization of tinnitus by tinnitus patients. *J Speech Hear Disord.* 1990;55:439–453.
3. Coles RR, Hallam RS. Tinnitus and its management. *Br Med Bull.* 1987;43:983–998.

4. Sismanis A. Pulsatile tinnitus. *Otolaryngol Clin North Am.* 2003;36:389–402.

5. Adams PF, Hendershot GE, Marano MA. Current Estimates from the National Health Interview Survey, 1996. National Center for Health Statistics, Centers for Disease Control and Prevention; 1999.

6. Fritsch MH, Wynne MK, Matt BH, Smith WL, Smith CM. Objective tinnitus in children. *Otol Neurotol.* 2001;22:644–649.

7. Moller AR. Pathophysiology of tinnitus. *Otolaryngol Clin North Am.* 2003;36:249–266.

8. Reed GF. An audiometric study of two hundred cases of subjective tinnitus. *Arch Otolaryngol.* 1960;71:84–94.

9. Waldvogel D, Mattle HP, Sturzenegger M, Schroth G. Pulsatile tinnitus–a review of 84 patients. *J Neurol.* 1998;245:137–142.

10. Newman CW, Jacobson GP, Spitzer JB. Development of the Tinnitus Handicap Inventory. *Arch Otolaryngol Head Neck Surg.* 1996;122:143–148.

11. Dobie RA. A review of randomized clinical trials in tinnitus. *Laryngoscope.* 1999;109:1202–1211.

Diagnostic Approach: Tinnitus

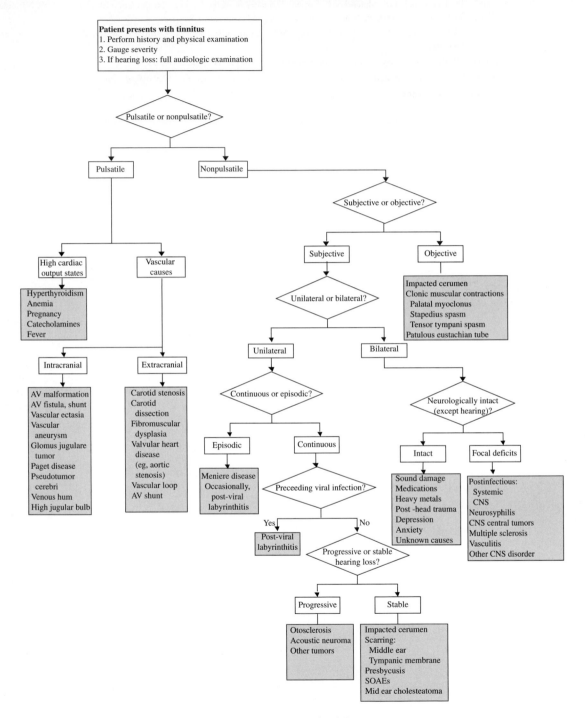

AV, arteriovenous; CNS, central nervous system; SOAEs, spontaneous otoacoustic emissions.

Sore Throat

19

Craig R. Keenan, MD

Sore throat was the sixth most common reason for seeking outpatient care in 2000, accounting for 2.1% of all ambulatory visits in the United States.[1] Although the term "sore throat" is frequently equated with pharyngitis (inflammation of the pharynx), sore throat often results from other causes. Most cases are benign and self-limited, but sore throat may be the presenting symptom for dangerous and potentially life-threatening conditions.

Identification and treatment of acute group A β-hemolytic streptococcal (GAS) pharyngitis ("strep throat") prevents the rare suppurative sequelae (peritonsillar abscess, parapharyngeal infection, retropharyngeal abscess, otitis media, sinusitis, and mastoiditis), reduces the transmission of GAS, and shortens the illness by 1–2 days.[2] However, even without antibiotics, most cases of GAS pharyngitis resolve uneventfully after 7–10 days. GAS pharyngitis can rarely cause acute rheumatic fever (ARF), and antibiotics have proved to reduce this risk. Because ARF is rare in the United States, it is estimated that 3000–4000 cases of GAS pharyngitis would need to be treated to prevent a single case.[3] Post-streptococcal glomerulonephritis is a very rare complication of GAS pharyngitis, but antibiotics have not been shown to reduce its incidence.[3]

The classic history for GAS pharyngitis is the sudden onset of sore throat, odynophagia, fever > 101 °F, abdominal pain, headache, nausea and vomiting. Cough, rhinorrhea, and diarrhea are absent. The classic physical findings include pharyngeal erythema with exudates, palatal petechiae, and anterior cervical adenopathy. Unfortunately, there is a broad overlap of clinical manifestations between GAS and nonstreptococcal pharyngitis. Even though only 5–15% of adults with sore throat have a positive GAS culture, about 75% of adult patients with acute sore throat receive antibiotics.[3,4] Thus, the desire to treat GAS infections has led to the overprescribing of antibiotics, and the proper exclusion of patients without GAS could lead to dramatic reductions in inappropriate antibiotic use.

KEY TERMS

Odynophagia	*Pain with swallowing.*
Dysphagia	*Difficulty initiating the swallowing process (oropharyngeal dysphagia) or difficulty in passage of a bolus from the upper esophagus to the stomach (esophageal dysphagia).*
Sore throat	*Pain in the throat region. Odynophagia is the usual symptom, but occasionally dysphagia also occurs.*
Pharyngitis	*Inflammation of the pharynx, including the tonsillar and adenoid lymphoid tissue.*
Trismus	*Inability to open the jaw. May result from processes affecting the motor branch of the trigeminal nerve, and from pressure or infection of the muscles of mastication.*

(continued)

> *(continued from previous page)*
>
> **Clinical prediction rule**   *A clinical tool that quantifies the individual contributions that various components of the history, physical examination, and basic laboratory results make toward the diagnosis, prognosis, or likely response to treatment in an individual patient.*

ETIOLOGY

The differential diagnosis for sore throat is extensive. The prevalence for all of the various causes has not been well established. Most non-GAS cases of infectious pharyngitis are benign, but there are important exceptions that are often missed. Clinicians must be aware of these symptom complexes and consider them in at-risk persons.

Several suppurative complications of oropharyngeal infections may present with sore throat. These are rare but life-threatening, so prompt recognition is important. There is usually a history of preceding oral infection or pharyngitis. These infections can spread to the peritonsillar space (peritonsillar abscess), parapharyngeal space (carotid sheath infection or suppurative jugular thrombophlebitis), submandibular space (Ludwig's angina), and retropharyngeal space.

Common noninfectious causes of sore throat are acid irritation of the pharynx and larynx due to gastroesophageal reflux disease (GERD),[5] postnasal drip (due to sinusitis or allergic rhinitis), and head and neck malignancies. In addition, 15–50% of patients complain of sore throat after surgeries.[6]

Differential Diagnosis	Associated organisms and conditions	Estimated % of infectious pharyngitis[8]
Infectious		
Bacterial pharyngitis	Group A streptococci	*15–30*
	Other streptococci	*5*
	Mycoplasma pneumoniae	*< 1*
	Moraxella catarrhalis	
	Chlamydia pneumoniae	
	Staphylococcus aureus	
	Neisseria meningitidis	
Viral pharyngitis	*Rhinovirus, coronavirus, adenovirus, parainfluenza*	*> 32*
Herpetic stomatitis, pharyngitis	*Herpes virus 1 and 2. May be sexually transmitted or seen in immunocompromised patients.*	*4*
Acute epiglottitis/ supraglottitis[b]	Haemophilus influenzae *and other*	
Gonococcal pharyngitis	*Sexually transmitted via oral sexual contact. Often asymptomatic but can cause acute pharyngitis.*	*< 1*
Infectious mononucleosis	*Epstein-Barr virus, cytomegalovirus. Syndrome with fatigue, fever, pharyngitis, splenomegaly (50%), posterior cervical lymphadenopathy, occasional rash*	*1*
Peritonsillar abscess[b]		
Parapharyngeal infections[b]		

Retropharyngeal infections[b]		
Necrotizing ulcerative gingivostomatitis (Vincent's angina)[b]	Anaerobes (including Fusobacterium nucleatum)	
Primary HIV infection	HIV. Syndrome with sore throat, fever, rash, diffuse lymphadenopathy, weight loss, fatigue, mucocutaneous ulcers. Usually occurs 2–4 weeks after HIV exposure and lasts 2 weeks.	< 1
Oropharyngeal candidiasis	Candida albicans. Seen in immunocompromised persons or in those who use inhaled corticosteroids.	
Influenza	Influenza viruses. Syndrome with sudden onset fever, myalgias, and sore throat. Measures to prevent spread sometimes important. Seasonal.	2
Diphtheria[b]	Corynebacterium diphtheriae. Rare due to high vaccination rates. Characteristic pharyngitis with gray pseudomembrane in throat on examination.	< 1
Herpangina	Coxsackievirus	< 1
Secondary syphilis	Treponema pallidum. Syndrome with fever, weight loss, sore throat, anorexia, malaise, headache, and rash.	
Toxic shock syndrome[b]	Streptococci or staphylococci	
Noninfectious		
Sinusitis	Postnasal drip, nasal congestion	
Allergic rhinitis	Rhinitis, postnasal drip, conjunctivitis	
Acute/subacute thyroiditis	Symptoms of hyperthyroidism or hypothyroidism	
Head and neck cancer	Laryngeal, tongue, oropharyngeal	
Lymphoma	Adenopathy, fever, night sweats, weight loss	
Gastroesophageal reflux	Heartburn, acid taste	
Esophageal spasm		
Cervical spondylosis		
Postoperative		
Post-irradiation		
Burn or irritant injuries	Smoking cocaine, drinking caustic agents	
Coronary artery disease	Angina may present as neck pain	

(continued)

Noninfectious

Glossopharyngeal
neuralgia

Systemic illnesses

Rheumatoid arthritis (Adult-onset Still disease)[7]	Accompanied by fever, rash, arthritis
Wegener's granulomatosis	
Sarcoidosis	

[a]Incidence unknown when not indicated.
[b]Potentially life-threatening.

INTERVIEW FRAMEWORK

- Use open-ended questions to determine the symptoms and chronology of the illness.
- If the patient reports fever, rhinorrhea, adenopathy, malaise, myalgias, or headache, think about an infectious cause. Direct your subsequent questions to determine the specific infectious cause and the severity of the illness:
  - Ask about alarm symptoms (eg, trismus, drooling, and shortness of breath).
  - Ask the questions below that can help include or exclude GAS pharyngitis.
  - Take a sexual history to assess whether the patient is at risk for sexually transmitted causes (herpes, gonorrhea, syphilis, acute HIV).
  - Perform a review of systems to detect other symptoms that may be related to a systemic disease masquerading as an infection (eg, patients with lymphoma or Still disease may have fevers).
- Always review the past medical and social history, including substances, tobacco, and medication use.

IDENTIFYING ALARM SYMPTOMS

The alarm symptoms suggest severe infections of the supraglottic, submandibular, peritonsillar, parapharyngeal, and retropharyngeal spaces. These extensive infections are life-threatening and usually require prompt surgical intervention.

Serious Diagnoses

Symptoms	Serious diagnoses	Potential complications
Sore throat, dysphagia, or odynophagia with any of the following: • Drooling • Respiratory distress • Inability to open mouth fully (trismus)	Acute epiglottitis or supraglottitis Peritonsillar abscess Parapharyngeal space infection Retropharyngeal space infection Submandibular space infection (Ludwig's angina) Superficial jugular thrombophlebitis	Airway obstruction Sepsis Spread to parapharyngeal, retropharyngeal spaces, with subsequent spread to pleura, mediastinum, carotid sheath, or jugular vein

- *Muffled voice*
- *Stiff neck*
- *Erythema of neck*

History of recent foreign body impaction or oropharyngeal procedure (trauma)	*Retropharyngeal abscess*	*Airway obstruction Sepsis Spread to mediastinum, pleural space, or pericardium*
Fever, rash, diffuse adenopathy, sore throat	*Primary HIV infection*	*Transmission of disease*
Recent cocaine smoking	*Mucosal burn injury to pharynx and larynx[8]*	*Respiratory obstruction*

FOCUSED QUESTIONS

If infection is likely and there are no alarm symptoms, focus on determining whether the patient has GAS pharyngitis. Many studies have evaluated the usefulness of historical and physical examination findings in differentiating GAS from other causes of acute pharyngitis.

Ebell and colleagues evaluated studies from children and adults to calculate the positive and negative likelihood ratios (LR+ and LR−) for elements of the history in each study.[2] The LR+ are all below 5, with most between 1 and 2; and LR− are mostly between 0.5 and 2.0. Thus, the presence or absence of each element alone is weak evidence for or against GAS pharyngitis, and does *not* appreciably change the pretest probability.

Symptom	LR+[a]	LR−[a]
Reported fever	*0.75–2.6*	*0.66–0.94*
Absence of cough	*1.1–1.7*	*0.53–0.89*
Absence of runny nose	*0.86–1.6*	*0.51–1.4*
Presence of myalgias	*1.4*	*0.93*
Presence of headache	*1.0–1.1*	*0.55–1.2*
Presence of nausea	*0.76–3.1*	*0.91*
Duration of symptoms < 3 days	*0.72–3.5*	*0.15–2.2*
Streptococcal exposure in previous 2 weeks	*1.9*	*0.92*

[a]The range of likelihood ratios from the studies are presented for each variable. If there was agreement among all studies, a single summary likelihood ratio is presented.

Others have created clinical prediction rules that incorporate both history and physical examination elements. The most widely accepted rule for adults is the Centor Clinical Prediction Rule.[9] Due to the limitations of the history alone, clinicians should apply this clinical prediction rule to help determine the likelihood of GAS pharyngitis. In patients with either 0–1 or 4 points, the associated LR considerably alters the pretest probability of GAS infection. Scores of 2–3 points do not appreciably affect the pretest probability.

Centor Clinical Prediction Rule[2,9]

Symptom or Sign	Points
History of fever	*1*
Absence of cough	*1*
Tonsillar exudates	*1*
Anterior cervical adenopathy	*1*
Total Score	***LR+ for GAS***
4 points	*6.3*
3 points	*2.1*
2 points	*0.75*
1 point	*0.3*
0 points	*0.16*

Of course, other questions must be directed toward the other potential causes. It is useful to determine whether the sore throat is chronic (> 2 weeks duration). The common causes of sore throat, which are mostly viral and bacterial infections, usually resolve in 2 weeks. Thus, chronic symptoms should lead clinicians to think about less common conditions that cause prolonged symptoms, including atypical infections (eg, infectious mononucleosis), noninfectious etiologies (eg, malignancy, allergic rhinitis, GERD, adult-onset Still disease, chronic sinusitis), or complications of acute infections (eg, peritonsillar abscess, parapharyngeal and retropharyngeal infections).

Questions	Think about
Do you work with children or have small children in your home?	*May increase risk of GAS infection in adults.*
Are you sexually active? *Do you perform oral sex on your partner?* *Do you use condoms or other barrier protection when performing oral, anal, or vaginal intercourse?* *Have you had any recent sexually transmitted diseases?*	*Oral sex predisposes to sexually transmitted causes, including herpes simplex and gonococcal pharyngitis, HIV, and syphilis.* *Unprotected sex puts persons at risk for HIV transmission and thus primary HIV infection.* *Patients with recent genital gonorrhea infections have a high incidence of gonococcal pharyngitis.*
Do you have swollen glands in your neck? Elsewhere in your body?	*Anterior cervical adenopathy suggests GAS.* *Posterior cervical adenopathy accompanies infectious mononucleosis.* *Lymphoma and other head and neck cancers can present with cervical adenopathy.* *Diffuse adenopathy is seen in systemic diseases such as primary HIV infection, infectious mononucleosis, lymphoma, sarcoidosis.*
Do you have a rash?	*Primary HIV infection, GAS infection (scarlet fever), secondary syphilis, infectious mononucleo-*

	sis, toxic shock syndrome, adult-onset Still disease. Neck erythema suggests submandibular space infection (Ludwig's angina).
Do you have a cough?	Makes GAS less likely, and suggests other infections, GERD, or malignancy.
Do you smoke or use smokeless tobacco?	Increases risk of head and neck cancers.
Do you have acid reflux disease? Do you have frequent heartburn? Do you frequently get an acid taste in you mouth?	GERD may cause sore throat, odynophagia, hoarseness, or cough.
Have you had recent surgery?	Postoperative sore throat (common).
Have you had a recent dental procedure or infection?	Submandibular space infection, Ludwig's angina.
Does the pain come on with exertion and resolve with rest?	Angina (coronary artery disease).
Have symptoms been going on for > 2 weeks?	Chronic sore throat may be due to head and neck cancers, lymphoma, postnasal drip from allergic rhinitis or chronic sinusitis, GERD, infectious mononucleosis, or Still disease. Also consider suppurative complications of bacterial infections.
Do you have HIV disease?	Predisposes to oropharyngeal candidiasis, recurrent herpes simplex infection, lymphoma.
Have you lost weight?	Infectious mononucleosis, primary HIV infection, head and neck malignancy, lymphoma, secondary syphilis.

DIAGNOSTIC APPROACH

There is no consensus on the best approach to the diagnosis and treatment of GAS pharyngitis.[10] The diagnostic algorithm is adapted from a recent clinical practice guideline for adults with acute pharyngitis.[3] By following it, inappropriate antibiotic use will be reduced. Although a small number of patients with GAS infection will go untreated using this algorithm, their prognosis remains excellent due to the rarity of suppurative complications and rheumatic fever.

CAVEATS

- Although dangerous conditions are rare in patients with sore throat, the clinician should always consider suppurative complications, head and neck malignancies, and primary HIV infection.
- Patients with diabetes, recent chemotherapy, or any immunocompromised states are more susceptible to suppurative complications of bacterial pharyngitis.
- The clinical decision rules and guidelines were developed in ambulatory, immunocompetent patients in the United States and Canada where the endemic rate of rheumatic fever is low. As such, they cannot be applied to immunosuppressed patients, patients with chronic or recurrent pharyngitis, or those with a history of rheumatic fever. Finally, such tools do not apply when there is a known outbreak or a high endemic rate of acute rheumatic fever.
- Patients with sore throats often expect antibiotics. Physicians should take the time to reassure their patients that antibiotics are unnecessary in most cases.

REFERENCES

1. Cherry DK, Woodwell DA. National Ambulatory Medical Care Survey: 2000 Summary. Advance Data from Vital and Health Statistics 2002; 328. Available at: http://www.cdc.gov/nchs/data/ad/ad328.pdf

2. Ebell MH, Smith MA, Barry HC, et al. Does this patient have strep throat? *JAMA.* 2000;284:2912–2918.

3. Cooper M, Hoffman JR, Bartlett JG, et al. Principles of appropriate antibiotic use for acute pharyngitis in adults: background. *Ann Intern Med.* 2001;134:509–517.

4. Linder JA, Stafford RS. Antibiotic treatment of adults with sore throat by community primary care physicians. A National Survey, 1989–1999. *JAMA.* 2001;286:1181–1186.

5. Tauber S, Gross M, Issing WJ. Association of laryngopharyngeal symptoms with gastroesophageal reflux disease. *Laryngoscope.* 2002;112:879–886.

6. McHardy FE, Chung F. Postoperative sore throat: cause, prevention, and treatment. *Anaesthesia.* 1999;54:444–453.

7. Nguyen KH, Weisman MH. Severe sore throat as a presenting symptom of adult onset Still's disease: a case series and review of the literature. *J Rheumatol.* 1997;24:592–597.

8. Bisno AL. Acute pharyngitis. *N Engl J Med.* 2001;344:205–211.

9. Centor RM, Witherspoon JM, Dalton HP, et al. The diagnosis of strep throat in adults in the emergency room. Med Decis Making 1981;1:239–246.

10. Bisno AL, Peter GS, Kaplan EL. Diagnosis of strep throat in adults: are clinical criteria really good enough? *Clin Infect Dis.* 2002;35:126–129.

Diagnostic Approach: Sore Throat

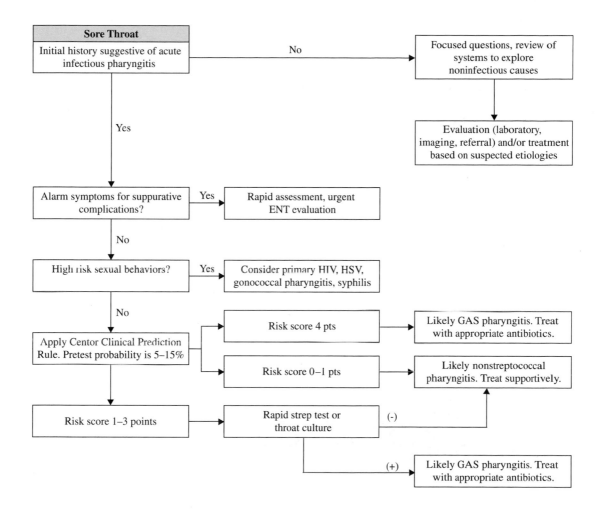

ENT, ear, nose, and throat; HSV, herpes simplex virus; GAS, group A β-hemolytic streptococcal.

SECTION IV
Dermatology

Inflammatory Dermatoses (Rashes)

20

Mona A. Gohara, MD, Julie V. Schaffer, MD, & Kenneth A. Arndt, MD

Dermatologists are not the only physicians who assess and treat patients with skin disorders. The results of the National Ambulatory Medical Care Survey (1990–1994)[1] showed that dermatologists saw only 40% of patients with diseases of the skin, hair, or nails. In the primary care setting, 25% of all visits were found to involve skin disorders. All health care providers should have a fundamental understanding of the skin, our body's largest organ.

KEY TERMS

Primary lesions

Bulla	A circumscribed, elevated lesion that measures ≥ 1 cm and contains serous or hemorrhagic fluid (ie, a large blister).
Macule	A circumscribed, nonpalpable discoloration of the skin that measures < 1 cm in diameter.
Nodule	A palpable, solid, round or ellipsoidal lesion measuring ≥ 1 cm; it differs from a plaque in that it is more substantive in its vertical dimension compared with its breadth.
Papule	An elevated, solid lesion that measures < 1 cm.
Patch	A circumscribed, nonpalpable discoloration of the skin that measures ≥ 1 cm.
Petechiae	Nonblanching reddish macules representing extravascular deposits of blood, measuring ≤ 0.3 cm (less than the size of a pencil eraser).
Plaque	A palpable, solid lesion that measures ≥ 1 cm.
Purpura	Nonblanching reddish macules or papules representing extravascular deposits of blood, measuring > 0.3 cm.
Pustule	A lesion that contains pus; may be follicular (centered around a hair follicle) or nonfollicular.
Vesicle	A circumscribed, elevated lesion that measures < 1 cm and contains serous or hemorrhagic fluid (ie, a small blister).
Wheal	A round or annular (ring-like), edematous papule or plaque that is characteristically evanescent, disappearing within hours; may be surrounded by a flare of erythema (ie, a hive).

(continued)

KEY TERMS

Secondary lesions

Atrophy	A depression in the skin resulting from thinning of the epidermis, dermis, and/or subcutaneous fat.
Crust	A collection of dried blood, serum, and/or cellular debris.
Erosion	A focal loss of epidermis; does not penetrate below the dermal-epidermal junction and, therefore, can heal without scarring.
Lichenification	Thickening of the epidermis resulting from repeated rubbing, appearing as accentuation of the skin markings.
Scale	Excess dead epidermal cells; scale may be fine, silvery, greasy, desquamative, or adherent.
Scar	Abnormal formation of connective tissue, implying dermal damage.
Ulcer	A focal loss of full-thickness epidermis and partial to full-thickness dermis, which often heals with scarring.

Other

Nikolsky sign	In the area adjacent to a bulla, application of lateral pressure on normal-appearing epidermis produces further shearing of the skin.

ETIOLOGY

Inflammatory skin eruptions ("rashes") represent a heterogeneous group of disorders with etiologies ranging from drug reactions to infections (viral, bacterial, or fungal) to autoimmune attacks on the skin. The pathogenesis of many primary inflammatory dermatoses (eg, psoriasis) is unknown. A small subset of inflammatory dermatologic conditions is regularly encountered in clinical practice. For example, cutaneous drug eruptions represent the most frequent reason for inpatient dermatology consultation as well as the most common form of adverse drug reaction.[2] In a recent retrospective study, Ibia et al[3] found that "rashes" developed in 7% of 6000 pediatric outpatients treated with oral antibiotics. Chronic inflammatory skin conditions often seen by physicians include psoriasis, atopic dermatitis, stasis dermatitis, and acne vulgaris.

Differential Diagnosis

Ask the following questions (with or without a brief examination of the skin) to determine the morphologic pattern of the eruption.

Question	Morphologic pattern
Do you have a rash consisting of many small red spots and/or bumps?	Exanthematous eruptions
Do you have scaly spots and/or bumps on your skin?	Papulosquamous dermatoses
Do you have red, itchy, oozy, crusty, and scaly skin?	Eczematous dermatoses

Have blisters developed on your skin?	*Vesiculobullous disorders*
Do you ever have bumps on your skin that are filled with fluid?	
Do you have "pus-bumps" or pimples on your skin?	*Pustular dermatoses*
Do you have red or purple spots or bumps that do not fade when you press on them? (ie, lesions are nonblanching)	*Purpuras*
Do you have areas of red, hot skin?	*Erythemas*
Do you have spots on your skin that look like targets?	
Do you have hives?	*Urticaria*
Do you have bumps deep in your skin?	*Subcutaneous nodules*

Morphologic pattern	*Possible diagnoses*
Exanthematous eruptions	• *Morbilliform drug eruption (maculopapular eruption; accounts for ~ 70% of exanthematous eruptions in adults)* • *Drug rash with eosinophilia and systemic symptoms (DRESS)* • *Acute graft-versus-host disease (GVHD)* • *Scarlet fever* • *Viral exanthems, such as measles (rubeola), rubella (German measles), roseola (exanthem subitum), and erythema infectiosum (fifth disease) account for 80–90% of exanthematous eruptions in children*
Papulosquamous dermatoses	• *Lichen planus* • *Pityriasis rosea* • *Psoriasis* • *Seborrheic dermatitis* • *Lupus erythematosus* • *Dermatomyositis* • *Tinea corporis/cruris/faciei (ringworm, jock itch)* • *Secondary syphilis (lues)*
Eczematous dermatoses	• *Atopic dermatitis* • *Allergic contact dermatitis (20% of contact dermatitis)* • *Irritant contact dermatitis (80% of contact dermatitis)* • *Venous stasis dermatitis* • *Autosensitization dermatitis (id reaction)* • *Systemic contact dermatitis*
Vesiculobullous disorders	• *Stevens-Johnson syndrome/toxic epidermal necrolysis (SJS/TEN)* • *Bullous pemphigoid* • *Pemphigus vulgaris*

(continued)

Morphologic pattern	Possible diagnoses
	• Porphyria cutanea tarda (PCT)
	• Dermatitis herpetiformis
	• Phytophotodermatitis
	• Herpes simplex viral infection (cold sores, fever blisters)
	• Varicella (chickenpox)
	• Zoster (shingles)
	• Staphylococcal scalded skin syndrome (SSSS)
	• Bullous impetigo
Pustular dermatoses	• Acute generalized exanthematous pustulosis (AGEP)
	• Generalized pustular psoriasis (von Zumbusch)
	• Acne vulgaris
	• Steroid acne
	• Acne rosacea
	• Periorificial dermatitis
	• Folliculitis
	• Cutaneous candidiasis
	• Disseminated gonococcal infection
Purpuras	• Thrombocytopenic purpura
	• Schamberg pigmented purpuric dermatosis
	• Actinic purpura
	• Scurvy (vitamin C deficiency)
	• Leukocytoclastic vasculitis
	• Polyarteritis nodosa
	• Cryoglobulinemia, type I (monoclonal)
	• Cholesterol emboli
	• Calciphylaxis
	• Purpura fulminans
	• Rocky Mountain spotted fever
	• Acute bacterial endocarditis
	• Ecthyma gangrenosum
Erythemas and urticaria	• Phototoxic reactions
	• Urticaria
	• Erythema multiforme
	• Sweet syndrome
	• Erysipelas
	• Cellulitis
	• Necrotizing fasciitis ("flesh-eating bacteria" syndrome)
	• Lyme disease (erythema migrans)
	• Toxic shock syndrome (TSS)
Subcutaneous nodules	• Erythema nodosum
	• Nodular vasculitis (erythema induratum)
	• Lipodermatosclerosis
	• Pancreatic panniculitis
	• α_1-antitrypsin deficiency panniculitis
	• Lupus panniculitis

GETTING STARTED

- Due to the unique accessibility of the skin as an organ, the diagnosis of dermatologic diseases is highly dependent on the physical examination. However, the history plays a key role in putting the skin findings in the context of the whole patient, understanding the evolution of the disease process, and eventually arriving at the correct diagnosis. The history is especially important when the eruption is in a later stage or not active at the time of the evaluation, or when only secondary lesions are present (eg, bullae have ruptured and left erosions with "collarettes" of scale; or all lesions are excoriated and crusted).

- To elicit the history of a dermatologic condition, start with open-ended questions such as "tell me about what has been going on with your skin," and listen to the patient's story.

- With regard to the physical examination, in addition to recognizing the primary lesion and any secondary changes (see above), several other observations can serve as clues to help further categorize an eruption:
  - Color (eg, pink, red, purple, or violaceous)
  - Palpation (eg, soft, firm, or hard)
  - Margination (well- or ill-defined borders)
  - Shape/configuration of lesions (eg, annular [ring-like], linear, retiform [branching])
  - Location/distribution of lesions (eg, symmetric versus asymmetric, grouped versus scattered)

- A complete skin examination includes inspection of the entire cutaneous surface (including the palms and soles); the nails; the hair/scalp; and the oral, conjunctival, and genital mucosa.

INTERVIEW FRAMEWORK

Gather general information	• *When did you first develop this rash?* • *Have you had any similar rashes in the past?* • *On what part of the body did it start? Where did it spread to next?* • *How long does each individual spot or bump last?* • *Do you think the rash is getting better or worse?* • *Is the rash itchy? Is it painful or tender when you touch it?* • *Is there anything that makes the rash better or worse (eg, sun exposure)?* • *Have you been putting anything at all on the rash, such as lotions or ointments?*
Obtain a drug history. An eruption may be a reaction to a medication (including prescription, nonprescription, and herbal remedies) or to anything else that may have been ingested, inserted, or inhaled.	• *Determine the date of onset of the eruption (many occur within 1–2 weeks of starting a drug, but some have a delayed onset or even develop after a drug is discontinued)* • *Make a "drug chart" including all agents the patient was taking at the time of onset as well as during the prior 3 months, and the date each agent was started and stopped.* • *Determine whether the patient has any history of reactions to medications, and if so, what these reactions were.*

IDENTIFYING ALARM SYMPTOMS

Although the vast majority of skin conditions are not life threatening, it is extremely important to recognize the warning signs of a potentially serious eruption.

Serious Diagnoses

Morphologic pattern	Serious diagnoses
Exanthematous eruptions	DRESS GVHD
Papulosquamous dermatoses	Erythrodermic psoriasis Systemic lupus erythematosus Dermatomyositis
Eczematous dermatoses	Erythrodermic dermatitis
Vesiculobullous disorders	SJS/TEN Pemphigus vulgaris Disseminated herpes simplex viral infection Disseminated zoster
Pustular dermatoses	Generalized pustular psoriasis Disseminated gonococcal infection
Purpuras	Leukocytoclastic vasculitis with systemic involvement Polyarteritis nodosa Calciphylaxis Purpura fulminans Rocky Mountain spotted fever Acute bacterial endocarditis Ecthyma gangrenosum
Erythemas	Urticaria/angioedema associated with anaphylaxis Erysipelas Necrotizing fasciitis TSS
Subcutaneous nodules	Pancreatic panniculitis

Alarm signs and symptoms	Serious causes	Benign causes
Painful skin	SJS/TEN Pemphigus vulgaris Pustular psoriasis Calciphylaxis Necrotizing fasciitis	SSSS Phototoxic reaction
Confluent erythema (bright red skin all over)	DRESS Acute GVHD TEN TSS	Severe morbilliform drug eruption SSSS AGEP Scarlet fever
Erythroderma (redness and scaling involving > 90% of the skin)	Drug eruption (20%) Severe psoriasis (20%) Cutaneous T-cell lymphoma (8%) Atopic dermatitis (9%)	(Erythroderma in itself is a potentially serious condition)

	Contact dermatitis (6%) Autosensitization dermatitis Seborrheic dermatitis (4%)	
Dusky or grayish-purple skin (signals impending necrosis)	*SJS/TEN* *Various causes of retiform purpura (including calciphylaxis, purpura fulminans, and polyarteritis nodosa)* *Ecthyma gangrenosum* *Necrotizing fasciitis*	
Widespread blistering or sloughing skin	*SJS/TEN* *Severe pemphigus vulgaris*	*SSSS*
Painful erosions of the mucous membranes	*SJS/TEN* *Pemphigus vulgaris*	*Erythema multiforme* *Herpes simplex viral infection with primary gingivostomatitis*
Palpable purpura (red or purple, nonblanching papules)	*Leukocytoclastic vasculitis with systemic involvement* *Rocky Mountain spotted fever*	*Leukocytoclastic vasculitis with involvement limited to the skin*
Facial swelling	*DRESS* *Acute cutaneous lupus erythematosus* *Dermatomyositis (particularly if periocular)* *Angioedema*	*AGEP*
Swollen mouth or tongue, difficulty swallowing, tingling of the top of the mouth, and/or itching of the palms and soles	*Anaphylaxis*	
High fever (> 40 °C)	*DRESS* *SJS/TEN* *Purpura fulminans* *Rocky Mountain spotted fever* *Acute bacterial endocarditis* *TSS*	*Scarlet fever* *Roseola* *AGEP*
Arthritis	*Systemic lupus erythematosus* *Disseminated gonococcal infection* *Leukocytoclastic vasculitis with systemic involvement* *Pancreatic panniculitis*	*Rubella (unless pregnant)* *Erythema infectiosum* *Psoriasis* *Leukocytoclastic vasculitis with involvement limited to the skin* *Erythema nodosum*
Shortness of breath or difficulty breathing	*Anaphylaxis*	

(continued)

Alarm signs and symptoms	Serious causes
Hypotension	*Purpura fulminans*
	Ecthyma gangrenosum
	Anaphylaxis
	TSS

FOCUSED QUESTIONS

Exanthematous eruptions	*Think*
Have you started any new medications in the past 2 weeks?	*Morbilliform drug eruption*
Have you had a bone marrow or peripheral blood stem cell transplant within the past 3 months or recently stopped post-transplant immunosuppressive medications?	*GVHD*
Have you recently had a sore throat, high fever, and headache?	*Scarlet fever*
Did you have cough, runny nose, and red eyes just before developing this rash?	*Measles*
Has your child just had a high fever for several days, during which he or she otherwise looked well?	*Roseola*
Did your child have bright red cheeks, followed by lacy redness on the arms that is most noticeable when he or she is hot?	*Erythema infectiosum*
Are your immunizations up to date?	*If not, consider measles or rubella*
Papulosquamous dermatoses	*Think*
Do you have itchy, purple, flat-topped bumps on your wrists or shins that you rub frequently?	*Lichen planus*
Do you have an itchy rash in areas exposed to the sun? Have you started a new medication within the past year?	*Lichenoid drug eruption*
Did you develop a single scaly pink spot on your trunk, followed by an eruption of multiple similar but smaller spots?	*Pityriasis rosea*
Do you have well-defined areas of thick, red skin covered with silvery scale on your elbows, knees, or scalp? Are the joints of your hands swollen and painful? Do you have a family history of psoriasis?	*Psoriasis ± psoriatic arthritis*
Have you had redness and greasy scaling of your eyebrows, around your nose, and in/around your ears for many years? Do you have dandruff?	*Seborrheic dermatitis*
Are you particularly sensitive to the sun? Have you noticed redness of your cheeks and the top of your nose in a "butterfly" shape?	*Systemic lupus erythematosus*
Do you have difficulty combing your hair or climbing stairs? Have you been ever been diagnosed with any kind of cancer?	*Dermatomyositis*
Do you have pets, particularly a kitten?	*Tinea corporis*

Do you have a history of a genital ulcer in the past 6 months?
Have you had multiple sexual partners in the past year?
Have you had unprotected sexual intercourse?

Secondary syphilis

Eczematous dermatoses

Think

Is your rash extremely itchy?
Have you had itchy rashes since childhood?
Do you or does anyone in your family have eczema, hay fever, or asthma?

Atopic dermatitis

Did you do yard work or other outdoor activities a day or 2 before the rash developed? Is the rash extremely itchy?

Allergic contact dermatitis due to poison ivy

Do you have an itchy rash on your lower legs?
Are your legs often swollen at the end of the day?
Do you have varicose veins?

Venous stasis dermatitis

Vesiculobullous disorders

Think

Did your skin suddenly become painful?
Do you have sores in your mouth?
Have you started a new medication in the past 2 months?

SJS/TEN

Did you have itchy pink bumps/spots before blisters developed?

Bullous pemphigoid

Did you have sores In your mouth before blisters developed on your skin?

Pemphigus vulgaris

Do you have fragile skin and blistering, particularly on the backs of your hands, which is worse after exposure to the sun?

Porphyria cutanea tarda

Do you have recurrent lesions of the lip or buttock that are preceded by a day of itching/tingling/burning?

Herpes simplex viral infection

Were your lesions preceded by several days of intense pain, pain with slight touch by clothing, or tingling?

Zoster

Is your child febrile, extremely irritable, and complaining that his skin hurts (especially in the folds)?

SSSS

Pustular dermatoses

Think

Do you a fever and painful skin?
Do you have a history of psoriasis?

Pustular psoriasis

Are you taking prednisone or other systemic corticosteroids?

Steroid acne

Do you use corticosteroid creams or ointments on your face?

Steroid rosacea or perioral dermatitis

Does your face flush easily when you drink hot liquids?

Acne rosacea

Have you been in a hot tub in the past week?

Pseudomonas folliculitis

Is your rash extremely itchy? Do you have HIV?

Eosinophilic folliculitis

Do you have diabetes or perspire excessively?
Has the area involved recently been under occlusion?

Cutaneous candidiasis

(continued)

Pustular dermatoses	***Think***
Are you taking antibiotics, prednisone, or other systemic corticosteroids?	*Cutaneous candidiasis*
Have you had multiple sexual partners in the past year? Have you had unprotected sexual intercourse? Do you have painful, swollen joints?	*Disseminated gonococcal infection*

Purpuras	***Think***
Do you have nosebleeds, bleeding gums, or excessive bleeding with your menses?	*Thrombocytopenic purpura*
Do you develop bruises and tearing with minimal trauma to your skin? Are you taking prednisone or other systemic corticosteroids?	*Actinic purpura*
Have you had fevers, pain or swelling of your joints, severe spasms of abdominal pain, or bloody stools or urine?	*Leukocytoclastic vasculitis/ Henoch-Schönlein purpura*
Have you started anticoagulant therapy within the past few months? Have you recently had a cardiac or other arterial catheterization or thrombolytic therapy?	*Cholesterol emboli*
Do you have renal failure? Are you on dialysis?	*Calciphylaxis*
Did you develop a severe headache, fever, and generalized achiness 2–4 days before your rash started? Have you had a tick bite or spent much time outdoors in the past 2 weeks?	*Rocky Mountain spotted fever*
Have you had high fevers and shaking chills? Have you used injection drugs?	*Acute bacterial endocarditis*

Erythemas and urticaria	***Think***
Have you recently been out in the sun? Are you taking any medications? (Doxycycline and ciprofloxacin are common culprits.)	*Phototoxic reaction*
Is your rash itchy? How long does each individual spot last? Have you started any new medications in the past week? Have you had a recent cold or sore throat?	*Urticaria (if individual lesions last < 24 hours)*
Have you had a recent cold sore/fever blister (ie, herpes simplex viral infection)? Have you ever had spots like this before?	*Erythema multiforme*
Did you have a sudden onset of fever, chills, and a headache? Is the red area spreading and extremely tender?	*Erysipelas*
Do you have diabetes? How much do you drink? Do you use intravenous drugs? Have you had cellulitis of this area before?	*Cellulitis*
Was the area extremely tender previously, but now you can't feel when it is touched?	*Necrotizing fasciitis*
Has the border of the lesion been expanding outward? Have you had a tick bite or spent much time outdoors in the past 2 weeks? Was the tick on your body for > 24 hours?	*Erythema migrans*

Have you recently undergone a surgical procedure, given birth, had a skin infection, or used contraceptive sponges or other vaginally inserted devices?	TSS
Do you have a fever, muscle aches, a sore throat, vomiting, or diarrhea?	
Subcutaneous nodules	**Think**
Do you have tender bumps on your shins that develop in crops and leave a bruise-like spot when they resolve?	*Erythema nodosum*
Have you had fevers and joint pains? (These symptoms may be associated with erythema nodosum, particularly in the setting of sarcoidosis)	
Have you recently had a sore throat or a diagnosis of strep throat?	
Do you take oral contraceptive pills?	
Do you have inflammatory bowel disease or chronic diarrhea?	
Have you recently traveled to the southwestern US? (Coccidioidomycosis is endemic in this area.)	

DIAGNOSTIC APPROACH

As noted above, the first step is to classify the morphologic pattern of the eruption. This entails careful visual inspection and palpation to identify the primary lesion and its distribution, with particular attention to whether or not the lesions blanch with pressure and whether any lesions contain fluid. Recognition of secondary changes, such as the presence of scale or crust, is also important, and clinicians should always pay particular attention to alarm features. Once clues from the history and physical examination have been used to determine the overall pattern of the eruption, the focused questions help highlight distinguishing features of the potential diagnoses within each category.

CAVEATS

- An early eruption of erythema multiforme that does not yet have obviously targetoid lesions may resemble a morbilliform drug eruption.
- Morbilliform drug eruptions often become purpuric on the lower extremities.
- Tinea corporis or faciei that has been treated with topical corticosteroids may have an atypical appearance and lack scale (tinea incognito).
- Asymmetric linear streaks or bizarre shapes often signal an external insult to the skin as seen in allergic and irritant contact dermatitis.
- Patients with venous stasis dermatitis, particularly those with venous ulcers that have been treated with topical antibiotics, often have a superimposed allergic contact dermatitis and may develop an autosensitization (id) eruption.
- Determination of whether bullae are tense or flaccid and whether the Nikolsky sign is positive can help classify vesiculobullous eruptions (see Diagnostic Approach: Inflammatory Dermatoses ["Rashes"]).
- Zoster involving the tip of the nose should raise concern about possible ocular involvement.
- Generalized pustular psoriasis may be precipitated by rapid withdrawal of systemic corticosteroids.
- Not all purpura is due to the same process that caused the lesion itself; secondary purpura often results from venous stasis (particularly on the lower legs), trauma (eg, due to scratching pruritic primary lesions), or thrombocytopenia (usually platelet count < 50,000/μL).

- Early lesions of leukocytoclastic vasculitis and Rocky Mountain spotted fever are often partially blanching.
- Tracing the edge of a lesion and noting migration/resolution within a few hours can help confirm the diagnosis of urticaria.
- When evaluating patients with a history of urticaria, it is important to determine whether they develop wheals upon stroking the skin (dermographism, a form of pressure-induced urticaria that could represent the cause of the eruption).
- Acute lipodermatosclerosis may mimic cellulitis; involvement of both legs and localization to the area above the medial malleolus are suggestive of the former diagnosis.

PROGNOSIS

It is not possible to categorically apply a prognosis to such a heterogeneous group of skin diseases. Although the majority of dermatologic disorders have an overall "benign" prognosis, it is important to remember that diseases such as pemphigus vulgaris, TEN, acute GVHD, and Rocky Mountain spotted fever may have a high mortality rate if not identified and treated properly. In addition, the psychological impact of skin disease is often profound.

REFERENCES

1. Feldman SR, Fleischer AB Jr, Wolford PM, White R, Byington R. Increasing utilization of dermatologists by managed care: an analysis of the National Ambulatory Medical Care Survey, 1990-1994. *J Am Acad Dermatol.* 1997;37:784–788.
2. Nigen S, Knowles SR, Shear NH. Drug eruptions: approaching the diagnosis of drug-induced skin diseases. *J Drugs Dermatol.* 2003;2:278–299.
3. Ibia EO, Schwartz RH, Wiedermann BL. Antibiotic rashes in children: a survey in a private practice setting. *Arch Dermatol.* 2000;136:849–854.

SUGGESTED READING

Bolognia J, Jorizzo J, Rapini R, eds. *Dermatology.* Elsevier, Ltd. 2003.

Callen J, ed. *Dermatologic Signs of Internal Disease.* Harcourt Brace Jovanovich. 2003.

Williams H, Bigby M, Diepgen T, et al (editors). *Evidence-based Dermatology.* BMJ Publishing Group. 2003.

Diagnostic Approach: Inflammatory Dermatoses ("Rashes")

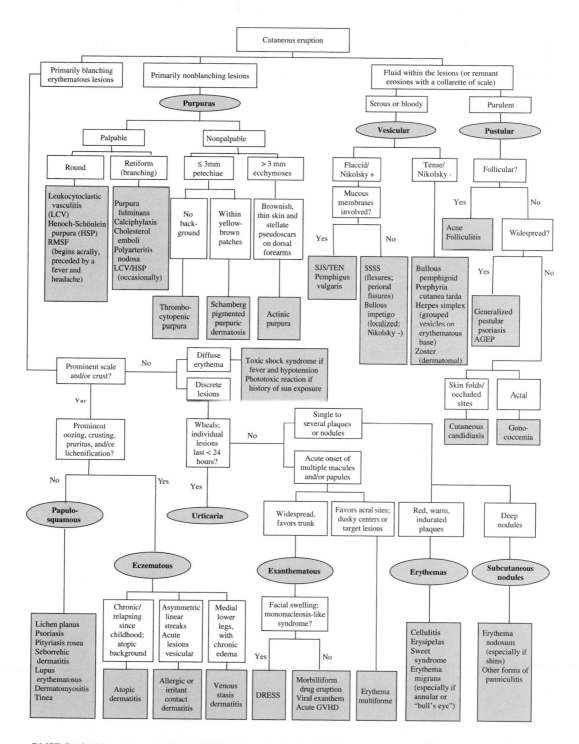

RMSF, Rocky Mountain spotted fever; DRESS, drug rash with eosinophilia and systemic symptoms; GVHD, graft-versus-host disease; SJS, Stevens-Johnson syndrome; TEN, toxic epidermal necrolysis; SSSS, staphylococcal scalded skin syndrome; AGEP, acute generalized exanthematous pustulosis.

SECTION V
Respiratory System

Cough

Pablo E. Molina, MD, & Antonio Anzueto, MD

Cough is the fifth most common complaint encountered by office-based health care practitioners.[1] Cough is a mechanical reflex that involves a deep inspiration, which increases lung volume; followed by muscle contraction against a closed glottis; and then sudden opening of the glottis. The cough reflex helps clear mucus, secretions, and foreign objects from the airway. Although cough may often only be a minor annoyance, it can also be a sign of severe underlying disease.

Acute cough is usually a self-limited condition lasting less than 3 weeks. The most frequent causes of acute cough include upper respiratory tract infections (ie, the common cold, acute viral or bacterial sinusitis, *Bordetella pertussis* infection); lower respiratory tract infections (ie, acute viral or bacterial bronchitis, community-acquired pneumonia); acute exacerbation of chronic obstructive pulmonary disease (COPD); allergic rhinitis, rhinitis due to environmental irritants; and irritation to the bronchial tree by cigarette smoke, fumes, or other chemical products such as cleaners. In elderly patients, acute cough may be the manifestation of left ventricular failure (chronic heart failure) or chronic aspiration.

Chronic cough is defined as persistent cough lasting longer than 3 weeks and is the most common reason for referral to a lung specialist.[2–4] While patients with acute cough usually have a benign cause, chronic cough may occasionally be a symptom of a life-threatening disease.

A careful cough history will allow clinicians to establish a correct diagnosis in most cases, will limit use of unnecessary and expensive diagnostic testing, and will lead to proper treatment to reduce the symptoms. Two general approaches to history taking exist. First, evaluate for alarm features that should prompt consideration of a serious cause of cough. Second, determine the duration of cough, which will narrow the differential diagnosis.[2–4]

KEY TERMS

Acute bronchitis	*Acute inflammation of the bronchial tree more frequently seen in patients without underlying lung disease and is produced by a viral infection.*
Acute cough	*Episodes of cough lasting less than 3 weeks.*
Asthma	*Disease characterized by episodic bronchospasm and excessive thick mucous secretions most frequently related to an allergic condition.*
Bronchiectasis	*Disorder characterized by dilated bronchial walls with chronic excessive sputum production.*
Chronic bronchitis	*Included in the spectrum of COPD. Presence of chronic productive cough for 3 months in each of 2 successive years.*
Chronic cough	*Persistent cough lasting longer than 3 weeks.*

(continued)

KEY TERMS

Chronic obstructive pulmonary disease (COPD)[5]	*Disease state characterized by airflow limitation that is not fully reversible. The airflow limitation is usually both progressive and associated with an abnormal inflammatory response of the lungs to noxious particles or gases.*
Gastroesophageal reflux disease (GERD)[6]	*Disorder characterized by reflux of the gastric contents into the esophagus, upper airway, and tracheobronchial tree (lung).*
Hemoptysis	*Cough with expectoration of bloody sputum or blood.*
Postnasal drip syndrome	*Syndrome characterized by abundant secretions from the upper respiratory tract, which drip into the oropharynx and tracheobronchial tree, causing cough.*

ETIOLOGY

The most common causes of chronic cough are postnasal drip syndrome, asthma, and GERD. Chronic cough may also be related to a patient's occupation or habits. Up to 25% of smokers have chronic cough related to the irritant effects of cigarette smoke, so-called "smoker's cough." Patients with heavy exposure to pollutants (sulfur dioxide, nitrous oxide, particulate matter) and dusts may also have chronic cough.[2–7]

Differential Diagnosis	Prevalence[a]
Chronic allergic rhinitis or postnasal drip syndrome	41%
Asthma	24%
GERD[6]	21%
COPD including chronic bronchitis	5%
Bronchiectasis	4%
Lung cancer	< 2%
Related to medication use (angiotensin-converting enzyme [ACE] inhibitors, β-blockers)	5–25%
Idiopathic and/or psychological cough	< 5%

[a]Among patients with chronic cough in the ambulatory setting.[3,4]

GETTING STARTED

- History is the most important aspect of the evaluation of cough.
- Let the patient talk about the cough in his or her own words.
- One quarter of patients with chronic cough may have more than one cause identified.
- The history taking should be performed completely even after a presumed cause is found.

Open-ended questions

Why did you come to see me today for the cough?

Tell me about when and how the cough began.

Do you have any other symptoms associated with the cough?

Tips for effective interviewing

- *Determine the patient's agenda for the visit.*
- *Listen to the story and do not interrupt.*
- *Consider several etiologies for cough during the interview.*
- *Reassure patients when possible.*

INTERVIEW FRAMEWORK

- The first goal is to determine whether the cough is associated with alarm symptoms that require immediate attention.
- Then, determine whether the cough is acute or chronic.
- In your review of systems, pay special attention to the upper and lower respiratory tract, cardiovascular system, and digestive tract (esophagus).
- Ask about smoking habits and environmental and occupational exposures.
- Take a detailed list of current and prior medications.
- Review the past medical history including history of previous allergies, asthma, sinusitis, recent respiratory infections, tuberculosis exposure, coronary artery disease, and esophageal disease.
- Inquire about cough characteristics using the following cardinal symptom features:
    –Onset
    –Duration
    –Frequency
    –Associated symptoms
    –Precipitating and/or alleviating factors
    –Change in frequency over time

IDENTIFYING ALARM SYMPTOMS[2]

- Serious causes of cough are rare.
- After the open-ended portion of the history, ask about alarm symptoms to assess for the possibility of a serious cause and determine the speed of subsequent evaluation.
- There are no published data available to calculate likelihood ratios for predicting serious causes for the symptoms listed below.

Alarm symptoms	Serious causes	Benign causes
Cough with hemoptysis	*Lung cancer* *Tuberculosis* *Pulmonary embolism* *Pneumonia*	*Acute viral or bacterial bronchitis* *COPD exacerbation*
Cough, fever, and purulent sputum production	*Pneumonia* *Lung abscess*	*Acute sinusitis*
Cough with wheezing and shortness of breath	*Asthma* *COPD exacerbation* *Heart failure*	*Acute bronchitis*

(continued)

Alarm symptoms	Serious causes	Benign causes
Cough with chest pain	Pulmonary embolism Acute coronary syndrome (angina pectoris)	COPD exacerbation
Cough with excessive chronic sputum production	Bronchiectasis Lung abscess Lung cancer	Chronic bronchitis Chronic sinusitis
Cough and unintentional weight loss	Lung cancer Tuberculosis Lung abscess	COPD
Cough, dyspnea, and lower extremity edema	Congestive heart failure Pulmonary embolism	

FOCUSED QUESTIONS

After hearing the patient's story and considering potential alarm symptoms, ask the following questions to narrow the differential diagnosis.

Questions	Think about
Do you have postnasal drip?	Allergic, vasomotor, or nonallergic rhinitis Acute nasopharyngitis Acute or chronic sinusitis
Do you have wheezing?	Asthma (cough-variant asthma presents as episodes of cough with or without wheezing); congestive heart failure, pulmonary embolism
Do you have heartburn? Have you noticed a food or acid/bitter taste in your mouth?	Chronic cough is the only symptom in 75% of patients with GERD. Gastric acid reflux to the lower third of the esophagus may trigger cough.
Have you had recent flu-like symptoms with significant cough?	Postinfectious cough should be considered in patients with persistent symptoms after a viral infection (ie, the flu).
When did you start your ACE inhibitor? Have you taken another ACE inhibitor in the past?	ACE inhibitor–induced cough is more common in females, is not dose-related, and can be produced by any formulation. Cough usually improves after a drug holiday of 1–4 days, based on the half-life of the compound.
Are you under severe stress? Do you know if your cough is present during sleep?	Idiopathic or psychogenic cough is a diagnosis of exclusion. Usually occurs in adolescents.
Quality	**Think about**
Do you have dry cough?	GERD Irritant cough Postviral infection Interstitial lung disease (pulmonary fibrosis)

Do you need to clear your throat frequently?	Postnasal drip syndrome Allergic, vasomotor, or nonallergic rhinitis

Time course — **Think about**

Is this cough worsening over time?	Bronchitis Asthma Congestive heart failure
Is your cough worse during a particular season?	Postnasal drip syndrome Asthma
Has your cough persisted after having flu-like symptoms?	Postinfectious cough Postnasal drip syndrome

Associated symptoms — **Think about**

Do you cough up any sputum?	Pneumonia Asthma Bronchitis Postnasal drip syndrome Bronchiectasis Sinusitis Smoker's cough Congestive heart failure
Does your sputum look purulent or yellow-green?	Bronchitis Sinusitis Pneumonia Bronchiectasis COPD exacerbation Tuberculosis Postnasal drip syndrome
Does your sputum look clear or whitish?	Asthma Postnasal drip syndrome Smoker's cough Bronchitis
Do you cough up large quantities of purulent sputum?	Bronchiectasis Pneumonia Lung abscess
Do you have cough with dyspnea on exertion?	Asthma Congestive heart failure COPD Pneumonitis
Is your cough associated with wheezing?	Asthma Congestive heart failure
Do you have associated hoarseness?	GERD Chronic laryngitis Laryngeal nodules/polyps Postnasal drip syndrome

(continued)

Associated symptoms	*Think about*
Do you have a burning feeling in your throat at night or early in the morning?	*GERD* *Allergic rhinitis (with mouth breathing)*
Do you have frequent heartburn or a sour taste in your mouth?	*GERD*
Do you feel frequent secretions in the back of your throat?	*Postnasal drip syndrome* *Sinusitis*
Is your cough seasonal?	*Asthma* *Postnasal drip syndrome* *Allergic rhinitis*
Have you ever been diagnosed with nasal allergies or allergic rhinitis?	*Postnasal drip syndrome*
Do you have chronic bad breath or halitosis?	*Chronic sinusitis*
Do you have chronic facial pain?	*Chronic sinusitis*
Do you have to sleep with more than one pillow (orthopnea) or do you wake up choking or very dyspneic (paroxysmal nocturnal dyspnea)?	*Congestive heart failure* *Sleep apnea*

Modifying factors	*Think about*
Do you get coughing spells during or after exercising?	*Asthma* *Postnasal drip syndrome* *Allergic or vasomotor rhinitis*
Do you get coughing spells when exposed to cold air or cold weather?	*Asthma* *Postnasal drip syndrome* *Allergic or vasomotor rhinitis*
Does your cough worsen when you lie down?	*Postnasal drip syndrome* *GERD* *Congestive heart failure* *Bronchiectasis* *Acute bronchitis*
Does your cough worsen at night?	*Asthma* *GERD* *Congestive heart failure*
Is your cough precipitated by changes in position?	*Bronchiectasis* *Congestive heart failure*
Does your cough improve with over-the-counter antihistamines?	*Allergic rhinitis* *Postnasal drip syndrome*

DIAGNOSTIC APPROACH[7]

The first step in evaluating a patient with cough is to assess for any of the alarm symptoms previously described. Then, the clinician must define the duration of the symptoms. While most cases of acute cough are related to viral infections and other benign diagnoses, serious causes of cough may also present acutely. Chronic cough (lasting longer than 3 weeks) is usually due to postnasal drip syndrome, allergic rhinitis, asthma, gastroesophageal reflux, chronic bronchitis, or drugs. Additional diagnostic procedures may be required to identify the cause of chronic cough.

Diagnostic studies to identify the cause of cough include chest radiography, sinus radiography, pulmonary function tests, barium esophagography, 24-hour esophageal pH monitoring, differential white blood cell count, and occasionally invasive procedures such as direct laryngoscopy or fiberoptic bronchoscopy.

CAVEATS

- Chronic cough is often caused by multiple and simultaneously contributing causes.
- Two of the most common causes of chronic cough are nonpulmonary diseases (GERD and postnasal drip syndrome).[4,6]
- GERD, postnasal drip syndrome, and asthma account for 90% of chronic cough in nonsmoking patients with normal chest radiographs.[3,4,6]
- Chronic cough occurs in 5–25% of patients taking ACE inhibitors.
- Patients with alarm symptoms (eg, lower extremity swelling, progressive dyspnea, orthopnea, wheezing, hemoptysis, or fever) should be evaluated rapidly.

PROGNOSIS

- Specific therapy is successful in eliminating chronic cough in most patients with asthma, postnasal drip syndrome, and gastroesophageal reflux.
- Resolution of chronic cough due to other etiologies depends on the therapy and prognosis of the underlying disease.[4]
- Complications of chronic cough include headache, pneumothorax, pneumomediastinum, syncope, urinary incontinence, trauma to chest muscles, rib fractures, and psychological fear of public appearances.

REFERENCES

1. Braman SS, Corrao WM. Chronic cough. Diagnosis and treatment. *Prim Care.* 1985;12:217–225.
2. Irwin RS, Curley FJ, French CL. Chronic cough. The spectrum and frequency of causes, key components of the diagnostic evaluation, and outcome of specific therapy. *Am Rev Respir Dis.* 1990;141:640–647.
3. Mello CJ, Irwin RS, Curley FJ. Predictive values of the character, timing and complications of chronic cough in diagnosing its cause. *Arch Intern Med.* 1996;156:997–1003.
4. Smyrnios NA, Irwin RS, Curley FJ, French CL. From a prospective study of chronic cough: diagnostic and therapeutic aspects in older adults. *Arch Intern Med.* 1998;158:1222–1228.
5. Pauwels RA, Buist AS, Calverley PM, et al. Global strategy for the diagnoses, management, and prevention of chronic obstructive pulmonary disease. NHLBI/WHO Global initiative for Chronic Obstructive Pulmonary Disease (GOLD) workshop summary. *Am J Respir Crit Care Med.* 2001;163:1256–1276.
6. Irwin RS, French CL, Curley FJ, et al. Chronic cough due to gastroesophageal reflux. Clinical diagnostic, and pathogenetic aspects. *Chest.* 1993;104:1511–1517.
7. Pratter MR, Bartter T, Akers S, Dubois J. An algorithmic approach to chronic cough. *Ann Intern Med.* 1993;119:977–983.

SUGGESTED READING

Goroll AH, Mulley AG. Primary Care Medicine. Chapter 4. *Evaluation of Chronic Cough.* 4th edition. Lippincott Williams & Wilkins; 2000:271–276.

Irwin RS, Madison M. The diagnosis and treatment of cough. *N Engl J Med.* 2000;343:1715–1721.

Mladenovic J. Primary Care Secrets. Chapter XII. *Cough and Sputum Production.* 2nd edition. Hanely & Belfus, Inc./Mosby. 1999:377–381.

Diagnostic Approach: Cough

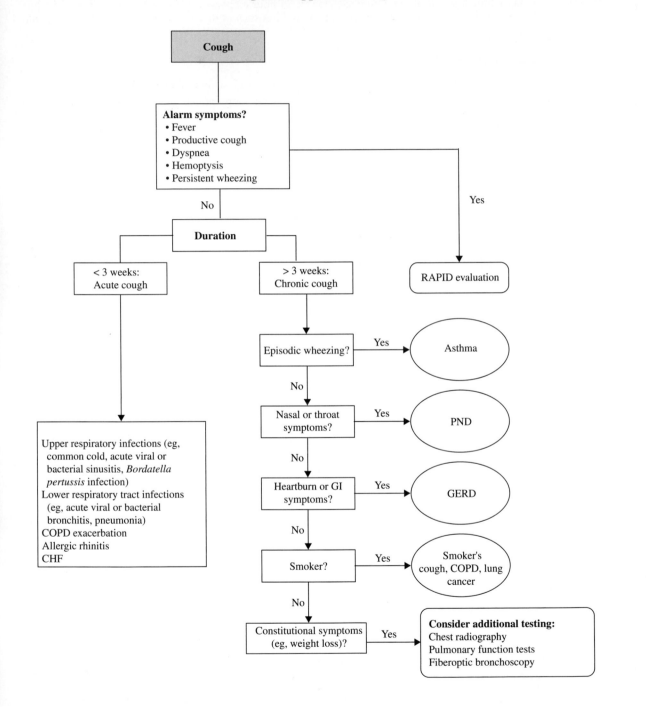

CHF, congestive heart failure; COPD, chronic obstructive pulmonary disease; GERD, gastroesophageal reflux disease;
GI, gastrointestinal; PND, postnasal drip syndrome.

Dyspnea

22

Catherine R. Lucey, MD

Shortness of breath, or dyspnea, is the sensation of uncomfortable breathing. This breathing discomfort may reflect an increased awareness of breathing or the sense that breathing is different, difficult, or inadequate. Dyspnea usually suggests pulmonary or cardiac disease but can also be the presenting symptom of metabolic derangements, hematologic disorders, toxic ingestions, psychiatric conditions, or simple deconditioning.

Dyspnea can be classified based on the primary physiologic derangement:

- Primary pulmonary causes
- Primary cardiac causes
- Neuromuscular disease
- Metabolic causes (anemia or acidosis)
- Functional dyspnea (panic disorders)
- Deconditioning

KEY TERMS

Cardiomyopathies	A heterogeneous group of conditions causing heart failure. Etiologies include coronary artery disease, cardiac valvular disease, hypertension, and others.
Dyspnea	The sensation of increased awareness of or increased difficulty with breathing.
Interstitial lung disease	A heterogeneous set of conditions characterized by hypoxia and evidence of interstitial abnormalities on chest radiographs. Examples include sarcoidosis, idiopathic pulmonary fibrosis, rheumatoid lung, and some occupational lung diseases.
Orthopnea	The feeling that breathing is easier when sitting up than when lying down. Orthopnea is typically described in terms of the number of pillows the patient must use to feel comfortable breathing.
Paroxysmal nocturnal dyspnea (PND)	Breathing difficulty that arises some time after the patient has lain down to rest or sleep. The patient often describes the need to sit up abruptly to breathe and frequently finds more relief sitting at an open window.
Platypnea	The sensation that breathing is more comfortable when lying down rather than sitting up.

ETIOLOGY

The purpose of breathing is to meet the metabolic demands of the body. Any condition that increases the work of breathing (eg, airway obstruction, changes in lung compliance, or respiratory muscle weakness) or increases respiratory drive (eg, hypoxia or acidosis) may result in dyspnea.[1] In addition, dyspnea may result from or be exacerbated by primary psychological conditions (eg, anxiety disorders).

The differential diagnosis of dyspnea depends on the duration of the symptom and the clinical setting. Conditions associated with acute dyspnea (developing over hours to a few days) are outlined under alarm conditions. There is no literature documenting the prevalence of different causes of acute dyspnea.

Conditions associated with more insidious development of dyspnea are outlined below. In patients referred to a pulmonary clinic for evaluation of chronic, unexplained dyspnea, 67% suffered from asthma, chronic obstructive pulmonary disease (COPD), interstitial lung disease, or myocardial dysfunction.[2]

Differential Diagnosis of Chronic Dyspnea

Cardiac

Cardiomyopathies

Myocardial ischemia

Primary pulmonary hypertension

Pericardial disease

Pulmonary

Asthma

COPD

Interstitial lung diseases

Chronic pneumonia

Chronic pulmonary emboli

Pulmonary neoplasm (primary or metastatic)

Pleural effusions

Miscellaneous

Deconditioning

Anemia

Neuromuscular disease

Psychiatric

Panic attack, anxiety disorders

GETTING STARTED

Begin by assessing the patient's stability. If the patient is unable to talk or complete a full sentence without pausing for a deep breath, move quickly to stabilize the patient. Return to the interview after the patient is more comfortable.

Open-ended questions	**Tips for effective interviewing**
Tell me about your problem with breathing.	Allow the patient to tell the story in his or her own words. You may need to help with close-ended questions.
How long has this shortness of breath been going on?	The differential diagnosis varies dramatically depending on the time course.

INTERVIEW FRAMEWORK

The clinician should focus on the following elements:

- Duration of symptoms
- Detailed description of the patient's dyspnea

- Associated signs and symptoms
- Risk factors for conditions causing dyspnea from the past medical, social, and family histories.

IDENTIFYING ALARM SYMPTOMS

Most causes of dyspnea are serious. Patients with chronic dyspnea who are able to talk comfortably may have serious underlying disease, but the physician has ample time to thoroughly evaluate the patient. Patients with acute or severe dyspnea require a more rapid diagnostic evaluation, since their condition may worsen quickly.

Causes of acute dyspnea	Comment
Congestive heart failure (acute or flash pulmonary edema)	Almost 50% of patients with flash pulmonary edema will require revascularization for coronary artery disease. Other causes include acute valvular insufficiency and severe hypertension.[3]
Acute pulmonary embolism (PE)	Ninety percent of patients with PE have dyspnea or tachypnea; 20% have dyspnea alone.[4]
Anaphylaxis	Up to 15% of residents in the US may be susceptible to anaphylaxis.[5] Fifty percent of patients will have dyspnea associated with anaphylaxis.[6]
Aspiration	Dyspnea due to aspiration generally begins abruptly within hours of the event.
Cardiac tamponade	Tamponade is associated with dyspnea, chest pain, and lightheadedness.
Acute pneumonia	The prevalence of pneumonia in healthy patients presenting with acute cough is approximately 6–7%.[7] The prevalence is higher in populations with comorbid illness.
Respiratory muscle weakness	Approximately 40% of patients with acute Guillain-Barré syndrome will require assisted ventilation because of muscular weakness.[8]
Spontaneous pneumothorax	The lifetime risk of spontaneous pneumothorax in men is 12% for heavy smokers and < 0.001% for nonsmokers.[9]
Metabolic acidosis (diabetic ketoacidosis, aspirin overdose, lactic acidosis)	Patients with a severe metabolic acidosis compensate by hyperventilating. This may cause dyspnea or tachypnea without dyspnea.

Alarm symptoms	Serious causes	Positive likelihood ratio (LR+)	Benign causes
Sharp, unilateral chest pain that increases with respiration	Spontaneous pneumothorax PE	66% of patients with PE will have pleuritic pain.[4]	Chest wall muscle spasm (Tietze syndrome)

(continued)

Alarm symptoms	Serious causes	Positive likelihood ratio (LR+)	Benign causes
Lip swelling, hives, or wheezing	Anaphylaxis or angioedema	88% of patients with anaphylaxis will have hives; 50% will have wheezing or dyspnea.[6]	
Substernal chest pressure	Acute myocardial ischemia or infarction		Esophageal spasm
Pink, frothy sputum	Cardiogenic pulmonary edema		
Fever and sputum production	Acute pneumonia	LR+ 1.7–2.1 for fever[10]	Bronchitis
Fever and signs of serious infection or shock	Acute respiratory distress syndrome		
Lower extremity weakness or neuromuscular weakness	Guillain-Barré syndrome Myasthenia gravis		
Known or suspected diabetes or renal failure	Diabetic ketoacidosis or metabolic acidosis		
Suicidality, known or suspected arthritis	Aspirin overdose		Panic disorder

FOCUSED QUESTIONS

To narrow the differential diagnosis of dyspnea, the physician should attempt to characterize the patient's dyspnea-related illness. The following questions should be used to outline the time course, precisely describe the dyspnea, and identify predisposing conditions and associated symptoms.

If answered in the affirmative	Think about
Time course	
Does your shortness of breath come and go while you are at rest?	Acute or recurrent PE
Risk factors and associated diseases	*Think about*
Do you smoke?	COPD Interstitial lung disease Coronary artery disease Lung cancer • Smoking is a major risk factor for COPD with LR+ 8.0–11.6.[11,12]
What is your occupation?	Occupational exposure to lung toxins (eg, asbestos) or chemicals associated with asthma may explain chronic dyspnea.

Have you been in a situation where you were sitting or lying still for a long period of time?	*PE*
Do you have cancer or lower extremity weakness?	*PE*
Are you taking birth control pills or estrogen?	*PE*
Do you have diabetes, high blood pressure, high cholesterol, or heart disease?	*Coronary artery disease, cardiomyopathy.* • *Although some patients have a heart attack or heart failure without risk factors, many will have at least 1 risk factor.*
Has anyone in your immediate family had a serious heart condition before the age of 55?	*A family history of premature coronary disease is present when a first-degree relative has significant coronary heart disease before age 55 for men or age 60 for women.*
Do you have any medical problems?	*Patients with known malignancy are at risk for metastases to the lungs, pleura, or pericardium, which may cause dyspnea. Chemotherapy can cause pulmonary fibrosis (bleomycin), heart failure (adriamycin), and anemia. Radiation therapy to the chest can cause constrictive pericarditis and accelerated coronary artery disease.* *Many collagen vascular diseases (eg, rheumatoid arthritis, ankylosing spondylitis) cause chronic interstitial lung disease.* *Neuromuscular diseases (eg, amyotrophic lateral sclerosis, myasthenia gravis) may predispose the patient to aspiration or may weaken respiratory muscles.*
Do you have any known allergies to foods, insects, or latex?	*Anaphylaxis (patients may know that they are allergic to insects, nuts, or shellfish but be unaware that recently ingested food contained these allergens)*
Have you started taking any new medications (eg, penicillin-related antibiotics, angiotensin-converting enzyme inhibitors) recently?	*Allergic reactions* *Angioedema*
Are you taking methotrexate (for rheumatologic disease) or nitrofurantoin (for urinary tract infections)?	*Interstitial lung disease (medication-induced)*

Quality

Think about

Is it hard to get a deep breath or is your breathing unsatisfying?	*COPD*[13]
Is your chest tight or does it take an increased amount of effort to breathe?	*Asthma*[13]
Do you feel as if you are smothering or suffocating?	*Congestive heart failure*[13]

(continued)

Quality	Think about
Do you feel that your breathing is rapid and/or shallow?	Interstitial lung disease[13]
Does your breathing only get heavy with activity?	Deconditioning[13]
Do you feel as if your throat is closing or that air can't get all of the way in to your lungs?	Panic disorder[13]

Modifying symptoms	Think about
Do you have shortness of breath when lying flat?	Orthopnea and PND are seen in patients with congestive heart failure.
Do you get short of breath with walking on a flat surface?	Patients with interstitial lung disease report shortness of breath with any exertion. In rheumatoid arthritis patients, the LR+ for this symptom was 11.5.[14]
Does lying on 1 side or the other cause increasing shortness of breath?	Unilateral pleural effusion (on the recumbent side)
Can you exercise for some distance before getting short of breath?	Exercise-induced asthma: symptoms begin after exercising for some time. Cardiomyopathy: symptoms begin after a short period of exercise (50–100 ft)

Associated symptoms	Think about
Do you have chest pain?	Myocardial infarction: a heaviness, pressure, or crushing substernal pain radiating to the jaw or left arm. Spontaneous pneumothorax: unilateral pleuritic pain. PE: unilateral or bilateral pleuritic pain. Cardiac tamponade: central chest heaviness
Do you have any itching or hives? Do you feel that your lips or tongue are swelling?	Anaphylaxis
Have you had a fever?	Acute pneumonia: 80% have fever[4] Acute PE: 20% have fever[10] Chronic pneumonia Inflammatory interstitial lung disease
Do you have cough?	Asthma: nonproductive cough Acute pneumonia Aspiration PE: nonproductive cough with occasional scant hemoptysis Flash pulmonary edema: cough with pink frothy sputum COPD: 3 months of productive cough per year; LR+ 4.0[12] Interstitial lung disease
Do you have any swelling in your legs or abdomen?	Deep venous thrombosis with PE: unilateral leg edema

	Cardiomyopathy: bilateral edema
	Pericardial disease: bilateral edema with abdominal swelling
	Severe right heart failure due to chronic lung disease with pulmonary hypertension: bilateral edema with abdominal swelling.
Have you lost any weight?	*Primary or metastatic lung cancer*
	Chronic pneumonia
Have you had any fainting spells?	*Primary or secondary pulmonary hypertension*
Do you have any rashes or joint pains?	*Interstitial lung diseases associated with systemic inflammatory conditions (eg, sarcoidosis).*
Do you have any weakness in your arms or legs or difficulty speaking or swallowing?	*Guillain-Barré syndrome*
	Myasthenia gravis
	Amyotrophic lateral sclerosis
	• Swallowing disorders predispose to aspiration
Do you feel lightheaded or weak when you stand up?	*Anemia*
Do you have any numbness or tingling in your fingertips? Did you feel a sense of impending doom or extreme fear?	*Panic attack or anxiety disorder*

CAVEATS

- The history and physical examination identify the etiology of dyspnea in approximately 67% of cases. The remainder will require more specific testing, such as chest radiographs or pulmonary function tests.[2]
- Although various types of dyspnea may occur with different diseases, platypnea is fairly specific for a right to left shunt, generally at the atrial level or in the pulmonary vasculature (eg, hepatopulmonary syndrome).
- Patients may have more than 1 cause of chronic dyspnea. For example, heavy smoking is a risk factor for both COPD and coronary artery disease. Patients with chronic lung or heart disease may also suffer from deconditioning. Adequate treatment of the patient requires identification of all causes of dyspnea, since the therapies may differ.
- Be particularly cautious about assuming anxiety is the cause of acute or chronic dyspnea, since patients with dyspnea caused by organic disease are often anxious.

PROGNOSIS

The prognosis of dyspnea depends on the etiology and severity of the underlying disease. Acute dyspnea is often reversible. Myocardial infarctions, pulmonary emboli, aspiration pneumonia, and asthma can generally be successfully treated once diagnosed. In contrast, chronic dyspnea may reflect disease that has progressed to an irreversible stage. Dyspnea associated with chronic pulmonary or cardiac disease may improve if the patient stops smoking and participates in cardiopulmonary exercise training/rehabilitation.[15]

REFERENCES

1. Dyspnea. Mechanisms, assessment, and management: a consensus statement. American Thoracic Society. *Am J Respir Crit Care Med.* 1999;159:321–340.

2. Pratter MR, Curley FJ, Dubois J, Irwin RS. Cause and evaluation of chronic dyspnea in a pulmonary disease clinic. *Arch Intern Med.* 1989;149:2277–2282.

3. Kramer K, Kirkman P, Kitzman D, Little WC. Flash pulmonary edema: association with hypertension and reoccurrence despite coronary revascularization. *Am Heart J.* 2000;140:451–455.

4. Stein PD, Terrin ML, Hales CA, et al. Clinical, laboratory, roentgenographic, and electrocardiographic findings in patients with acute pulmonary embolism and no preexisting cardiac or pulmonary disease. *Chest.* 1991;100:598–603.

5. Neugut AI, Ghatak AT, Miller RL. Anaphylaxis in the United States: an investigation into its epidemiology. *Arch Intern Med.* 2001;161:15–21.

6. Zweiman B, O'Dowd LC. Anaphylaxis. UptoDate. 2004. Available at http://www.uptodate.com

7. Emerman CL, Dawson N, Speroff T, et al. Comparison of physician judgment and decision aids for ordering chest radiographs for pneumonia in outpatients. *Ann Emerg Med.* 1991;20:1215–1219.

8. Sharshar T, Chevret S, Bourdain F, Raphael JC. Early predictors of mechanical ventilation in Guillain-Barré syndrome. *Crit Care Med.* 2003;31:278–283.

9. Bense L, Eklund G, Wiman LG. Smoking and the increased risk of contracting spontaneous pneumothorax. *Chest.* 1987;92:1009–1012.

10. Metlay JP, Kapoor WN, Fine MJ. Does this patient have community-acquired pneumonia? Diagnosing pneumonia by history and physical examination. *JAMA.* 1997;278:1440–1445.

11. Straus SE, McAlister FA, Sackett DL, Deeks JJ for the CARE-COAD1 Group. The accuracy of patient history, wheezing and laryngeal measurements in diagnosing obstructive airway disease. *JAMA.* 2000;283:1853–1857.

12. Holleman DR, Simel DL. Does the clinical examination predict airflow limitation? *JAMA.* 1995;273:313–319.

13. Mahler DA, Harver A, Lentine T, et al. Descriptors of breathlessness in cardiorespiratory diseases. *Am J Respir Crit Care Med.* 1996;154:1357–1363.

14. Dawson JK, Graham DR, Kenny J, Lynch MP. Accuracy of history, examination, pulmonary function tests and chest radiographs in predicting high-resolution computed tomography-diagnosed interstitial lung disease. *Br J Rheumatol.* 1997;36:1342–1343.

15. Sassi-Dambron DE, Eakin EG, Ries AL, et al. Treatment of dyspnea in COPD. A controlled clinical trial of dyspnea management strategies. *Chest.* 1995;107:724–729.

Diagnostic Approach: Dyspnea

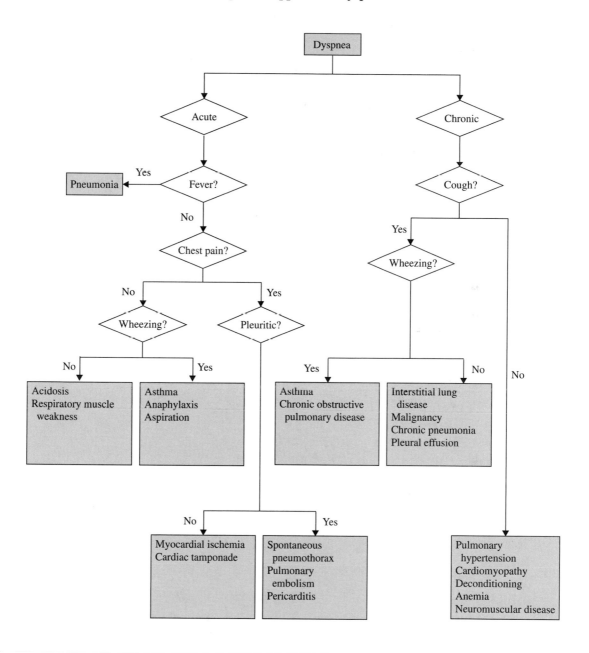

Hemoptysis

23

Juan A. Garcia, MD, & Jay I. Peters, MD

Hemoptysis is the expectoration of blood or blood-stained sputum. Patients with hemoptysis usually seek medical attention promptly due to the frightening sight of blood and its association with lung cancer. The clinical presentation of massive hemoptysis is always dramatic and the consequences can be grave. Hemoptysis implies that the blood originates below the larynx.[1] However, patients may have difficulty differentiating hemoptysis from bleeding from the upper gastrointestinal tract or bleeding from the upper airway. Based on the amount of blood expectorated, hemoptysis can be classified as scant or mild, submassive or moderate, and massive or severe.[2–4]

KEY TERMS[2–4]

Cryptogenic or idiopathic hemoptysis	No cause is found after extensive diagnostic evaluation.
Scant (mild) hemoptysis	Less than 20 mL in 24 hours. Blood streaks, usually noted with expectorated phlegm.
Submassive (moderate) hemoptysis	Between 20 and 200 mL in 24 hours.
Massive (severe) hemoptysis	More than 200–600 mL in 24 hours.

ETIOLOGY

There are more than 100 causes of hemoptysis. Older literature reports tuberculosis, bronchiectasis, and lung cancer as the most common causes of hemoptysis.[5] More recent series report that, in developed countries, bronchitis, cryptogenic hemoptysis, and pneumonia are the most common etiologies along with lung cancer and bronchiectasis, while TB has been declining.[4–7] Bronchitis is still considered the most common cause of hemoptysis, but it rarely causes massive hemoptysis. Massive hemoptysis is a true medical emergency that requires intensive care with immediate evaluation for the underlying cause.[8–11]

Differential Diagnosis[4–7]	Prevalence
Bronchitis	*20–40%*
Lung cancer	*15–30%*
Bronchiectasis	*10–20%*
Cryptogenic	*10–20%*
Pneumonia	*5–10%*
Tuberculosis	*5–15%*

GETTING STARTED

- To determine the likely etiology of hemoptysis, consider the amount of blood expectorated, the patient's age, smoking history, and past medical history.
- Establish if patient has hemoptysis versus bleeding from the upper airway or gastrointestinal tract.
- Estimate the amount of hemoptysis and duration of symptoms.
- Review past medical history.
- Review medications, including aspirin and nonsteroidal anti-inflammatory drugs, anticoagulants (warfarin and heparin), and chemotherapeutic agents (which may cause thrombocytopenia)
- Differentiate between hemoptysis and hematemesis.[1,12]

Questions	Remember
Tell me how much blood you coughed up.	*Let patients use their own words.*
Was the amount more than a tablespoon (30 mL)?	*Avoid leading questions.*
Was the amount more than a can of soda (240 mL)?	

Distinguishing Between Hemoptysis and Hematemesis

Hemoptysis	Hematemesis
• *Episode preceded by tingling of throat or chest and then a desire to cough*	• *Coughing is not usually reported*
• *Nausea/vomiting absent*	• *Nausea/vomiting present*
• *Frothy sputum*	• *Sputum not frothy (Low pH)*
• *Blood-tinged sputum persists for days*	• *No blood tinged sputum*
• *History of lung disease*	• *History of gastric or liver disease*
• *Symptoms related to significant blood loss uncommon*	• *Symptoms related to significant blood loss common (eg, orthostatic dizziness)*
• *Asphyxia possible*	• *Asphyxia unusual*

INTERVIEW FRAMEWORK

The most important step is to assess for alarm symptoms. Some patients with massive hemoptysis will be unable to give an adequate history.

IDENTIFYING ALARM SYMPTOMS

Massive or severe hemoptysis is considered a life-threatening emergency that requires immediate admission for observation and diagnostic evaluation. Respiratory distress may be related to the amount of hemoptysis, but can also result from poor pulmonary reserve due to comorbid medical conditions.

Serious Diagnoses	Approximate prevalence[a]
Cancer	*40%[b]*

Infections   20% (most commonly tuberculosis or lung abscess)
• Lung abscess
• Pneumonia
• Tuberculosis
• Fungal infections

Alveolar hemorrhage syndrome (Wegener's   < 5%
granulomatosis, microscopic polyangiitis,
systemic lupus erythematosus [SLE], Behçet
syndrome, Goodpasture syndrome, crack
cocaine inhalation, etc)

[a]Among patients with massive hemoptysis; prevalence may vary with geographic location and patient population.
[b]Bronchiectasis is less serious but accounts for 30–40% of cases.

FOCUSED QUESTIONS

Questions	Think about
History of present illness (HPI)	
Do you have scant to moderate hemoptysis with increased sputum production?	Bronchitis
Do you have hoarseness? Do you have a personal history of cancer? Do you smoke? If so, how much?	Cancer
Have you had severe or recurrent pneumonia (including tuberculosis)? Do you chronically produce large amounts of purulent sputum?	Bronchiectasis
Do you have fever? Have your symptoms lasted a few days or less? Are you producing purulent sputum?	Pneumonia, lung abscess
Do you have cough, fever, dyspnea, arthralgias, skin rash?	SLE, other collagen vascular disease
Do you have hematuria, sinusitis, otitis, skin lesions?	Wegener's granulomatosis
Have you had tuberculosis in the past? Have you been exposed to patients with active tuberculosis? Are you HIV positive?	Tuberculosis
Do you have acute chest pain with dyspnea? Do you have a recent history of immobilization or surgery?	Pulmonary embolism or infarct

(continued)

Past medical and surgical histories	*Think about*
Do you have a history of	
• *Cancer?*	*Primary or metastatic lung cancer*
• *Deep venous thrombosis or pulmonary embolism?*	*Anticoagulant-related bleeding* *Pulmonary embolism or infarct*
• *Cardiovascular disease (arrhythmias, valvular heart disease, ischemic heart disease, congestive heart failure)?*	*Anticoagulant-related bleeding*
• *Hemoptysis with exertion?*	*Mitral stenosis*
• *Chronic liver disease?*	*Coagulopathy* *Thrombocytopenia* *Upper gastrointestinal bleeding*
• *Peptic ulcer disease?*	*Upper gastrointestinal bleeding*
• *Renal disease?*	*Wegener granulomatosis, Goodpasture syndrome, SLE*
• *Transplantation?*	*Bacterial, fungal, or mycobacterial pulmonary infections*
• *HIV infection?*	*Bacterial, fungal, or mycobacterial pulmonary infections* *Kaposi sarcoma*
• *Vascular surgeries or tracheotomy?*	*Aortoenteric fistula*
• *Bleeding tendencies?*	*Hemophilia, other coagulation disorders* *Medications*
• *Chronic obstructive pulmonary disease?*	*Lung cancer*
Other	**Think about**
Have you recently traveled to areas or countries where tuberculosis is endemic (Latin America, South Asia, India, Russia, New York)?	*Tuberculosis*
Do you use injection drugs?	*Infections (endocarditis)* *Crack-induced alveolar hemorrhage* *Crack-induced pulmonary infarct*
Do you have any occupational exposures?	*Possible exposure to toxic inhalants* *Cancer*

CAVEATS

- Every patient with hemoptysis should have chest radiography and/or computed tomography of the chest.
- No cause will be found after extensive investigation in up to 20% of cases.
- Consider the possibility that some patients may be malingering.
- Bronchoscopy should be considered in patients with the following characteristics: age over 40, tobacco use, prior history of cancer, and hemoptysis lasting more than 1 week.
- If computed tomography of the chest (with thin cuts) or bronchoscopy is negative, consider ear, nose, and throat evaluation for upper airway bleeding source.

PROGNOSIS

The prognosis depends on the amount of hemoptysis, the underlying etiology, and the patient's comorbid conditions. Hemoptysis due to bronchitis is usually self-limited but it may recur; prognosis is favorable. Hemoptysis due to lung cancer, opportunistic infection, and alveolar hemorrhage syndromes has a guarded prognosis. Early mortality for the various alveolar hemorrhage syndromes ranges from 25% to 50%.[13] Massive hemoptysis carries a mortality rate of 13–58%.[8,10]

REFERENCES

1. Israel R, Poe R. Hemoptysis. *Clin Chest Med.* 1987;8:197–205.
2. Lenner R, Schilero G, Lesser M. Hemoptysis: diagnosis and management. *Comp Ther.* 2002;28:7–13.
3. Corder R. Hemoptysis. *Emerg Med Clin North Am.* 2003;21:421–435.
4. Hirshberg B, et al. Hemoptysis: etiology, evaluation, and outcome in a tertiary referral hospital. *Chest.* 1997;112:440–444.
5. Johnston H, Reisz G. Changing spectrum of hemoptysis. *Arch Intern Med.* 1989;149:1666–1668.
6. Santiago S, Tobias J, Williams A. A Reappraisal of the Causes of Hemoptysis. *Arch Intern Med.* 1991;151:2449–2451.
7. McGuinness G, et al. Hemoptysis: prospective high-resolution CT/bronchoscopic correlation. *Chest.* 1994;105:155–162.
8. Ong T, Eng P. Massive hemoptysis requiring intensive care. *Intens Care Med.* 2003;29:317–320.
9. Endo S, et al. Management of massive hemoptysis in a thoracic surgical unit. *Eur J Cardiothorac Surg.* 2003;23:467–472.
10. Jean-Baptiste E. Clinical assessment and management of massive hemoptysis. *Crit Care Med.* 2000;28:1642–1647.
11. Johnson J. Manifestations of hemoptysis. *Postgrad Med.* 2002;112:101–113.
12. Sapira J. In: *Art & Science of Bedside Diagnosis,* 2nd ed. Lippincott Williams & Wilkins; 2000.
13. Shwarz M. The Diffuse Alveolar Hemorrhage Syndromes. Available at http://www.uptodate.com. Accessed 9/14/03

Diagnostic Approach: Hemoptysis

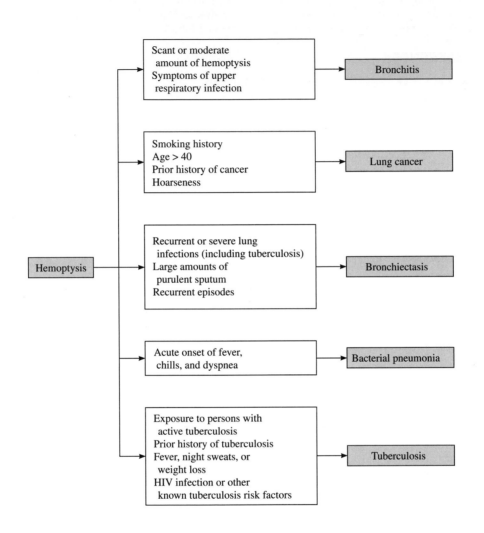

SECTION VI
Cardiovascular System

Chest Pain

24

Sumanth D. Prabhu, MD

Chest pain is a commonly encountered symptom in both the emergency department and the outpatient clinic, resulting from a spectrum of etiologies from minor illness to life-threatening disease. Perhaps the most pressing determination is whether chest pain is due to acute cardiac ischemia or to nonischemic cardiovascular or noncardiac causes. Each of these categories encompasses etiologies that are potentially serious. In view of this, the initial evaluation, consisting of the history, physical examination, and electrocardiogram (ECG), is exceedingly important for determining the severity and acuity of the clinical presentation, and for guiding the proper selection of additional diagnostic and therapeutic modalities. Of these, the history remains the cornerstone of patient assessment.

KEY TERMS[1]

Angina pectoris	Discomfort in the chest and/or adjacent areas (jaw, shoulder, back, arm), usually, but not always, due to myocardial ischemia
Typical angina	Substernal chest discomfort with the following features: • Characteristic quality (described as "pressure," "squeezing," or "heaviness," but almost never sharp or stabbing) and duration (typically minutes) • Provoked by exertion or emotional stress • Relieved by rest or nitroglycerin (within several minutes).
Atypical angina	Chest discomfort that meets 2 of the typical angina characteristics.
Noncardiac chest pain	Chest pain that meets 1 or none of the typical angina characteristics.
Canadian Cardiovascular Society (CCS) Angina Classification System	Clinical grading system based on degree of limitation of ordinary physical activity: Class I: No limitation Class II: Slight limitation Class III: Marked limitation Class IV: Angina occurs with any physical activity or at rest.
Myocardial infarction (MI)	Prolonged severe anginal discomfort associated with myocardial necrosis.
Pleuritic chest pain	Sharp chest pain that increases with inspiration or cough.
Unstable angina (UA)	Angina presenting as rest angina, severe new-onset angina (CCS class III or IV), or acceleration of previously diagnosed effort angina (to at least CCS class III).

ETIOLOGY

Chest pain may arise from cardiac, noncardiac, or psychogenic causes. Cardiovascular causes may be subdivided into ischemic and nonischemic etiologies. Myocardial ischemia results from an imbalance between myocardial oxygen supply and demand, such that demand exceeds supply. Ischemic chest pain or angina is most often secondary to obstructive atherosclerotic coronary artery disease (CAD). However, angina is also a feature of valvular heart disease (eg, aortic stenosis), severe hypertension, hypertrophic cardiomyopathy, severe pulmonary hypertension (with right ventricular ischemia), and coronary spasm. Angina may also be precipitated by extracardiac conditions, such as severe anemia, hypoxia, hyperthyroidism, and hyperviscosity. In all of these conditions, chest pain occurs due to a perturbation of the normal oxygen supply/demand relationship (ie, increased demand and/or decreased supply), even in the absence of CAD. Nonischemic cardiovascular chest pain may accompany aortic dissection, pericarditis, or mitral valve prolapse. Noncardiac chest pain may occur with esophageal and other gastrointestinal (GI) conditions, pulmonary disease, and musculoskeletal and psychiatric disorders. Esophageal pain often resembles angina in quality and frequently cannot be differentiated from cardiac ischemia. Given the diversity of etiologies for chest pain, and the extent of testing required to exclude each possibility, it is difficult to determine the prevalence of every cause. In patients presenting to the emergency department with chest pain, the reported frequency of acute ischemia ranges from 16% to 28%.[2–4] In patients discharged from the coronary care unit with noncardiac chest pain, more than 75% had evidence of esophageal disorders.[5]

Differential Diagnosis	Prevalence[a]
Cardiovascular, ischemic	
Stable angina, UA, MI	**16–28%[2–4]**
Coronary atherosclerosis	
Coronary artery spasm	
Aortic stenosis	
Hypertrophic cardiomyopathy	
Dilated cardiomyopathy	
Tachycardia (ventricular/supraventricular)	
Sympathomimetic toxicity (eg, cocaine)	
Severe hypertension	
Severe pulmonary hypertension	
Severe anemia, hypoxia, hyperviscosity	
Hyperthyroidism, hyperthermia	
Cardiovascular, nonischemic	
Aortic dissection	**0.003%[6]**
Pericarditis	
Mitral valve prolapse	
Noncardiovascular	**72–84%[2–4]**
GI	
Esophageal (spasm, reflux, esophagitis)	
Biliary disease (cholecystitis, choledocholithiasis)	
Peptic ulcer	
Pancreatitis	

Pulmonary

   Pulmonary embolism (PE)

   Pneumothorax

   Pneumonia

   Pleuritis

Musculoskeletal

   Sternoclavicular arthritis

   Costochondritis

   Cervical spine disorders

   Herpes zoster

Psychogenic

   Anxiety disorders (hyperventilation, panic attacks)

   Depression

   Somatiform disorders

   Secondary gain

[a]Among emergency department patients; prevalence is unknown when not indicated.

GETTING STARTED

- Remember, acute chest pain may result from potentially life-threatening conditions. Thus, the history should be performed in a targeted and expeditious fashion.
- Initially, ask open-ended questions so the patient can describe the chest pain. Once a primary description is obtained, quickly move on to more focused questioning for possible underlying etiologies.
- Definitive diagnosis often requires a physical examination, ECG, and additional laboratory testing. However, the history serves as the primary guide for medical decision-making.

Questions	Remember
Are you having chest pain right now? If not, when was the last time you had it? How long has this been going on?	• *Determine whether symptoms are acute or chronic and recurring.*
Describe your current chest pain (or a typical prior episode) to me.	• *Listen to the patient's description.*
Does the chest pain prevent you from doing things you would normally do?	• *Assess the impact of chest pain on the patient's physical activity.*

INTERVIEW FRAMEWORK

- Determine whether symptoms represent an ongoing acute episode, which is more likely to be unstable disease, or chronic and recurring episodes, which more often reflect stable disease.

- Characterize the chest pain using the following components:
  - Quality
  - Location
  - Radiation
  - Duration
  - Time course
  - Precipitating/relieving factors
  - Associated symptoms
- Ascertain the presence of associated conditions and risk factors for CAD:
  - Diabetes
  - Smoking
  - Hypertension
  - Hyperlipidemia
  - Family history of premature CAD
  - Postmenopausal status
  - Peripheral vascular disease
  - Cocaine abuse
- Predict the probability of underlying CAD using pain type, age, gender, and risk factors.

IDENTIFYING ALARM SYMPTOMS

Chest pain by itself is an alarm symptom since it can be due to serious causes that require prompt attention. By far, the most common serious cause is acute cardiac ischemia, which includes stable angina, UA, and MI. Albeit less common, other serious conditions to be considered include aortic dissection, PE, spontaneous pneumothorax, pneumonia, and acute GI processes (eg, cholecystitis, pancreatitis) with referred pain.

Serious Diagnoses	Prevalence[a]
Acute myocardial ischemia	16–28%[2–4]
• *MI*	5–6%[2,4]
• *UA*	9–16%[2,4]
• *Stable angina and other cardiac conditions*	2–7%[2,4]
Aortic dissection	0.003%[6]
PE	
Spontaneous pneumothorax	
Pneumonia	
Acute GI pathology	

[a]Among patients with chest pain seeking care at an emergency department; prevalence is unknown when not indicated.

In general, the suspicion for these serious diagnoses is raised by the results of careful questioning regarding the character and pattern of the pain, associated symptoms, and associated medical conditions. A primary distinction is the differentiation of anginal pain from noncardiac chest pain.

Alarm symptoms	Serious causes	Likelihood ratio (LR)[a]	Benign causes
Typical angina that is prolonged or occurs at rest OR Atypical angina that is prolonged or occurs at rest, with high probability of CAD (see below)	MI UA	2.7[7]	Esophageal disease Musculoskeletal chest pain Nonischemic chest pain (eg, mitral valve prolapse) Psychogenic chest pain
New-onset or acceleration of effort chest pain (to at least CCS III), typical or atypical with high CAD probability	UA		Esophageal disease Musculoskeletal chest pain Nonischemic chest pain Psychogenic chest pain
Chest pain with prior history of MI	MI UA	2.3[7]	Nonischemic chest pain
Chest pain with diaphoresis (especially profuse diaphoresis)	MI UA PE Aortic dissection	2.0[7]	
Chest pain with nausea/vomiting	MI UA	1.9[7]	Acute GI pathology
Chest pain radiation to left arm	MI UA	2.3[7]	Pericarditis Cervical spine disorders
Chest pain radiation to right shoulder	MI UA	2.9[7]	Pericarditis Biliary colic Cervical spine disorders
Chest pain radiation to both arms	MI UA	7.1[7]	Pericarditis Cervical spine disorders
Sudden onset chest pain and acute dyspnea	PE MI Spontaneous pneumothorax	3.6[8]	Pleuritis Musculoskeletal chest pain
Chest pain with hemoptysis	PE Pneumonia	2.4[8]	Tracheobronchitis
Chest pain with fever	Pneumonia Acute GI pathology		Pleuritis Tracheobronchitis Pericarditis
Chest pain with syncope (hypotension)	MI PE Arrhythmia Pericardial tamponade	3.1[7]	Vasovagal syncope

(continued)

Alarm symptoms	Serious causes	Likelihood ratio (LR)[a]	Benign causes
Chest pain with palpitations	MI Tachyarrhythmia		
Chest pain with history of Marfan's syndrome	Aortic dissection	4.1[6]	
Sudden onset of severe "tearing" or "ripping" chest pain	Aortic dissection	10.8[6]	
Severe persistent chest pain radiating to the back	Aortic dissection Aortic aneurysm		Pericarditis Pancreatitis Peptic ulcer
Severe migrating chest and back pain	Aortic dissection	7.6[6]	

[a]Each LR applies to the adjacent serious cause.

The following features significantly *decrease* the likelihood of MI[7]:

- Pleuritic chest pain (LR 0.2)
- Chest pain reproduced by palpation (LR 0.2–0.4)
- Sharp or stabbing chest pain (LR 0.3)
- Positional chest pain (LR 0.3)

The *absence* of sudden onset chest pain *decreases* the likelihood of acute aortic dissection (LR 0.3).[9]

Estimating the Pretest Probability (%) of CAD[1,10]

Age	Nonanginal Chest Pain		Atypical Angina		Typical Angina	
	Men	*Women*	*Men*	*Women*	*Men*	*Women*
30–39 yr	*3–35*	*1–19*	*8–59*	*2–39*	*30–88*	*10–78*
40–49 yr	*9–47*	*2–22*	*21–70*	*5–43*	*51–92*	*20–79*
50–59 yr	*23–59*	*4–25*	*45–79*	*10–47*	*80–95*	*38–82*
60–69 yr	*49–69*	*9–29*	*71–86*	*20–51*	*93–97*	*56–84*

First number within each range is the probability or prevalence of CAD in patients without risk factors (diabetes, smoking, and hyperlipidemia). Second number is the probability with risk factors. All groups have normal ECGs.

As evident from this data, CAD prevalence rises with age. Men with typical angina generally have a high likelihood of CAD, even without risk factors in the older age groups. Women with nonanginal chest pain generally have a low prevalence of CAD.

FOCUSED QUESTIONS

Chest pain should be characterized according to the components listed below, and alarm symptoms should be assessed. The pain can be labeled as typical or atypical angina or as noncardiac chest pain. The pain type, together with the patient's age, gender, and cardiac risk factors, allow a reasonable estimation of the probability of underlying CAD.

Quality

Does it feel like

- *Pressure, squeezing, burning, or strangling?*
- *Tightness or heaviness, "a band across the chest"?*

- *Deep, heavy aching (visceral pain)?*

- *Indigestion, a need to belch?*

- *Severe tearing or ripping pain?*
- *Sharp and stabbing?*

- *Dull, persistent ache lasting hours or days localized (< 3 cm) to cardiac apex (inframammary area)?*

Location

Is the pain diffuse, poorly localized, retrosternal?

Is pain localized over skin or superficial structures, such as costochondral joints, that is reproduced by palpation?

Is pain localized (< 3 cm), region of left nipple (circumscribed by 1 finger)?

Radiation

Does pain radiate to medial aspect of left shoulder/arm, right shoulder/arm, both arms?

- *Lower jaw, neck, teeth?*
- *Interscapular region, back?*

- *Epigastrium?*

Think about

Myocardial ischemia
Esophageal disease (spasm, reflux)
[Pulmonary hypertension (with right ventricular ischemia) can present with chest pressure]

[Herpes zoster (prior to rash) can present as a tight band around chest]

Myocardial ischemia
Esophageal disease, peptic ulcer

Aortic dissection

Pericarditis, pleuritis
PE, pneumothorax
Musculoskeletal pain
Psychogenic pain

Psychogenic pain

Think about

Myocardial ischemia
PE

Musculoskeletal pain
Costochondritis

Noncardiac pain (musculoskeletal, psychogenic, gaseous distention of the stomach)

Think about

Myocardial Ischemia
Pericarditis
Cervical spine disease
Cholecystitis (to right shoulder)

Myocardial ischemia

Aortic dissection
Thoracic aortic aneurysm
Pericarditis
Esophageal disease
Pancreatitis
Peptic ulcer
Myocardial ischemia

Esophageal disease
Pancreatitis
Peptic ulcer

(continued)

Radiation	***Think about***
• *Epigastrium?*	*Biliary tract disease*
	Myocardial ischemia
Duration, time course	***Think about***
How long does it last?	
• *Brief (2–20 minutes)*	*Angina pectoris*
	Esophageal disease
	Musculoskeletal pain
	Psychogenic pain
• *Very brief (< 15 seconds)*	*Noncardiac pain*
	Musculoskeletal pain
	Hiatal hernia
	Psychogenic pain
• *Prolonged (> 20 minutes to hours)*	*UA/MI*
	Esophageal disease
	Pulmonary disorders
	Pericarditis
	Aortic dissection
	Musculoskeletal disease
	Herpes zoster
	Acute GI pathology
	Psychogenic pain
Precipitating factors	***Think about***
What brings pain on	
• *Exertion (classically in the cold or against a wind, especially after a heavy meal)?*	*Angina pectoris*
• *Emotional stress, fright?*	*Angina pectoris*
	Psychogenic pain
• *Eating, meals?*	*Esophageal pain*
	Peptic ulcer
	Angina pectoris
• *Lying down or bending after meals?*	*Esophageal reflux*
• *Bending or moving the neck?*	*Cervical/upper thoracic spine disease*
• *Respiration or cough (pleuritic pain)?*	*PE*
	Pneumothorax
	Pericarditis, pleuritis
	Musculoskeletal pain
• *Changes in body position (positional pain)?*	*Pericarditis*
	Musculoskeletal pain
	Pancreatitis
Relieving factors	***Think about***
What relieves the pain?	
• *Rest or sublingual nitroglycerin (usually within 1 to 5 minutes)?*	*Angina pectoris*
	Esophageal spasm

• Sitting up and leaning forward?	*Pericarditis* *Pancreatitis*
• Antacids, food?	*Esophagitis, peptic ulcer*
• Holding the breath at deep expiration?	*Pleuritis*
Associated symptoms	**Think about**
Do you have any of the following symptoms?	
• Nausea and vomiting?	*Acute myocardial ischemia or MI* *Acute GI pathology*
• Diaphoresis?	*Acute myocardial ischemia or MI* *PE* *Aortic dissection*
• Dyspnea?	*Acute myocardial ischemia or MI* *PE* *Pneumothorax* *Pneumonia*
• Syncope/hypotension?	*Acute myocardial ischemia or MI* *Massive PE* *Aortic stenosis* *Arrhythmia*
• Waterbrash (acid reflux into the mouth)?	*Esophageal disease*
• Hemoptysis?	*PE, pneumonia*
• Fever?	*Pneumonia* *Pleuritis* *Pericarditis*

DIAGNOSTIC APPROACH

The first step is to determine the acuity of the symptoms. Although there may be overlap, chronic and recurring episodes without any change in symptom pattern are less likely to be emergent and may be evaluated in the outpatient setting. Such diagnoses will include stable angina, GI pain, and musculoskeletal pain. In contrast, an acute or ongoing chest pain episode is more likely to represent an urgent situation and should be evaluated in the emergency department or inpatient setting. These diagnoses will include UA, MI, aortic dissection, PE, pericarditis, and pneumothorax. In both situations, alarm symptoms and the probability of underlying CAD should be assessed. It is important to keep in mind, however, that in addition to the history, proper decision-making will also necessitate a targeted physical examination, ECG, and other laboratory testing, as appropriate. See Diagnostic Approach: Acute Chest Pain.

CAVEATS

- Angina is often precipitated by effort or physical activity. Thus, it is important to determine whether functional limitations preclude proper assessment of effort-related chest pain or, conversely, whether effort-related chest pain is limiting the patient's physical activity.
- In clinical practice, myocardial ischemia is the most common serious cause of chest pain encountered. In the majority of patients, this is due to obstructive epicardial CAD.
- Angina is almost never sharp or stabbing, pleuritic, or positional. The following features suggest causes other than angina: (1) very brief pain lasting less than 15 seconds; (2) dull, localized (< 3 cm) pain, especially in the inframammary region; (3) localized, superficial chest pain reproduced by palpation; (4) radiation to the upper jaw or below the umbilicus.

- In patients with typical angina but low probability of CAD, consider conditions that can produce myocardial ischemia in the absence of significant CAD (eg, systemic or pulmonary hypertension, aortic stenosis, hypertrophic cardiomyopathy, severe anemia, hyperthyroidism).
- Typical angina in an otherwise healthy athlete should raise the possibility of hypertrophic cardiomyopathy, especially if associated with dizziness or presyncope.
- Chest pain associated with PE, although typically pleuritic, may resemble angina due to associated pulmonary hypertension and attendant right ventricular ischemia.
- Be aware of gender differences in chest pain presentation. Atypical angina is more common in women than men. Women with chronic stable angina are more likely to have pain at rest, sleep, or during mental stress than men.

PROGNOSIS

The prognosis of the patient with chest pain is highly variable and depends on the underlying etiology. Obviously, patients with chest pain due to potentially life-threatening illnesses such as MI, PE, and aortic dissection have a much more guarded prognosis than do patients with esophageal, musculoskeletal, or psychogenic pain. Thus, prompt and targeted evaluation of all patients presenting with chest pain is essential. Specialized chest pain centers with protocol-driven assessment and short-stay observation units can help risk-stratify such patients, and efficiently identify those with acute myocardial ischemia versus nonischemic causes.

REFERENCES

1. Gibbons RJ, Chatterjee K, Daley J, et al. ACC/AHA/ACP-ASIM guidelines for the management of patients with chronic stable angina: a report of the American College of Cardiology/American Heart Association Task Force on Practice Guidelines (Committee on Management of Patients With Chronic Stable Angina). *J Am Coll Cardiol.* 1999;33:2092–2197.
2. Baxt WG, Shofer FS, Sites FD, Hollander JE. A neural network aid for the early diagnosis of cardiac ischemia in patients presenting to the emergency department with chest pain. *Ann Emerg Med.* 2002;40:575–583.
3. Pozen MW, D'Agostino RB, Selker HP, Sytkowski PA, Hood WB Jr. A predictive instrument to improve coronary-care-unit admission practices in acute ischemic heart disease. A prospective multicenter clinical trial. *N Engl J Med.* 1984;310:1273–1278.
4. Tatum JL, Jesse RL, Kontos MC, et al. Comprehensive strategy for the evaluation and triage of the chest pain patient. *Ann Emerg Med.* 1997;29:116–125.
5. Panju A, Farkouh ME, Sackett DL, et al. Outcome of patients discharged from a coronary care unit with a diagnosis of "chest pain not yet diagnosed." *CMAJ.* 1996;155:541–546.
6. von Kodolitsch Y, Schwartz AG, Nienaber CA. Clinical prediction of acute aortic dissection. *Arch Intern Med.* 2000;160:2977–2982.
7. Panju AA, Hemmelgarn BR, Guyatt GH, Simel DL. The rational clinical examination. Is this patient having a myocardial infarction? *JAMA.* 1998;280:1256–1263.
8. Miniati M, Monti S, Bottai M. A structured clinical model for predicting the probability of pulmonary embolism. *Am J Med.* 2003;114:173–179.
9. Klompas M. Does this patient have an acute thoracic aortic dissection? *JAMA.* 2002;287:2262–2272.
10. Pryor DB, Shaw L, McCants CB, et al. Value of the history and physical in identifying patients at increased risk for coronary artery disease. *Ann Intern Med.* 1993;118:81–90.

SUGGESTED READING

American College of Emergency Physicians. Clinical policy for the initial approach to adults presenting with a chief complaint of chest pain, with no history of trauma. *Ann Emerg Med.* 1995;25:274–299.

Campeau L. Grading of angina pectoris [letter]. *Circulation.* 1976;54:522–523.

Diamond GA, Forrester JS. Analysis of probability as an aid in the clinical diagnosis of coronary artery disease. *N Engl J Med.* 1979;300:1350–1358.

Douglas PS, Ginsburg GS. The evaluation of chest pain in women. *N Engl J Med.* 1996;334:1311–1315.

Paterson WG. Canadian Association of Gastroenterology Practice Guidelines: management of noncardiac chest pain. *Can J Gastroenterol.* 1998;12:401–407.

Diagnostic Approach: Acute Chest Pain

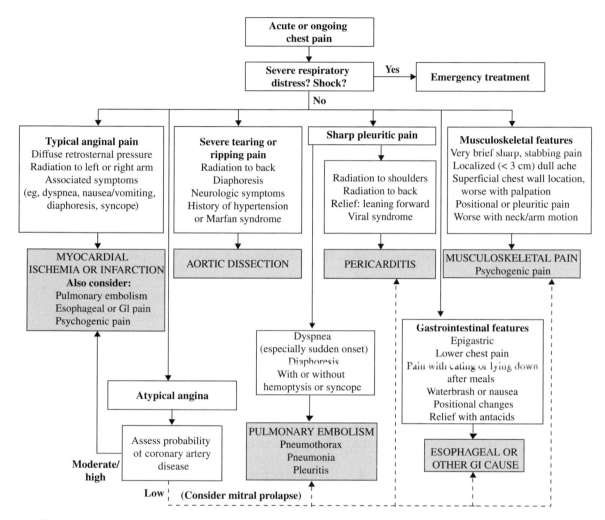

GI, gastrointestinal.

Palpitations

25

Kathryn A. Glatter, MD, & Melissa Robinson, MD

Palpitation is one of the most common symptoms encountered by primary care physicians.[1–4] Palpitation refers to an abnormal sense of one's own heartbeat. This may mean the sensation of skipped or irregular beats, increased heart rate, or unusually forceful contractions of the heart. Accompanying symptoms may include shortness of breath, dizziness, nausea, fatigue, chest pain, and syncope or presyncope. Both life-threatening cardiac disorders and common psychiatric diseases may cause palpitations. A careful patient history is an essential part in elucidating the cause.

KEY TERMS

Arrhythmia	*Any deviation from the normal cardiac rhythm. Examples include ventricular tachycardia (VT), ventricular fibrillation, supraventricular tachycardia (SVT), atrial fibrillation, and others.*
Dizziness	*Poorly defined sensation of lightheadedness or similar symptoms. Patients with palpitations commonly experience dizziness but it is not the primary symptom. (See Chapter 6.)*
Presyncope	*Sensation that one may "pass out," but actual loss of consciousness is averted.*
Syncope	*Transient loss of consciousness with spontaneous recovery.*
Tachycardia	*Any cardiac rhythm with a rate > 100.*

ETIOLOGY

Many patients will have an obvious cause of their symptoms. Examples include a diabetic patient with palpitations each time she forgets to eat (hypoglycemia) or a severely anemic patient who experiences palpitations with exertion. The etiology of palpitations depends on the patient population. In a prospective study of 190 patients seeking medical attention at primary care clinics or emergency departments, cardiac disorders comprised nearly half of the final diagnoses. In this study and others, at least 15% of individuals have no definable cause of their palpitations despite extensive testing.[2–4]

A significant number of patients with palpitations suffer from somatization or other psychiatric disorders. Persons with palpitations score higher on psychiatric tests for panic disorder, hypochondriasis, and anxiety than persons without palpitations.[2]

Causes	Frequency
Cardiac (including arrhythmias and valvular disease)	*43.2%*
Psychiatric (including panic disorder or anxiety)	*30.5%*
Miscellaneous (including thyrotoxicosis and medications)	*10.0%*
Unknown	*16.3%*

GETTING STARTED

- Take a detailed history focusing on when palpitations occur, associated symptoms, triggers of episodes, and what makes the palpitations stop. Caffeine, stress, and exercise are common precipitants.
- Review previous cardiac or other diagnostic tests, especially Holter monitoring or cardiac imaging (echocardiography).
- Assess the seriousness of the palpitations by making sure the patient is not currently hypotensive or tachycardic, which would mandate urgent therapy.

Questions	**Tips for effective interviewing**
Tell me about your palpitations.	• *Ask open-ended questions.*
What starts your symptoms? Can you make them stop?	• *Inquire about other cardiac symptoms (see below).*
Have you fainted with the palpitations? Do you get chest pain or shortness of breath?	• *Allow the patient to describe the symptoms in his or her own words as much as possible.*

INTERVIEW FRAMEWORK

- First determine whether the palpitations may be due to a life-threatening arrhythmia (eg, ventricular arrhythmias associated with myocardial infarction).
- Ask the patient to describe the actual sensation he or she is feeling. Recognize that patients may not accurately describe what they are feeling. A "racing heartbeat" may be mistakenly ascribed to noncardiac conditions, such as asthma (shortness of breath).
- Obtain a quantitative description of the palpitations including frequency, duration, and temporal relationship to other activities.
- Take a detailed medical history, family history, and social history. Probe for depression and anxiety since these findings are often associated with palpitations.
- Focus on common words used to describe palpitations:
  –Fluttering or racing heartbeat
  –Skipped beats
  –Irregular heartbeat
  –Pounding or thumping heart
  –Heart stops beating

IDENTIFYING ALARM SYMPTOMS

- Palpitations associated with syncope, chest pain, or shortness of breath may indicate a serious underlying rhythm disorder (arrhythmia) or other cardiac condition (eg, cardiomyopathy or valvular heart disease).
- The following descriptors suggest an arrhythmia:
  –Heart fluttering
  –Irregular heartbeat
  –Heart stopping

Serious Diagnoses

Most causes of palpitations are not life-threatening. However, ventricular arrhythmias that can cause sudden death occur in patients with cardiomyopathy, heart failure, or myocardial infarction. Otherwise, benign atrial arrhythmias (eg, SVT or atrial fibrillation) can be serious when occurring with a rapid rate. Finally, palpitations associated with syncope can frequently lead to injury and must be addressed promptly.

Alarm symptoms[a]	Consider
Chest pain	Myocardial infarction
Syncope or presyncope	Cardiac arrhythmia
	Valvular heart disease (aortic stenosis, hypertrophic cardiomyopathy)
Shortness of breath	Cardiac arrhythmia
	Myocardial infarction
	Pulmonary embolism

[a]Panic attack can cause all of these alarm symptoms but should be considered only after more serious conditions have been excluded.[5]

FOCUSED QUESTIONS

If answered in the affirmative	Think about
Do the palpitations last only seconds?	SVT
	Paroxysmal atrial fibrillation
Do the palpitations begin and end abruptly?	Arrhythmia
Does caffeine provoke your symptoms?	SVT
	Premature ventricular contractions (PVCs)
Do the palpitations stop if you hold your breath or strain?	SVT
Do you feel sweaty, shaky, or anxious with these episodes?	Arrhythmia
	Anxiety or panic disorder
Do you have hyperthyroidism?	Atrial fibrillation
Have you had a prior myocardial infarction?	VT
Do you smoke, have diabetes, or use illicit drugs?	Risk factors for heart disease and ventricular arrhythmias
Do you take over-the-counter cold medications?	May trigger SVT
Do you consider yourself a sad, anxious, or depressed person?	Anxiety disorder

Time course	Think about
How long do the episodes last?	
• Seconds?	Paroxysmal arrhythmia
• Minutes to hours?	SVT
	Atrial fibrillation
• Days?	Panic disorder

(continued)

Associated symptoms	Think about
Do you have	
• Chest pain or pressure?	Myocardial ischemia or infarction Arrhythmia
• Shortness of breath?	Arrhythmia
• Syncope or presyncope?	Arrhythmia Valvular disease
• Anxious feeling?	Arrhythmia Panic disorder
• Sweating, trembling, or shaking? • Fear of losing control or dying? • Feeling of choking? • Nausea or dizziness? • Numbness or tingling?	Panic disorder
Modifying symptoms	**Think about**
Does caffeine trigger your symptoms?	SVT PVCs
Do you have an impending sense of doom?	Panic disorder Myocardial infarction
Does it feel like your heart speeds up and stops?	Bradyarrhythmia
Have you taken your pulse during these episodes?	
• Fast heart rate during episodes (> 100)	
– Feel heart fluttering	SVT
– Heart racing	Tachyarrhythmia PVCs
• Slow heart rate during episodes (< 60)	
– Feel heart stops beating	Bradyarrhythmia
– Presyncope	Heart block Atrial fibrillation
Can you "tap out" the pattern of your heartbeat during one of these episodes?	
Is the rhythm irregular?	Atrial fibrillation

DIAGNOSTIC APPROACH

The key to discovering the etiology of palpitations lies with the history. Frequently, the patient's description of the episodes (or skillful use of focused questioning) will guide the clinician to the diagnosis.

Define what triggers palpitations

SVT is often triggered by caffeine, exercise, or anxiety. In contrast, atrial fibrillation often has no clear trigger but may be associated with comorbid illnesses such as hypertension, diabetes mellitus, hyperthyroidism, or pericarditis. VT often has no clear trigger but is associated with heart failure, cardiomyopathy, or previous myocardial infarction. Patients with panic attacks may describe anxiety or sweating.

Associated symptoms with palpitations

Episodes of SVT may be associated with presyncope, syncope, or shortness of breath. Patients rarely experience chest pain during SVT. The person may feel no symptoms during atrial fibrillation or feel dizzy if the ventricular response is rapid. During VT, the patient may experience syncope or chest pain, as during a myocardial infarction. Those with panic attacks may report extreme nervousness and nausea.

Physical examination during palpitations

The heart rate and blood pressure during the episodes may give clues to the etiology (eg, fast heart rates may suggest an arrhythmia whereas slow heart rates point toward sick sinus syndrome). The cardiovascular examination may also shed light onto the cause but is beyond the scope of this text.

Cardiac evaluation of palpitations

Cardiac diagnostic testing is often required in the evaluation of palpitations, depending on the patient's symptoms, medical history, and other clinical factors. Commonly used tests include 12-lead electrocardiography, Holter or cardiac event monitoring for arrhythmia detection, exercise stress testing, and echocardiography to evaluate cardiac function.

CAVEATS

- Some patients may be unable to precisely describe their symptoms.
- Many patients will have no clear etiology established for the palpitations.
- If no cause has been found after a thorough evaluation, consider panic or anxiety disorder as a possible diagnosis.

PROGNOSIS

The prognosis for palpitations depends on the underlying etiology but is generally excellent.[6,7] Certain patients (eg, ventricular arrhythmia due to previous myocardial infarction or cardiomyopathy) may have an increased risk of sudden death and so require more extensive evaluation by a cardiologist.

Up to 75% of patients experience recurrent palpitations a year after initial presentation.[7] However, most do not report that these recurrent symptoms are disabling. Palpitations may disappear spontaneously or become manageable without formal intervention as patients learn to avoid certain behaviors that trigger the episodes (eg, avoiding caffeine ingestion). The key for the clinician is to be systematic in the evaluation of this often nonspecific complaint to identify the cause of the palpitations, and to treat them, when possible.

REFERENCES

1. Weber BE, Kapoor WN. Evaluation and outcomes of patients with palpitations. *Am J Med.* 1996;100:138–148.
2. Barsky AJ, Cleary PD, Coeytaux RR, Ruskin JN. The clinical course of palpitations in medical outpatients. *Arch Intern Med.* 1995;155:1782–1788.
3. Barsky AJ, Cleary PD, Barnett MC, Christiansen CL, Ruskin JN. The accuracy of symptom reporting by patients complaining of palpitations. *Am J Med.* 1994;97:214–221.
4. Zimetbaum P, Josephson ME. Evaluation of patients with palpitations. *N Engl J Med.* 1998;338:1369–1373.
5. *Diagnostic and Statistical Manual of Mental Disorders* (DSM–IV): Washington DC: American Psychiatric Association, 1994.
6. Ehlers A, Mayou RA, Sprigings DC, Birkhead J. Psychological and perceptual factors associated with arrhythmias and benign palpitations. *Psychosom Med.* 2000;62:693–702.
7. Zeldis SM, Levine BJ, Michelson EL, Morganroth J. Cardiovascular complaints: correlation with cardiac arrhythmias on 24-hour ECG monitoring. *Chest.* 1980;78:456–462.

SUGGESTED READING

Barksy AJ. Palpitations, arrhythmias and awareness of cardiac activity. *Ann Intern Med.* 2001;134:832–837.

Josephson ME, Wellens HJJ. Differential diagnosis of supraventricular tachycardia. *Cardiol Clin.* 1990;8:411–442.

Smith GR, Monson RA. Patients with multiple unexplained symptoms: their characteristics, functional health, and health care utilization. *Arch Intern Med.* 1986;146:69–72.

Syncope

26

John Wolfe Blotzer, MD, & Mark C. Henderson, MD

Syncope is sudden, brief loss of consciousness and postural tone with spontaneous, complete recovery as a consequence of transient global cerebral hypoperfusion. Syncope is a common symptom, most often caused by a vasovagal episode. Syncope may be associated with injury due to loss of consciousness or risk of sudden death from the underlying cause. It accounts for up to 3% of emergency department visits and 6% of hospital admissions.

There are myriad causes of syncope. The historian must distinguish syncope from other symptoms such as dizziness, presyncope, vertigo, and vague complaints such as "lightheadedness" or "giddiness" (see Chapter 6).

KEY TERMS

Neurocardiogenic syncope, neural reflex syncope, vasodepressor syncope	*Interchangeable terms for syncopes primarily involving neural or reflex mechanisms. Examples include vasovagal, situational, and carotid sinus syncope.*
Situational syncope	*Syncope associated with certain activities (eg, micturition, defecation, coughing, and swallowing)*
Vasovagal syncope	*The common faint, the most common neural reflex disorder causing syncope.*

ETIOLOGY[1-7]

Most patients with a simple fainting spell, or vasovagal syncope, do not seek medical attention. Etiologies of syncope vary depending on the clinical setting, study population, definition of syncope, and rigor of the diagnostic evaluation. For instance, psychiatric disease generally causes "pseudosyncope," not syncope; nevertheless it is classified as syncope in a number of studies. In general, syncope may be classified into the following major categories:

- Reflex-mediated
- Orthostatic hypotension
- Neurologic disease
- Medication-induced
- Cardiac syncope (due to organic heart disease and arrhythmias) and
- Due to an unknown cause.

In a recent study of patients in Switzerland who sought medical attention at an emergency department, the causes were as follows: vasodepressor (37%), orthostatic hypotension (24%), carotid sinus hypersensitivity (1%), neurologic (5%), arrhythmias (7%), pulmonary embolism (1%), acute coronary syndromes (1%), aortic stenosis (1%), psychiatric (1.5%), unknown (14%), and miscellaneous (1.5%).[6] Recent studies have classified fewer and fewer patients with syncope as having an unknown cause probably due to more extensive diagnostic evaluation. In a recent study of electrophysiology patients, causes were vasovagal (47%), situational (0.7%), carotid sinus hypersensitivity (7.9%), autonomic dysfunction/orthostatic hypotension (5.6%), cerebrovascular disease (1.9%), bradyarrhythmias (13.6%), supraventricular tachyarrhythmias (9.8%), ventricular tachyarrhythmias (12.1%), long QT or hypertrophic cardiomyopathy (1.1%), and unknown (19.8%). Furthermore, 18.4% were considered to have multiple potential causes.[6] The institutionalized elderly are especially apt to have multifactorial syncope.[8]

Differential Diagnosis	Prevalence[1-6]
Reflex-mediated	
• *Vasovagal syncope*	*8–47%*
• *Situational syncope*	*1–8%*
• *Carotid sinus syncope*	*0–7.9%*
Orthostatic hypotension *(including volume loss, autonomic insufficiency, endocrine [adrenal insufficiency, pheochromocytoma], medications)*	*4–24%*
Neurologic disease *(including vertebrobasilar transient ischemic attack, basilar migraine, subclavian steal, and glossopharyngeal syncope)*	*0–5%*
Medications	*1–7%*
Cardiac syncope	
• *Organic heart disease (including aortic stenosis, hypertrophic cardiomyopathy, pulmonary embolism, pulmonary hypertension, atrial myxoma, myocardial infarction, critical coronary artery disease [left main coronary artery or equivalent], pericardial tamponade, and aortic dissection)*	*1–8%*
• *Arrhythmias (bradyarrhythmias and tachyarrhythmias including sinus node disease, second- or third-degree heart block, pacemaker malfunction, ventricular tachycardia, torsades de pointes, and supraventricular tachycardia; may also be due to medications that prolong the QT interval)*	*4–38%*
Unknown	*13–41%*
Psychiatric	*0–5%*
Miscellaneous *(including hypoglycemia, hyperventilation, etc)*	*0–7%*

GETTING STARTED

- In addition to the patient, it is critically important to interview any observers of the episode.
- Remember that syncope is a medical term. The patient will describe a faint, falling out, passing out, dizziness, a spell, or a black out.
- Take a thorough family history, past medical history, and current medication history.

Questions	Tips for effective interviewing
Please describe for me everything you remember about your (most recent) episode.	• *Allow the patient to tell the entire story in his or her own words.*
Has this ever happened before?	• *Avoid interrupting.*
Describe exactly what you were doing prior to the episode.	• *Respond to the patient's emotions, as losing consciousness can be very frightening.*
Describe everything you remember witnesses telling you they observed during your episode.	• *Respond to the patient's concerns.*

INTERVIEW FRAMEWORK

- Determine whether the patient experienced true syncope (abrupt loss of consciousness, loss of postural reflexes, spontaneous and complete return to consciousness without intervention) rather than another type of "dizziness" or seizure (see Chapter 6).
- If the episode was witnessed, interview the witness(es).
- Determine the circumstances surrounding the episode—eg, body position (standing, sitting, or supine), activity, and environment.
- Determine whether there were any premonitory symptoms before the loss of consciousness (especially important for vasovagal syncope).
- Determine features common to all episodes.
- Assess for alarm symptoms (see below).
- Determine whether there is underlying heart disease (confers a worse prognosis).
- Classify syncope into 1 of the following subtypes:
  - –Reflex-mediated
  - –Orthostatic hypotension
  - –Neurologic
  - –Medication-induced
  - –Cardiac syncope (organic heart disease or arrhythmias).

IDENTIFYING ALARM SYMPTOMS

- Although the etiology of most syncope is vasovagal and has a benign prognosis, syncope may herald sudden death or be the presenting manifestation of a life-threatening illness, such as myocardial infarction, aortic dissection, pulmonary embolism, ventricular tachyarrhythmias, or complete heart block. Patients with cardiac syncope are at increased risk for death, which is related to the underlying heart disease and not the syncope per se. For instance, exertional syncope from aortic stenosis suggests very advanced disease (with mean survival of 2 years unless the valve is replaced).
- In a recent preliminary study of emergency department patients with syncope or near syncope, the presence of 1 of 5 clinical variables predicted serious short-term outcomes.[9] Of these, 2 risk factors were historical: shortness of breath or a history of congestive heart failure (the other 3 were abnormal electrocardiogram, systolic blood pressure < 90 mm Hg, and a hematocrit less than 30%).

Serious Diagnoses	Prevalence[a]
Structural cardiovascular disease (valvular stenosis, pericardial tamponade, aortic stenosis, acute coronary syndromes, left atrial myxoma, hypertrophic cardiomyopathy, aortic dissection, arrhythmogenic right ventricular dysplasia)	
Arrhythmias (tachyarrhythmias, bradyarrhythmias, heart block)	*In a study of ambulatory patients who died while being monitored, the causative arrhythmia was ventricular tachycardia in 62%, ventricular fibrillation in 8%, torsades de pointes in 13%, and bradycardia in 17%.[10]*
Pulmonary hypertension	
Pulmonary embolism	

(continued)

Serious Diagnoses

Major volume loss (acute gastrointestinal hemor-rhage, massive diarrhea, dehydration)

Vertebrobasilar transient ischemic attack

Severe autonomic insufficiency

^aPrevalence is unknown when not indicated.

Alarm symptoms	Serious causes	Benign causes
Age greater than 45	*Cardiac syncope*	
History of heart disease	*Cardiac syncope*	
Family history of heart disease or sudden death	*Long QT syndromes* *Hypertrophic cardiomyopathy*	
Chest pain or dyspnea	*Myocardial infarction* *Unstable angina (left main coronary artery disease or equivalent)* *Aortic dissection* *Pericardial tamponade* *Pulmonary embolism*	*Panic disorder*
Syncope with exertion	*Aortic stenosis* *Pulmonic stenosis* *Hypertrophic cardiomyopathy* *Pulmonary hypertension* *Ventricular fibrillation or tachycardia* *Severe coronary artery disease*	
Absence of nausea or vomiting	*Arrhythmia*	
Absence of prodrome[11] (especially in patients with heart disease)	*Arrhythmia*	
Palpitations	*Arrhythmia*	
Syncope in the supine position	*Arrhythmia*	
Diplopia, dysarthria, vertigo, or facial numbness	*Vertebrobasilar (brainstem) transient ischemic attack*	

FOCUSED QUESTIONS[11–14]

See Chapter 6 for examples of questions to evaluate lightheadedness, dizziness, presyncope, or vertigo. See algorithm entitled, Initial Diagnostic Approach: Suspected Syncope.

A common clinical conundrum is the differentiation between syncope and seizure.

Distinguishing Seizures from Syncope[12]

Questions	Probable diagnosis	Positive Likelihood ratio (LR+)
Do you wake up with a cut tongue after your episodes?	Seizure	*LR+ 16.5*
Do you have a sense of déjà vu or jamais vu before your episodes?	Seizure	*LR+ 3.4*
Is emotional stress associated with losing consciousness?	Seizure	*LR+ 3.8*
Has anyone ever noted your head turning during an episode?	Seizure	*LR+ 13.5*
Has anyone ever noted that you: • *Are unresponsive, have unusual posturing, or jerking limbs during an episode?* • *Have no memory of your episodes afterwards?*	Seizure	• *LR+ 3.0 (unresponsiveness), LR+ 12.9 (unusual posturing), LR+ 5.6 (jerking limbs)* • *LR+ 4.0 (no memory of episode)*
Has anyone ever noticed that you are confused after an episode?	Seizure	*LR+ 3.0*
Did bystanders notice you were blue during the episode?	Seizure	*LR+ 5.8*
Did you experience muscle pain after the episode?	Seizure	*LR+ 3.4*
Have you ever had lightheaded spells?	Syncope	*LR+ 0.27 (for seizure)*
At times do you sweat before your spells?	Syncope	*LR+ 0.17 (for seizure)*
Do you experience shortness of breath before your spells?	Syncope	*LR+ 0.08 (for seizure)*
Is prolonged sitting or standing associated with your spells?	Syncope	*LR+ 0.05 (for seizure)*

Vasovagal syncope or the "common faint" is the most common form of syncope. Its diagnosis is usually established by a detailed medical history. There is usually a trigger such as prolonged standing, pain including medical instrumentation (5–15% prevalence of syncope in healthy blood donors), unpleasant sights, or extreme emotion. Typical prodromal symptoms include nausea, vomiting, sweating, feeling cold, and feeling tired. Carotid sinus syncope is the second most common form of neurally mediated syncope and is suggested by a history of a close relationship between the syncopal episode and mechanical manipulation or pressure on the neck, particularly in an elderly patient.

Use focused questions to determine the circumstances just prior to the episode, the onset of the episode, what bystanders observed during the episode (eg, duration), and background information on past medical and family history. Answers to these questions help narrow the differential diagnosis.

Questions	**Think about**
Do you have heart disease or heart failure?	Cardiac syncope
Do you have a family history of sudden death?	Arrhythmias Long QT syndrome Brugada syndrome
Do you have chest or neck pain with your episodes?	Coronary artery disease Glossopharyngeal neuralgia
Does exercise bring on your symptoms?	Valvular stenosis Pulmonary hypertension Subclavian steal Severe coronary artery disease
Do you pass out with changes in position?	Atrial myxoma or thrombus
Do you lose consciousness in the supine position?	Arrhythmia
Do you notice palpitations or a fast heart rate before your episodes?	Arrhythmia
Are you taking any medication?	Medication-induced (see *Drugs associated with syncope or presyncope*). Hypoglycemic agents typically produce more prolonged symptoms, incompatible with syncope.
Do you have a history of seizures?	Epilepsy
Do you have a history of stroke or transient ischemic attack?	Cerebrovascular disease (vertebrobasilar transient ischemic attack)
Do you have a history of diabetes with neuropathy?	Autonomic neuropathy
Do you have a history of Parkinson disease or other autonomic neuropathy?	Parkinsonism Subacute combined atrophy
Do your episodes occur after coughing, urinating, defecating, swallowing, etc?	Situational syncope
Do your episodes occur during a migraine attack?	Basilar artery migraine
Do you have throat or facial pain with your episode?	Glossopharyngeal neuralgia
Do your episodes occur in hot crowded environments? With prolonged standing? After experiencing intense pain; fear or emotion; or unexpected sights, sounds, or smells?	Vasovagal syncope
Do you notice nausea, vomiting, or feeling cold or fatigued before the episode?	Vasovagal syncope
Are you pale during or after the episode?	Vasovagal syncope
Do you injure yourself during the episodes?	Seizure Arrhythmia
Do you have black tarry stools, bloody stools, or hematemesis?	Orthostatic hypotension from gastrointestinal bleeding (see Chapter 33)

Do you have severe diarrhea, frequent urination, or prolonged vomiting?	Volume depletion
Do your episodes occur within 1 hour of eating meals?	Postprandial hypotension
Do you have diabetes, alcoholism, or chronic renal failure?	Autonomic insufficiency
Do your symptoms occur with abrupt neck movements especially looking upward or with pressure on the neck?	Carotid sinus syncope

Drugs Associated with Syncope or Presyncope[15,16]

Cardiovascular

β-blockers

Vasodilators (α-blockers, calcium channel blockers, nitrates, hydralazine, angiotensin-converting enzyme inhibitors)

Antiarrhythmics

Diuretics

Centrally acting antihypertensives (clonidine, methyldopa)

Other antihypertensives (guanethidine)

Central nervous system

Antidepressants (tricyclics, monoamine oxidase inhibitors)

Antipsychotics (phenothiazines)

Sedatives (barbiturates, ethanol)

Antiparkinsonian agents

Anticonvulsants

Narcotic analgesics

Anxiolytic agents (benzodiazepines)

Drugs that prolong the QT interval[a]

Cardiovascular (disopyramide, dofetilide, ibutilide, procainamide, quinidine, sotalol, bepridil, amiodarone)

Cisapride

Calcium channel blockers (lidoflazine, not marketed in the United States)

Anti-infective agents (clarithromycin, erythromycin, halofantrine, pentamidine, sparfloxacin)

Antiemetic agents (domperidone, droperidol)

Antipsychotic agents (chlorpromazine, haloperidol, mesoridazine, thioridazine, pimozide)

Antihistamines (terfenadine and astemizole, no longer marketed in United States)

Methadone

Arsenic trioxide

[a]Further details can be found at http://www.torsades.org

DIAGNOSTIC APPROACH[17–20]

There are 3 key questions in the evaluation of a patient with syncope:

1. Does the patient really have syncope?
2. Does the patient have underlying heart disease?
3. Are there historical features that suggest a specific diagnosis?

The answers to these questions come from a detailed medical history obtained from the patient and any eyewitnesses. Based only on history and physical exam, the etiology of syncope can be established in at least 45% of cases.[17] Adding electrocardiography to the initial evaluation increases diagnostic yield to greater than 50% and may add prognostic information. The algorithm entitled, Diagnostic Approach: Syncope is a modified version of the one proposed by the Clinical Efficacy Project of the American College of Physicians and the Task Force on Syncope of the European Society of Cardiology.

CAVEATS

- Establish that the patient has suffered true loss of consciousness, not one of the other causes of dizziness.
- Seizures and metabolic disorders (eg, hypoglycemia, alcohol or other intoxications, etc) are suggested by a much longer episode.
- Older patients are more likely to have a serious (cardiac) cause.
- The elderly often have multifactorial syncope. Do not stop taking the history after finding a single plausible explanation for the patient's symptoms.
- Syncope can be diagnosed by history alone in 45–55% of cases.

PROGNOSIS

Prognosis of syncope is related to the underlying cause. Reflex-mediated syncope has an excellent prognosis unless the provocative event is a serious cause (eg, myocardial infarction). Vasovagal syncope requires only reassurance and patient education to sit or lie down at the first warning of prodromal symptoms. Cardiovascular causes are associated with increased mortality and require appropriate treatment for the specific condition. Primary autonomic insufficiency is usually treated supportively. Secondary autonomic insufficiency from diabetes mellitus is difficult to treat. The prognosis of other secondary causes of autonomic insufficiency (eg, chronic renal failure, amyloidosis, paraneoplastic, Chagas disease) depends on the underlying disease. Lastly, most patients with a simple faint (vasovagal syncope) never bother to even seek medical attention and have an excellent prognosis.

REFERENCES

1. Day SC, Cook EF, Funkenstein H, Goldman L. Evaluation and outcome of emergency room patients with transient loss of consciousness. *Am J Med.* 1982;73:15–23.
2. Silverstein MD, Singer DE, Mulley A. Patients with syncope admitted to medical intensive care units. *JAMA.* 1982;248: 1185–1189.
3. Eagle KA, Black HR. The impact of diagnostic tests in diagnosing syncope. *Yale J Biol Med.* 1983;56:1–8.
4. Ben-Chetrit E, Flugelman M, Eliakim M. Syncope: a retrospective study of 101 hospitalized patients. *Isr J Med Sci.* 1985; 21:950–953.
5. Martin GJ, Adams SL, Martin HG, et al. Prospective evaluation of syncope. *Ann Emerg Med.* 1984;13:499–504.
6. Sarasin FP, Louis-Simonet M, Carballo D. Prospective evaluation of patients with syncope: a population based study. *Am J Med.* 2001;111:177–184.
7. Chen LY, Gersh BJ, Hodge DO, et al. Prevalence and clinical outcomes of patients with multiple potential causes of syncope. *Mayo Clin Proc.* 2003;78:414–420.
8. Lipsitz LA, Pluchino FC, Wei YC, Rowe JW. Syncope in institutionalized elderly: the impact of multiple pathologic conditions and situational stress. *J Chronic Dis.* 1986;39:619–630.

9. Quinn JV, Stiehl IG, McDermott DA, et al. Derivation of the San Francisco Syncope Rule to predict patients with short-term serious outcomes. *Ann Emerg Med.* 2004;43:224–232.

10. Bayes de la Luna A, Coumel P, Leclercq JF. Ambulatory sudden death: mechanisms of production of fatal arrhythmia on the basis of data from 157 cases. *Am Heart J.* 1989;117:151–159.

11. Alboni P, Brignole M, Menozzi C, et al. Diagnostic value of history in patients with syncope with or without heart disease. *J Am Coll Cardiol.* 2001;37:1921–1928.

12. Sheldon R, Rose S, Ritchie D, et al. Historical criteria that distinguish syncope from seizures. *J Am Coll Cardiol.* 2002;40:142–148.

13. Calkins H, Shyr Y, Frumin H, Schork A, Morady F. The value of the clinical history in the differentiation of syncope due to ventricular tachycardia, atrioventricular block, and neurocardiogenic syncope. *Am J Med.* 1995;98:365–373.

14. Oh JH, Hanusa BH, Kapoor WN. Do symptoms predict cardiac arrhythmias and mortality in patients with syncope? *Arch Intern Med.* 1999;159:375–380.

15. Roden DM. Drug-induced prolongation of the QT interval. *N Engl J Med.* 2004;350:1013–1022.

16. Henderson MC, Prabu SD. Syncope, current diagnosis and treatment. *Curr Probl Cardiol.* 1997;22:242–296.

17. Linzer M, Yang EH, Estes NA 3rd, et al. Diagnosing syncope. Part 1: Value of history, physical examination, and electrocardiography: Clinical Efficacy Assessment Project of the American College of Physicians. *Ann Intern Med.* 1997;126:989–996.

18. Linzer M, Yang EH, Estes NA 3rd, et al. Diagnosing syncope. Part 2: Unexplained Syncope: Clinical Efficacy Assessment Project of the American College of Physicians. *Ann Intern Med.* 1997;126:76–86.

19. Brignole M, Alboni P, Benditt D, et al. Task Force on Syncope, European Society of Cardiology. Guidelines on management (diagnosis and treatment) of syncope. *Eur Heart J.* 2001;22:1256–1306. http://www.escardio.org/scinfo/Tforceguidelines.htm#Syncope

20. Goldschlager N, Epstein AE, Grubb BP, et al. Etiologic considerations in the patient with syncope and an apparently normal heart. Practice Guidelines Subcommittee, North American Society of Pacing and Electrophysiology. *Arch Intern Med.* 2003;163:151–162.

SUGGESTED READING

Benditt DG, Blanc J-J, Brignole M, Sutton R. *The Evaluation and Treatment of Syncope. A Handbook for Clinical Practice.* New York, Blackwell Publishing, Inc./Futura Division, 2003.

Grubb BP, Olshansky B (editors). *Syncope: Mechanisms and Management.* Armonk NY, Futura Publishing Company, 1998.

Kapoor WN. Syncope. *N Engl J Med.* 2000;343:1856–1862.

Schnipper JL, Kapoor WK. Diagnostic evaluation and management of patients with syncope. *Med Clin North Am.* 2001;85:423–456.

Initial Diagnostic Approach: Suspected Syncope

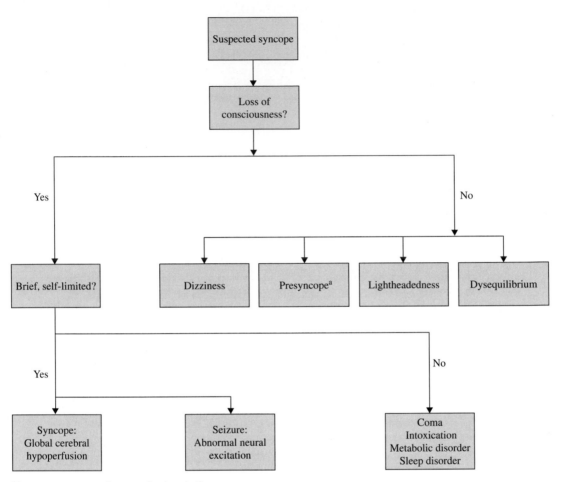

^aPresyncope may require an evaluation similar to syncope.

Diagnostic Approach: Syncope

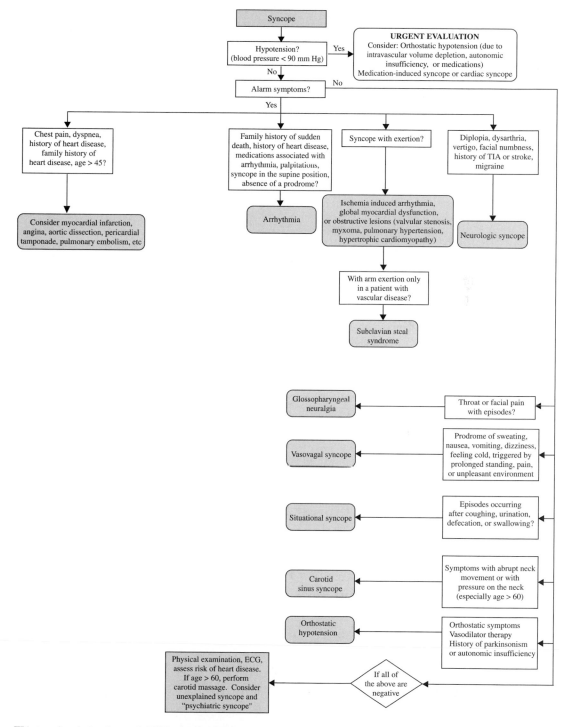

TIA, transient ischemic attack; ECG, electrocardiogram.

Edema

27

Jeff Wiese, MD

Edema is the accumulation of fluid in the interstitial space between cells. It is categorized into 5 subtypes based on the Starling law of fluid flow across a membrane:

$$\text{Edema} = K\,[(P_{in} - P_{out}) - (Onc_{in} - Onc_{out})]$$

where, K = vessel permeability
P_{in} = intravascular hydrostatic pressure
P_{out} = interstitial hydrostatic pressure
Onc_{in} = intravascular oncotic pressure
Onc_{out} = interstitial oncotic pressure.

Fluid is kept in the intravascular space by the capillary walls that selectively allow small amounts of fluid to leave the vascular space to deliver water, oxygen, and nutrients to the body cells. Under normal circumstances, only a small amount of fluid leaves the vascular space, and this small volume is returned to the vascular space via lymphatic drainage. The permeability constant of the capillary membrane regulates how much fluid leaks out (K). The high protein concentration in the blood also prevents excessive fluid from leaving the intravascular space by osmotically retaining water in the vessels where the protein is held (Onc_{in}).

Edema results when the pressure in the vessels (P_{in}) overrides the semipermeable capillary membrane, pushing more volume into the extravascular space. Although the Starling law indicates that both a high intravascular pressure and a low extravascular pressure may cause edema ($P_{in} - P_{out}$), there are no clinical conditions that cause edema by a low extravascular pressure.

Edema can also arise when the lymphatic drainage of the tissues is obstructed, the permeability of the capillary membranes is increased (K), or the concentration of protein in the blood is decreased (Onc_{in}). Increased protein concentration in the interstitium (Onc_{out}) is rarely a cause of edema, although excess fat in the interstitium may draw and hold water into the interstitial space causing edema (lipedema).

The most efficient method of diagnosing the etiology of edema is to sequentially consider each of these 4 forces that augment fluid leaving the intravascular space and entering the interstitial space.

KEY TERMS

Anasarca	Edema involving all aspects of the body: upper and lower extremities and the face.
Ascites	Collection of fluid in the peritoneal cavity.
Lipedema	Edema caused by fluid retained in the interstitial space by lipids in the dermis.
Lymphedema	Edema caused by obstruction of lymphatic drainage of the tissues.
Myxedema	Edema resulting from hypothyroidism (see below).
Pretibial myxedema	Not technically edema, the swelling on the anterior shins is due to coalescing of subcutaneous plaques due to Graves disease antibodies infiltrating dermal tissue.

ETIOLOGY

The etiology of edema depends on the clinical setting.

Differential Diagnosis	Prevalence
Venous stasis; varicose veins	30%
Congestive heart failure	30%
Lipedema	10%
Cirrhosis	10%
Nephrotic syndrome	5%
Hypothyroidism	5%
Venous stasis; venous thrombosis/obstruction	3%
Medications	3%
Anaphylaxis	1%
Lymphatic obstruction	1%
Protein losing enteropathy	1%
Malnutrition	1%

GETTING STARTED

- Review medication list prior to seeing the patient and validate during the interview.
- Avoid leading questions. It may be necessary to follow-up with a few close-ended questions directed at the most likely disorder.

Questions

When did the swelling begin? How has the swelling progressed since that time?

Do you have a history of heart, kidney, liver, or thyroid disease?

Tell me about your diet.

Remember

- *Let patients use their own words.*
- *Avoid interrupting.*
- *Listen to the patient's description for diagnostic clues.*
- *Try to assemble the patient's description into a chronologic story as you obtain the history.*

INTERVIEW FRAMEWORK

- Assess for alarm symptoms.
- Ask about symptoms of heart failure.
- Ask about alcohol use and risk factors for viral hepatitis.
- Ask about risk factors for venous stasis and vascular injury.
- Take a thorough dietary history.
- Determine the temporal pattern and duration of symptoms, accompanying symptoms, and precipitating factors.

IDENTIFYING ALARM SYMPTOMS

With the exception of anaphylaxis, edema is rarely a life-threatening condition. Congestive heart failure can be life-threatening, but the risk is due to pulmonary congestion from the heart failure and not the edema itself. A deep venous thrombosis is considered life-threatening because it can lead to pulmonary embolism.

Serious Diagnoses

- Congestive heart failure
- Anaphylaxis
- Fulminant liver failure
- Deep venous thrombosis leading to pulmonary embolism

Alarm symptoms	Consider
New medication *Exposure to latex or chemicals*	*Anaphylaxis*
Chest discomfort, shortness of breath, orthopnea or paroxysmal nocturnal dyspnea *Loss of consciousness (syncope)* *Feeling like going to pass out, especially when walking (presyncope)*	*Valve rupture* *Cardiac ischemia* *Outflow tract obstruction (eg, aortic stenosis, hypertrophic cardiomyopathy, primary pulmonary hypertension, or atrial myxoma)* *Pulmonary embolism*
Alcohol abuse *Unprotected sex (hepatitis B and C)* *Use of injection drugs (hepatitis C)* *Use of illicit drugs (eg, mushrooms or Ecstasy)* *Abdominal swelling (ascites)*	*Fulminant liver failure*
Sedentary position for a prolonged time (eg, bedridden, long travel)? *Smoking* *History of blood clots* *Use of oral contraceptives*	*Pulmonary embolism*

FOCUSED QUESTIONS

Considering each pathophysiologic category separately is the best method for determining the cause of edema.

Increased Permeability

Increased permeability affects all tissue beds equally; **edema of the upper and lower extremities (and face) suggests increased permeability as the etiology.**

Questions	Think about
What medications are you taking, and how long have you taken each? *Do you take over-the-counter medications?*	***Anaphylaxis:*** *All medications can cause edema by way of anaphylaxis. Histamine is released in response to the allergen, and this increases vessel permeability causing edema. Anaphylaxis may develop even after months of taking a medication.*
Are you taking an angiotensin-converting enzyme (ACE)-inhibitor or calcium channel blocker?	***ACE-inhibitor– or calcium channel blocker–induced edema:*** *ACE is responsible for degrading circulating bradykinin, which is released naturally from tissue injury to promote extravasation of fluid (and white blood*

(continued)

Questions	Think about
	cells) at sites of injury. High circulating bradykinin levels can cause unwarranted edema. Calcium channel blockers cause edema by an unknown mechanism.
Do you feel tired, have dry skin, coarse hair, or intolerance to cold?	**Hypothyroidism:** *Hypothyroidism causes increased vessel permeability and increased circulating volume due to excess antidiuretic hormone (ADH) production (triiodothyronine [T_3] inhibits ADH release).*
Does the edema come and go suddenly? Do you note hives or trouble breathing when you experience the edema?	**Hereditary angioedema:** *Hereditary angioedema is due to a deficiency in C1 esterase. Without this enzyme, C1 accumulates, stimulating the complement cascade that eventually results in excess histamine release and angioedema. Hereditary angioedema almost always involves the lips, face, and occasionally the airway.*
Have you been bitten by a pit viper?	**Pit viper bites:** *Pit viper venom induces bradykinin from the bite, and inhibits the ACE responsible for its degradation. See above.*

Increased Intravascular Pressure

Increased intravascular pressure is due to either volume overload or an obstruction of venous blood to the heart. Because pressure is greatest in the lower extremities due to gravity, edema due to increased intravascular pressure always begins in the lower extremities and ascends superiorly to the site of the obstruction. Venous pressure is higher in the left leg because the left iliac vein must cross under the aorta to join the vena cava. Edema due to increased intravascular pressure almost always begins in the left leg, eventually involving both legs.

A. Volume Overload

Questions	Think about
Have you noticed a decrease in your urinary output?	*Renal failure*
What types of food do you eat?	*Excessive sodium is contained in the following foods: potato chips, salted peanuts, fast food, canned foods, and Chinese food. Be certain to ask how much salt the patient adds to his or her foods.*
Is the patient receiving intravenous medications?	*Some medications come as the anion portion of a salt, and must be combined with a cation such as sodium for solubility (ie, Na+ Penicillin-). The sodium concentration can be considerable, especially for every 4-hour dosing of a medication (eg, ticarcillin).*
What intravenous fluids is the patient receiving?	*The recommended sodium intake per day is less than 3 g. One liter of normal saline is 0.9% sodium, or 9 g. Be certain the patient is not left on normal saline by mistake.*
Do you work outdoors or in hot climates?	**Steroid- or glucocorticoid-induced edema:** *In hot climates, many people will have minor lower extremity edema by the end of the day due to elevated aldosterone levels (stimulated by the loss of volume due to sweating). At the end of the*

	day when fluid is repleted, the elevated sodium content causes fluid retention and edema. The edema resolves as the patient is prone overnight.
Are you taking steroids?	Steroids, like endogenous cortisol, also stimulate the aldosterone receptor resulting in sodium and water retention.
Do you have weakness, fatigue, or abdominal stria?	**Cushing's syndrome:** Excess cortisol stimulates the aldosterone receptor causing sodium and water retention.

B. Venous or Lymphatic Obstruction

The best method is to start at the aortic root and work backwards, remembering that any valvular obstruction or incompetence will result in increased pressure in the venous system distal to the obstruction. All abnormalities from the aortic root to the left atrium will cause shortness of breath, as blood is "backed up" into the lungs.

Questions	**Think about**
Have you had chest pain, felt like passing out, or felt short of breath?	**Aortic stenosis:** Stenosis of the aortic valve impairs forward blood flow, resulting in pooling of the blood in the lungs causing dyspnea. The elevated left ventricular pressure increases myocardial work and impairs subendocardial blood flow, resulting in cardiac ischemia and chest pain. The lack of blood flow to the brain results in syncope.
Are you short of breath? Do you use injection drugs?	**Aortic insufficiency:** The incompetent valve increases left ventricular pressure, and thus pulmonary vein pressure causing dyspnea. The most common cause of acute aortic insufficiency is infection of the aortic valve (endocarditis).
Do you have a history of ischemic heart disease? Have you recently been pregnant? Have you received chemotherapy in the past? Are you short of breath?	**Cardiomyopathy:** Cardiomyopathy is a decrease in left ventricular function due to myocytes that are damaged from end-stage hypertension, ischemic heart disease, diabetes, chemotherapeutic agents, viral infections, or postpartum cardiomyopathy. The decreased left ventricular function elevates venous pressure in the lungs (dyspnea) and the systemic veins (edema).
Do you have a history of ischemic heart disease? Do you use injection drugs? Did you have rheumatic fever as a child?	**Mitral regurgitation or stenosis:** The most common cause of mitral stenosis is rheumatic heart disease. The most common causes of mitral insufficiency are dilation of the left ventricle due to heart failure (the dilating ventricle pulls the valve leaflets apart), myocardial infarction involving the papillary muscles (connecting the mitral valve to the left ventricle), or infection of the valve.
Did you have rheumatic fever as a child? Have you taken the dietary supplement phenfluramine?	**Pulmonic stenosis or insufficiency**

(continued)

Questions	Think about
Do you use injection drugs? *Did you have rheumatic fever as a child?*	***Tricuspid stenosis or insufficiency:*** *The most common causes of tricuspid stenosis or insufficiency is endocarditis or rheumatic heart disease.*
Have you had tuberculosis? *Have you been diagnosed with lung or breast cancer?* *Do you smoke?*	***Constrictive pericarditis:*** *Constrictive pericarditis impairs the right ventricle from expanding to accommodate venous blood being returned to the heart. The most common causes include tuberculosis or lung or breast cancer.*
	Cardiac tamponade: *Tamponade is collection of fluid between the pericardium and the heart that impairs the right heart from accommodating venous volume.*
Do you have a history of tuberculosis or lung cancer? *Are your face and arms swollen more than your legs?*	***Superior vena cava syndrome:*** *Superior vena cava syndrome results from a mass (infectious or malignant) that encases the superior vena cava preventing venous blood from returning to the heart. The edema is localized to the arms and face.*
Have you noticed abdominal swelling?	***Abdominal mass or pregnancy:*** *An abdominal mass that obstructs the inferior cava will prevent venous volume from returning to the right heart.*
Do you have a history of blood clots? *Do you smoke?* *Have you been in a prolonged state of immobility (airplane ride, bedridden)?* *Do you take oral contraceptives?* *Do you have a past diagnosis of cancer?*	***Deep venous thrombosis:*** *The Virchow triad of risk factors for intravascular thrombosis includes stasis, hypercoagulability, and vessel injury. The most common causes of hypercoagulability include smoking, estrogen use, and genetic predisposition (factor V Leiden, Prothrombin mutation 20210, antithrombin III deficiency).*
Is the edema localized to the left leg?	***May-Thurner disease:*** *May-Thurner syndrome is compression of the left iliac vein as it crosses under the aorta to get to the inferior vena cava. Definitive diagnosis is made with an ascending venogram.*
Have you noticed prominent veins on your legs?	*Varicose veins*
Do you have yellow nails? *Do you have a history of cancer?* *Have you traveled to tropical areas?*	***Lymphatic obstruction:*** *The most common cause of lymphatic insufficiency is a malignancy obstructing lymph flow. The yellow nail syndrome is a genetic syndrome composed of yellow nails and lymphatic insufficiency. Parasitic infection may also obstruct the lymphatic chain (elephantiasis).*

Decreased Oncotic Pressure

Decreased oncotic pressure results from a deficiency in albumin, either due to inadequate production or accelerated loss.

Questions	Think about
Describe your diet.	*Malnutrition (Kwashiorkor) only occurs in severely malnourished patients.*

Have you had diarrhea?	**Protein losing enteropathy:** *This is due to impairment of the bowel's ability to absorb protein. The increased oncotic pressure in the bowel lumen causes diarrhea.*
How much alcohol do you drink? Have you had viral hepatitis? Have you had liver disease?	**Cirrhosis:** *Damage to the liver tissue impairs its ability to convert absorbed protein to albumin. See Chapter 34 for questions that may reveal the cause of the liver failure and other symptoms associated with liver failure.*
Have you noticed frothy urine? Do you have a history of kidney disease? Do you have diabetes or hypertension?	**Nephrotic syndrome:** *Nephrotic syndrome is loss of the protein in the urine. The most common causes in adults are diabetes, hypertension, minimal change disease, and focal segmental glomerulosclerosis.*

PROGNOSIS

Most cases of edema are benign and will resolve without therapy. The prognosis for other cases depends on the etiology.

CAVEATS

- Peripheral edema is graded on a 1 to 4 scale based on the pit recovery time (PRT). To assess the PRT, apply pressure with 1 finger over the area of edema for 5 seconds. Release the pressure and assess the time required for the pit to return to normal. Each 1 point on the scale corresponds to 30 seconds of PRT (1+ edema = < 30 seconds PRT; 2+ edema = 30–60 seconds PRT, etc.). The higher the PRT, the greater the likelihood that the edema is due to increased hydrostatic pressure (ie, CHF).
- The distribution of edema may provide a clue as to its cause. Mild to moderate heart failure results in edema involving the legs, feet, and toes. Severe congestive heart failure leads to edema involving the legs and feet but sparing the toes. The inadequate cardiac output in severe heart failure causes peripheral vascular constriction to maintain core mean arterial pressure. This vascular constriction decreases blood flow to the toes, decreasing venous volume, and thus edema in the toes. Edema involving the legs but sparing the feet is lipedema, or fluid retained by fat in the interstitial space. Since there is no fat on the top of the feet, the feet are spared. Decreasing intravascular volume with diuretics will not mobilize the fluid of lipedema, but will only serve to dehydrate the patient.

SUGGESTED READING

Adler O, Kalidindi S, Butt A, Hussain KM. Chordae tendineae rupture resulting in pulmonary edema in a patient with discrete subvalvular aortic stenosis—a case report and literature review. *Angiology.* 2003;54:613–617.

Blankfield RP, et al. Etiology and diagnosis of bilateral leg edema in primary care. *Am J Med.* 1998;105:192–197.

Cho S, Atwood JE. Peripheral edema. *Am J Med.* 2002;113:580–586.

Elwell RJ, Spencer AP, Eisele G. Combined furosemide and human albumin treatment for diuretic-resistant edema. *Ann Pharmacother.* 2003;37:695–700.

Fishel RS, Are C, Barbul A. Vessel injury and capillary leak. *Crit Care Med.* 2003;31(8 Suppl):S502–511.

Macdonald JM, Sims N, Mayrovitz HN. Lymphedema, lipedema, and the open wound: the role of compression therapy. *Surg Clin North Am.* 2003;83:639–658.

Sica DA. Calcium channel blocker-related peripheral edema: can it be resolved? *J Clin Hypertens.* 2003;5:291–294, 297.

Sica DA. Metolazone and its role in edema management. *Congest Heart Fail.* 2003;9:100–105.

Szuba A, Shin WS, Strauss HW, Rockson S. The third circulation: radionuclide lymphoscintigraphy in the evaluation of lymphedema. *J Nucl Med.* 2003;44:43–57.

Yoshida S, Sakuma K, Ueda O. Acute mitral regurgitation due to total rupture in the anterior papillary muscle after acute myocardial infarction successfully treated by emergency surgery. *Jpn J Thorac Cardiovasc Surg.* 2003;51:208–210.

Diagnostic Approach: Edema

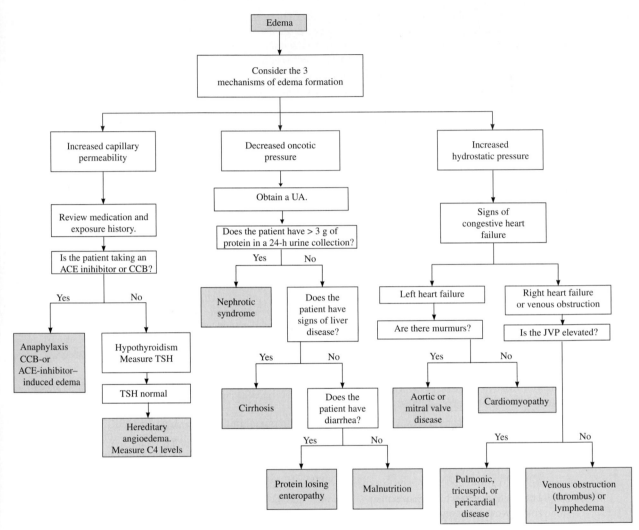

ACE, angiotensin-converting enzyme; CCB, calcium channel blocker; TSH, thyroid-stimulating hormone; UA, urinalysis; JVP, jugular venous pressure.

SECTION VII
Gastrointestinal System

Abdominal Pain

28

Joseph Ming Wah Li, MD

Abdominal pain is a commonly encountered clinical problem, accounting for nearly 10% of all visits to emergency departments. Nearly 25% of all patients evaluated for abdominal pain in such settings require hospitalization. What is the reason for such a high rate of hospitalization? The etiology of abdominal pain is often, at least initially, uncertain. Many other patients leave the emergency setting without a definite diagnosis. The frequency of this clinical problem and the associated diagnostic uncertainty mandate a further discussion of abdominal pain. A better understanding of the historical features associated with different causes of abdominal pain will expedite appropriate diagnosis and treatment.

KEY TERMS

Acute abdomen
An abdominal condition that requires immediate surgical intervention.[1,2] Patients with an acute abdomen represent only a fraction of those with acute abdominal pain.

Acute abdominal pain
Acute abdominal pain has an onset over minutes but can persist for days.[3] Sometimes, very severe abdominal pain is described as acute, which is appropriate only if the pain is a new problem. An acute exacerbation of chronic abdominal pain should not be described as acute abdominal pain.

Biliary colic
Pain caused by acute transient obstruction of the cystic duct, usually due to the passage of a gallstone. Patients commonly describe the pain as occurring "in waves." This may be due to peristaltic contractions against a fixed obstruction.

Chronic abdominal pain
Abdominal pain that is present for at least 6 months without a diagnosis despite an appropriate evaluation.

Nonspecific abdominal pain
Pain poorly localized to a specific area of the abdomen. It is often inadequately explained by any specific diagnosis.

Peritoneum
The membrane derived from embryonic mesoderm, which covers the viscera and lines the walls of the abdominal and pelvic cavities. The part of the peritoneum that lines the viscera is called the visceral peritoneum. The parietal peritoneum lines the abdominal and pelvic cavities. Autonomic nerves innervate the visceral peritoneum while spinal somatic nerves innervate the parietal peritoneum.[1]

Referred pain
Referred pain is experienced distant from the site of origin.[4] The referral of visceral pain to distant sites is not well understood but may involve both somatic and visceral input to the dorsal horn of the spinal cord.

(continued)

KEY TERMS

Somatic pain

Somatic pain emanates from the parietal peritoneum. The somatic nerves innervating the parietal peritoneum contain A-delta neurons.[1] These nerves are fast transmitters and typically produce very sharp, localized pain.

Visceral pain

Pain emanating from the visceral peritoneum. The visceral peritoneum contains C fibers, which transmit slowly, resulting in poorly localized, dull, achy pain.[1] The innervation of the visceral peritoneum is bilateral, resulting in pain that often refers to the midline. Visceral pain often results from distention of an organ (eg, inflamed gallbladder, impacted kidney stones, or small bowel obstruction).

ETIOLOGY

The prevalence of the various causes of acute abdominal pain depends on the age of the patient. The epidemiology of chronic abdominal pain has not been well studied.

Differential Diagnosis	Prevalence[a]		
	Total (%)	> 60 years old (%)	< 60 years old (%)
Abdominal pain, nonspecific	34.9	9.6–22.5	43
Aortic aneurysm, ruptured	1.3	3	0.1
Appendicitis, acute	12–26	3.5–6.7	25
Biliary			
• Cholangitis			
• Cholecystitis		26–40.8	
• Cholelithiasis	5.1	8.9	2.6
Colon, other diseases		3.5–3.7	
• Colitis			
Diverticulitis	3.9	3.4–8.5	0.8
Gastroenteritis	0.3	0	0.6
Gynecologic	1.1	0.2	1.7
Hernia, incarcerated		4.8–9.6	
Inflammatory bowel disease	0.8	1.1	0.7
Ileus		7.3–10.7	
Intestinal obstruction	14.8	28	6.1
Malignancy, abdominal	3	5.5–13.2	1.4
Pancreatitis	2.4	1.9–5.1	1.5
Peptic ulcer disease	3.3	3.3–8.4	2.5
Pelvic inflammatory disease			
Sickle cell crisis			
Testicular			

• Epididymitis			
• Testicular torsion			
Trauma, abdominal	3.1	0.4	4.9
Urologic	5.9	3.2	7.6
• Bladder distention			
• Cystitis			
• Nephrolithiasis			
• Pyelonephritis			
Vascular occlusion, mesenteric	0.6	1.5	0

[a]In patients presenting to the emergency department with acute abdominal pain[5,6]; prevalence is unknown when not indicated.

GETTING STARTED

- Allow patients to describe their symptoms in their own words.
- Avoid leading questions. Initiate the discussion with open-ended questions.
- Complete the history-taking with closed-ended questions directed at the most likely disorder.
- Review the list of medicines the patient is taking prior to seeing the patient and validate during the interview. Remember to ask about over-the-counter and herbal medicines.
- Inquire about alcohol and illicit drug use.

Questions	**Remember**
I'm sorry to hear that you're having abdominal pain. Can you tell me more about it?	• *Allow the patient to describe his or her story without interruption.*
When did your abdominal pain begin?	• *Listen carefully for details that may help formulate a differential diagnosis.*
I can tell that this abdominal pain is very uncomfortable for you; I'd like to ask you some questions so I can understand what is causing your pain.	• *Reassurance will put the patient at ease and facilitate the interview.*

INTERVIEW FRAMEWORK

- Determine whether this is acute or chronic abdominal pain (or an acute exacerbation of chronic abdominal pain). The differential diagnosis differs depending on the acuity of the pain.
- Assess for alarm symptoms.
- Identify the primary location of the pain (if possible), and determine whether the pain has moved to another location[4]:

  Right upper quadrant (RUQ) pain
  Epigastric pain
  Left upper quadrant (LUQ) pain
  Right flank pain
  Periumbilical pain
  Left flank pain

Right lower quadrant (RLQ) pain
Hypogastric pain (midline below the umbilicus)
Left lower quadrant (LLQ) pain
Diffuse abdominal pain

- Inquire about abdominal pain characteristics using the cardinal symptom features (PQRST):

Provocation	*What makes the pain worse or better?*
Quality	*What is the character of the pain?*
Radiation	*Does the pain radiate?*
Severity	*Rate the pain on a scale from 0 to 10 (with 0 being no pain and 10 being the worst pain possible).*
Timing/Treatment	*How long have you had the pain? Has the pain been persistent or intermittent over this period of time? What has been done to treat the pain?*

IDENTIFYING ALARM SYMPTOMS

There are many potentially serious causes of abdominal pain. Identification of these diagnoses requires detailed questioning aimed at identifying the characteristic features of the disease.

Serious Diagnoses	Comment
Abdominal aortic aneurysm (AAA)	• *Most AAAs are asymptomatic until rupture.* • *Abdominal or back pain suggests expansion of the AAA.* • *The first symptom of an AAA may be thrombosis or embolization to a distal site.* • *Only 50% of patients survive a ruptured AAA.*
Adnexal torsion	*Presents as sudden onset of pain in the lower abdomen on the affected side. Urinary urgency, nausea, and vomiting may accompany the pain.*
Adrenal insufficiency, acute	*Hypotension is the most concerning feature; often accompanied by abdominal pain, fever, confusion, fatigue, nausea, and vomiting.*
Aortic dissection, thoracic	• *Acute abdominal pain occurs in 22% of dissections of the ascending aorta (Stanford Classification type A) and in 43% of those involving the aorta distal to the origin of the left subclavian artery (Stanford Classification type B).* • *40–50% of untreated patients with dissection of the proximal aorta die within 48 hours. For those who survive beyond 48 hours, 1-year mortality is 90%.[10]* • *Patients present with sharp, "tearing" pain in the chest, back, or abdomen. The pain is maximal at its onset, as opposed to the crescendo nature of acute myocardial infarction. The pain may move inferiorly over time, which likely corresponds to extension of the aortic dissection.*
Appendicitis	• *Lifetime risk in general population is 7%.[3]* • *Patients often initially develop constant, nonspecific periumbilical or diffuse abdominal discomfort. Over a matter of*

hours, the pain localizes to the RLQ. Localized tenderness may not develop in patients with a retrocecal appendix since the appendix is not in contact with the parietal peritoneum. Patients often report constipation, although some will have diarrhea.

Biliary process

• *Cholangitis*

Charcot's triad (fever, RUQ abdominal pain, and jaundice) occurs in 50–75% of patients with cholangitis.

• *Cholecystitis*

• *75% of patients have nausea and vomiting.[3]*
• *Most commonly, persistent and severe RUQ and epigastric pain may occur. It can radiate to the right shoulder or back.*

Bowel obstruction

• *50% of patients have had prior abdominal surgery.[3]*
• *Patients typically have crampy, periumbilical pain, which occurs in paroxysmal waves every few minutes.*

Celiac sprue

The most common symptoms include diarrhea, flatulence, weight loss, abdominal discomfort, and bloating.

Diabetic ketoacidosis

• *Mortality ranges from 2–5% in developed countries to 6–24% in developing countries.*
• *Nearly 50% of patients have abdominal pain.*

Diverticulitis

• *Symptoms include LLQ pain (70%), nausea and vomiting (20–62%), constipation (50%), diarrhea (25–35%), and urinary symptoms (10–15%).*
• *Right-sided colonic diverticulitis is less common in western countries but accounts for up to 75% of diverticulitis in Asians.*

Endometriosis

• *Approximately 50% of teenage women who undergo laparoscopy for evaluation of pelvic pain or dysmenorrhea have endometriosis.*
• *Symptoms include pelvic pain, rectal pain, dysmenorrhea and dyspareunia. Aching pain tends to begin several days before menses and worsens until menses abates. Some patients are asymptomatic. The presence or extent of endometriosis does not correlate with symptoms.*

Familial Mediterranean Fever

• *Symptoms include recurrent attacks of abdominal pain (due to serositis) and fever lasting several days.*
• *65% of first attacks begin before age 10 and 90% before age 20.*

Hernia, incarcerated

• *The lifetime risk of developing a groin hernia is 25% in men and < 5% in women.*
• *96% of groin hernias are inguinal and 4% are femoral.*
• *Inguinal hernias are more common in men (9:1) and occur more frequently on the right side.*
• *Femoral hernias are more common in women (4:1); 40% of femoral hernias present with incarceration or strangulation.*
• *The most common symptom is a sensation of "heaviness" with activities that increase intra-abdominal pressure (ie, straining or lifting). Pain should raise concern for incarceration. Peritoneal signs often accompany bowel strangulation.*

(continued)

Serious Diagnoses	Comment
Hypercalcemia	• Up to 20% incidence of peptic ulcer disease (PUD) and nephrolithiasis among patients with primary hyperparathyroidism. Both conditions can cause acute abdominal pain. • Hypercalcemia causes different kinds of abdominal pain, depending on the complication (ie, constipation, nephrolithiasis, or pancreatitis).
Inflammatory bowel disease	
• Crohn's disease	• The symptoms of Crohn's disease are much more variable than ulcerative colitis; 80% of patients have small bowel involvement, usually in the distal ileum. • Common symptoms include abdominal pain, fever, weight loss, and diarrhea with or without bleeding. Up to 10% of patients do not have diarrhea.
• Ulcerative colitis	• Symptoms are due to inflammation of the mucosal surface of the colon, which almost always involves the rectum. The disease may extend proximally and continuously to involve other parts of the colon. Bloody diarrhea is the principal symptom. Defecation may relieve the lower abdominal cramps.
Intestinal ischemia, acute	• Patients complain of sudden onset of crampy abdominal pain. • Acute intestinal ischemia may be due to occlusive disease in either the arterial or venous system. • Arterial mesenteric ischemia accounts for over 60% of acute intestinal ischemia. Risk factors include atherosclerosis, low cardiac output states, recent myocardial infarction, and cardiac valvular disease. • Symptoms of colitis may occur if the inferior mesenteric artery is compromised. • Left unrecognized, ischemia may lead to bowel infarction, analogous to myocardial infarction.
Intestinal ischemia, chronic	• Typical patient is a smoker with atherosclerotic vascular disease. • Nearly 50% of patients have either peripheral vascular disease or coronary artery disease. • Patients typically complain of dull, crampy periumbilical pain within 1 hour of eating a meal. Symptoms usually subside over the ensuing hours until the next meal.
Irritable bowel syndrome	• Common idiopathic disorder characterized by chronic abdominal pain and bloating typically relieved by a bowel movement, passage of mucus, change in the number of bowel movements or stool consistency (harder or softer), and episodic diarrhea alternating with constipation (see Chapter 29). • Symptoms usually worsened by stress.
Malignancy, occult	• 33% of patients with renal cell carcinoma present with flank pain or abdominal mass. • 70% of patients with pancreatic cancer have abdominal pain.

Myocardial infarction or ischemia	• *Myocardial infarction can cause dull epigastric discomfort and is sometimes confused with PUD.*
Nephrolithiasis	• *Nephrolithiasis may be asymptomatic. Renal stones most commonly cause pain when they pass from the pelvis into the ureter. The pain is typically paroxysmal, related to stone movement and subsequent ureteral contractions. The pain migrates as the stone moves through the ureter (see Chapter 39).*
Pancreatitis, acute	• *Abdominal pain occurs in nearly 100% of patients. The pain typically starts in the epigastrium and radiates to the back. The pain resolves after the acute attack.* • *Nausea and vomiting occurs in 90% of patients.*
Pancreatitis, chronic	• *Abdominal pain may initially be episodic but often becomes continuous with intermittent exacerbations.* • *Presenting signs include exocrine and endocrine dysfunction, including steatorrhea and glucose intolerance.*
Pelvic inflammatory disease	• *The abdominal pain usually occurs bilaterally in the lower abdominal quadrants. The pain often begins during or shortly after the beginning of menses. In 33% of patients, the onset of pain is accompanied by abnormal uterine bleeding. Coitus and sudden movements may worsen the pain. Up to 10% of patients have perihepatitis, which presents with RUQ pain (Fitz-Hugh–Curtis syndrome). Only about 50% of patients are febrile. Many women have minimal symptoms.*
PUD	• *Patients may have a wide range of symptoms, none of which are sensitive or specific. These include "burning" epigastric pain and fullness, postprandial belching, bloating, anorexia, nausea, and vomiting. Pain due to a duodenal ulcer classically occurs several hours after a meal when the stomach is empty; whereas gastric ulcer usually causes severe pain soon after a meal. Pain caused by a duodenal ulcer is typically more responsive to antacid therapy or food than is pain caused by a gastric ulcer.*
Porphyria, acute intermittent (AIP)	• *AIP is the most common and most severe of the porphyrias diseases due to enzymatic deficiencies in the heme biosynthetic pathway.* • *Abdominal pain is the most common symptom and often the first sign of an acute attack.* • *Occurs most commonly in young postpubertal women.*
Pregnancy, ectopic	• *Symptoms include lower quadrant abdominal pain (99%), amenorrhea (74%), and vaginal bleeding (56%).*[3] • *50% of patients are asymptomatic before rupture.*
Pulmonary infarct	• *Abdominal pain, when present, is pleuritic and typically occurs in the upper quadrants.*
Sickle cell crisis	• *Acute hepatic crisis occurs in 10% of patients, resulting in RUQ pain.*

(continued)

Serious Diagnoses	Comment
Testicular torsion	• *Predominantly occurs in neonates and postpubertal boys, but nearly 40% occur in patients older than 21 years.* • *Sudden scrotal pain is the most common symptom.*
Vasculitis	• *Vasculitis may occur in the setting of inflammatory bowel disease, especially Crohn's disease.* • *Antiphospholipid antibody syndrome may present with abdominal pain due to intestinal ischemia.* • *25% of patients with polyarteritis nodosa have abdominal pain.* • *Churg-Strauss syndrome presents with a classic triad of symptoms: allergic rhinitis, asthma, and peripheral eosinophilia. A vasculitis of the small and medium-sized vessels often occurs.* • *Abdominal pain occurs in nearly 50% of people with Henoch-Schönlein purpura, a small vessel vasculitis, which more commonly affects children than adults. The classic tetrad includes rash, abdominal pain, arthralgia, and renal disease.* • *Behçet's disease is more common among men in the Middle East and women in Asia. Symptoms include recurrent oral and genital ulcers, uveitis, skin lesions, and arthritis. A multisystem vasculitis may occur.* • *Takayasu arteritis, most common in young Asian women, primarily affects the aorta and its branches but can present with intestinal ischemia.*

After asking open-ended questions, ask specifically about the presence of alarm symptoms. The patient's response will help guide further diagnostic evaluation.

Alarm symptoms	Serious causes	Positive likelihood ratio (LR+)[a]	Negative likelihood ratio (LR−)[a]	Benign causes
Cardiovascular symptoms				
Nausea and vomiting	*Myocardial infarction*	*1.9[7]*		*Gastroenteritis*
Constitutional symptoms				
Fever	*Appendicitis* *Cholangitis*	*1.94[8]*	*0.58[8]*	*Viral syndrome*
	Cholecystitis *Diverticulitis*	*1.5[9]*	*0.9[9]*	
Gastrointestinal symptoms				
Acholic stools *Tea-colored urine*	*Biliary obstruction*			*Dehydration causes concentrated urine, not to be confused with bilirubinuria*

Black-colored stools Bloody stools Hematemesis	Gastrointestinal bleeding			Iron supplements may cause dark stools
Constipation	Bowel obstruction Hypercalcemia			Dehydration
Nausea or vomiting	Appendicitis Bowel obstruction Cholecystitis Hernia, incarcerated or strangulated Pancreatitis	$0.69-1.2^8$ $1.0-1.5^9$	$0.7-1.12^8$ $0.6-1.0^9$	Gastroenteritis
Pain before vomiting	Appendicitis	2.76^8		
Migration of periumbilical pain to the RLQ	Appendicitis	3.18^8	0.5^8	
RLQ pain	Appendicitis	$7.31-8.46^8$	0.28^8	Mesenteric adenitis
RUQ pain	Cholecystitis	$1.5-1.6^9$	$0.4-0.7^9$	
Miscellaneous				
Jaundice	Biliary obstruction Cholangitis			
Neurologic deficit, focal	Aortic dissection	$6.6-33^{10}$	$0.71-0.87^{10}$	
Pain, abrupt onset	Aortic dissection	1.6^{10}	0.3^{10}	
Pain, abrupt and tearing in nature	Aortic dissection	2.6^{10}		
Pain, migratory	Aortic dissection	$1.1-7.6^{10}$	$0.6-0.97^{10}$	
Pain, tearing quality	Aortic dissection	$1.2-10.8^{10}$	$0.4-0.99^{10}$	

[a]Each LR applies to the adjacent serious cause.

FOCUSED QUESTIONS

After listening to the patient describe his or her abdominal pain with consideration to possible alarm symptoms, the following questions will help narrow the differential diagnosis.

Questions (Remember "PQRST")	Think about
Provoke	
Does eating worsen the pain?	Pancreatitis, gastric ulcer, mesenteric ischemia
Does eating alleviate the pain?	Duodenal ulcer, gastroesophageal reflux disease

(continued)

Questions (Remember "PQRST")	Think about
Quality or associated symptoms	
Is the pain associated with nausea and vomiting?	Pancreatitis, bowel obstruction, biliary colic
Is the pain "tearing"?	Aortic dissection
Is the pain "crampy"?	Distention of a hollow tube (ie, bowel, bile duct or ureter)
Is the pain associated with emesis of undigested food?	Esophageal obstruction
Is the pain associated with emesis of undigested food with acidic, digestive juices from the stomach but no bile?	Gastroparesis or gastric outlet obstruction
Is the emesis bloody?	Gastroesophageal reflux disease, esophageal or gastric varices, PUD, gastric cancer, aortoenteric fistula
Radiation	**Think**
Does the pain radiate to the back?	Pancreatitis, duodenal ulcer, gastric ulcer
Does the pain radiate to the right shoulder?	Biliary colic
Does the pain radiate to the left shoulder?	Splenomegaly or splenic infarction
Does the pain radiate to the left arm?	Myocardial ischemia
Severity	**Think**
Did the pain in your right lower abdomen suddenly improve from an 8 or 9 to a 2 or 3? (on a scale of 0 to 10)	Perforated appendix
Did the pain hurt the most at its onset?	Aortic dissection
Timing/Treatment	**Think**
Is the pain continuous with intermittent waves of worsening pain?	Biliary colic, renal colic, small bowel obstruction
Are there multiple waves of pain that increase in intensity, then stop abruptly for short periods of time?	Small bowel obstruction
Did you recently take antibiotics?	Colitis due to Clostridium difficile
Does the pain occur once monthly around 2 weeks after the beginning of your menses, occasionally associated with vaginal spotting?	Mittelschmerz

CAVEATS

- Although nonspecific abdominal pain accounts for up to 33% of patients with acute abdominal pain, it remains a diagnosis of exclusion. Consider a broad differential diagnosis before arriving at such a conclusion.

- The signs and symptoms of acute abdominal pain can change markedly over a period of minutes to hours. Serial abdominal examinations can increase the diagnostic yield.
- The severity of abdominal pain may be underestimated in the elderly, the very young, patients with diabetes mellitus, and immunocompromised patients (ie, patients receiving long-term corticosteroid therapy).
- Many patients cannot provide a history that readily fits into a specific diagnostic category. Barriers, including a different native language, emotional distress, or psychiatric illness, may delay a rapid and accurate diagnosis. Under such circumstances, it is important to recognize that the history may be incomplete. The use of laboratory and imaging studies should supplement the appropriate diagnostic evaluation.

PROGNOSIS

While most hospitals and clinics have sophisticated imaging and laboratory technologies, it is expensive and inefficient to order an abdominal CT scan on every patient with acute abdominal pain. Paradoxically, imaging may also delay a thorough history and physical examination, which might otherwise have led to the appropriate diagnosis. Triage based on history and physical examination is important because abdominal pain may result from a wide range of disorders with markedly different prognoses.

The prognosis of appropriately treated gastroesophageal reflux disease is very good. The prognosis for appendicitis depends on age. The overall mortality rate for patients who receive appropriate therapy is less than 1%, but is 5–15 times higher in the elderly.[8] A delay in diagnosis may underlie this mortality difference, which highlights the importance of rapid and thoughtful diagnostic evaluation of patients with acute abdominal pain.

REFERENCES

1. Martin RF, Rossi RL. The acute abdomen: an overview and algorithms. *Surg Clin North Am.* 1997;77:1227–1243.
2. Jung PA, Merrell RC. Acute abdomen. *Gastroenterol Clin North Am.* 1988;17:227–244.
3. Stone R. Acute abdominal pain. *Lippincotts Prim Care Pract.* 1998;2:341–357.
4. Kelso LA, Kugelmas M. Nontraumatic abdominal pain. *AACN Clin Issues.* 1997;8:437–448.
5. Irvin T. Abdominal pain: a surgical audit of 1190 emergency admissions. *Br J Surg.* 1989;76:1121–1125.
6. Fenyo G. Acute abdominal disease in the elderly: Experience from two series in Stockholm. *Am J Surg.* 1982;143:751–754.
7. Panju A, Hemmelgarn B, Guyatt G, Simel D. Is this patient having a myocardial infarction? *JAMA.* 1998;280:1256–1263.
8. Wagner JM, McKinney WP, Carpenter JL. Does this patient have appendicitis? *JAMA.* 1996;276:1589–1594.
9. Trowbridge RL, Rutkowski NK, Shojania KG. Does this patient have cholecystitis? *JAMA.* 2003;289:80–86.
10. Klompas M. Does this patient have an acute thoracic aortic dissection? *JAMA.* 2002;287:2262–2272.

SUGGESTED READING

American College of Emergency Physicians: Clinical policy for the initial approach to patients presenting with a chief complaint of nontraumatic acute abdominal pain. *Ann Emerg Med.* 1994;23:906–922.

Lukens T, Emerman C, Effron D. The natural history and clinical findings in undifferentiated abdominal pain. *Ann Emerg Med.* 1993;22:70–76.

Silen W. *Cope's Early Diagnosis of the Acute Abdomen.* 19th edition. New York: Oxford University Press; 1996.

Diagnostic Approach: Abdominal Pain

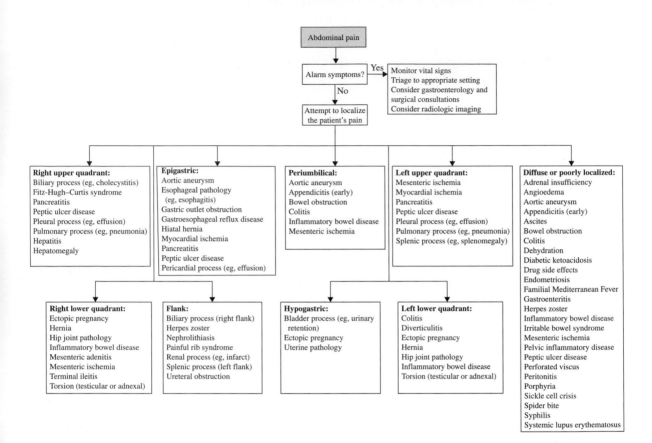

Abdominal pain

Alarm symptoms? — Yes → Monitor vital signs
Triage to appropriate setting
Consider gastroenterology and
surgical consultations
Consider radiologic imaging

No

**Attempt to localize
the patient's pain**

Right upper quadrant:
Biliary process (eg, cholecystitis)
Fitz-Hugh–Curtis syndrome
Pancreatitis
Peptic ulcer disease
Pleural process (eg, effusion)
Pulmonary process (eg, pneumonia)
Hepatitis
Hepatomegaly

Epigastric:
Aortic aneurysm
Esophageal pathology
 (eg, esophagitis)
Gastric outlet obstruction
Gastroesophageal reflux disease
Hiatal hernia
Myocardial ischemia
Pancreatitis
Peptic ulcer disease
Pericardial process (eg, effusion)

Periumbilical:
Aortic aneurysm
Appendicitis (early)
Bowel obstruction
Colitis
Inflammatory bowel disease
Mesenteric ischemia

Left upper quadrant:
Mesenteric ischemia
Myocardial ischemia
Pancreatitis
Peptic ulcer disease
Pleural process (eg, effusion)
Pulmonary process (eg, pneumonia)
Splenic process (eg, splenomegaly)

Diffuse or poorly localized:
Adrenal insufficiency
Angioedema
Aortic aneurysm
Appendicitis (early)
Ascites
Bowel obstruction
Colitis
Dehydration
Diabetic ketoacidosis
Drug side effects
Endometriosis
Familial Mediterranean Fever
Gastroenteritis
Herpes zoster
Inflammatory bowel disease
Irritable bowel syndrome
Mesenteric ischemia
Pelvic inflammatory disease
Peptic ulcer disease
Perforated viscus
Peritonitis
Porphyria
Sickle cell crisis
Spider bite
Syphilis
Systemic lupus erythematosus

Right lower quadrant:
Ectopic pregnancy
Hernia
Hip joint pathology
Inflammatory bowel disease
Mesenteric adenitis
Mesenteric ischemia
Terminal ileitis
Torsion (testicular or adnexal)

Flank:
Biliary process (right flank)
Herpes zoster
Nephrolithiasis
Painful rib syndrome
Renal process (eg, infarct)
Splenic process (left flank)
Ureteral obstruction

Hypogastric:
Bladder process (eg, urinary
 retention)
Ectopic pregnancy
Uterine pathology

Left lower quadrant:
Colitis
Diverticulitis
Ectopic pregnancy
Hernia
Hip joint pathology
Inflammatory bowel disease
Torsion (testicular or adnexal)

Constipation

29

Auguste H. Fortin VI, MD, MPH, & Sonal M. Patel, MD

Constipation is a common digestive symptom, with a prevalence of 2–28%, depending on the definition used.[1–3] The classic definition—fewer than 3 bowel movements per week—has been expanded to acknowledge patients' broader use of the term: in a survey of healthy young adults, 52% defined constipation as straining to pass fecal material, 44% thought it was the process of passing hard stools, and 34% believed it was the inability to have a bowel movement at will. Only 32% believed that constipation was the infrequent passage of stool.[4] A recent consensus meeting[5] defined chronic constipation as:

At least 12 weeks, which need not be consecutive, in the preceding 12 months of 2 or more of:

1. Straining during greater than 25% of defecations
2. Lumpy or hard stools in greater than 25% of defecations
3. Sensation of incomplete evacuation in greater than 25% of defecations
4. Sensation of anorectal obstruction/blockage in greater than 25% of defecations
5. Manual maneuvers to facilitate greater 25% of defecations (eg, digital evacuation, support of the pelvic floor) and/or
6. Fewer than 3 defecations per week.

Some patients may describe themselves as constipated even though having 1 or more bowel movements a day, while others with fewer than 3 per week may not. Constipation leads to 2.5 million physician visits per year[6] and more than $800 million expenditure on laxatives.[7] There is an increased prevalence of constipation among the elderly and female population. Other risk factors include limited physical activity, low socioeconomic status, and low caloric intake. In a national Canadian survey, 34% of persons with constipation had seen a physician for their symptoms.[8]

Constipation can signal serious disease, although most people with this symptom have a benign, functional disorder. Effective history-taking can help guide further evaluation. Knowing the alarm features that can indicate serious causes of constipation and using a sensitive interviewing style will help you appropriately diagnose the cause of this often-embarrassing symptom.

KEY TERMS

Constipation-predominant IBS	*A form of irritable bowel syndrome (IBS) wherein constipation alternates with periods of normal bowel function.*
Defecatory disorders	*During defecation the puborectalis and external anal sphincter muscles fail to relax in response to increased rectal pressure, leading to constipation (eg, pelvic floor dyssynergia, anismus, outlet obstruction, rectal prolapse).*

(continued)

KEY TERMS

Functional illness	*Nonorganic, ie, not caused by a structural defect. This term attempts to artificially separate bodily from psychological contributions to illness.*
Idiopathic chronic constipation	*Chronic constipation in the absence of any organic cause.*
Irritable bowel syndrome	*A gastrointestinal syndrome without organic cause, characterized by chronic abdominal pain and bloating relieved by a bowel movement, feelings of incomplete evacuation and/or passage of mucus, change in the number of bowel movements or change in stool consistency (harder or softer), episodic diarrhea that classically alternates with bouts of constipation, and periods of normal bowel function. It is usually worsened by stress.*
Normal transit constipation	*Also known as functional constipation. Normal stool transit through the colon, with normal stool frequency, but a perception of constipation (eg, constipation predominant irritable bowel syndrome).*
Organic illness	*Associated with detectable structural changes in an organ. Term attempts to artificially separate bodily from psychological contributions to illness.*
Slow transit constipation	*Delayed passage of feces through the colon. May be due to colonic hypomotility or hypermotile, disorganized peristalsis causing retropulsion of stool.*
Somatization	*The expression of psychological distress through physical symptoms such as constipation.*

ETIOLOGY

Many illnesses and medications can cause constipation. Acute-onset constipation is more likely due to an organic cause or medication side effect, while most patients with chronic constipation have a functional condition affecting the colon, anorectum, or both. The pathophysiology of idiopathic chronic constipation, particularly the brain's influence on gut function, is poorly understood. Idiopathic chronic constipation (as well as other functional gastrointestinal disorders) is associated with depression, anxiety, somatization, and a history of sexual abuse.[9–11] In gastroenterologic specialty settings, approximately 40% of patients with idiopathic chronic constipation report a history of sexual abuse. This is about twice both the prevalence reported by patients with organic gastroenterologic disorders and the estimated national prevalence.[9–11]

There is little data on the epidemiology of constipation in patients presenting to primary care providers. One study classified people with chronic constipation according to their responses in a structured telephone interview.[3] Although the group interviewed was not a nationwide representative sample, the overall prevalence of constipation was 14.7%. Of the respondents, approximately 33% were classified as having "functional" (normal transit) constipation; another 33% were classified as having defecatory disorder. About 15% were classified as having IBS. Approximately 25% were classified as having a combination of IBS and "outlet" defecatory disorder. Nearly 50% of the respondents with constipation had been symptomatic for 5 or more years. Of those with "functional" constipation, 8.3% had a medical condition (eg, diabetes mellitus, parkinsonism, multiple sclerosis) or took a medication (eg, opiate analgesics) that may have been the cause of the constipation.

Constipation in infants and children has a different differential diagnosis[7]; this chapter focuses on constipation in adolescents and adults.

Differential Diagnosis

Anorectal obstruction

Anal fissure

Colon cancer

Fecal impaction

Ileus

Megarectum

Strictures (diverticular, postradiation or postischemic)

Thrombosed hemorrhoids

Defecatory disorders

Pregnancy

Metabolic and endocrine conditions

Diabetes mellitus

Hypercalcemia

Hyperparathyroidism

Hypokalemia

Hypomagnesemia

Hypothyroidism

Lead poisoning

Pregnancy

Uremia

Neurogenic disorders

Autonomic neuropathy

Chagas disease

Hirschsprung disease

Neurofibromatosis

Central nervous system disorders

Multiple sclerosis

Parkinsonism

Spinal cord tumor or injury

Cerebrovascular accident

Muscular and connective tissue disorders

Amyloidosis

Systemic sclerosis

Myotonic dystrophy

Medication side effect

Antacids (aluminum- and calcium-containing)

Anticholinergics

Antidiarrheals

Antidepressants

Antipsychotics

Antispasmodics

Calcium supplements

Cholestyramine

Clonidine

Iron supplements

Levodopa

Nonsteroidal anti-inflammatory drugs

Opiate analgesics

Sympathomimetics

Verapamil

Colorectal motility dysfunction

Slow transit constipation

Constipation-predominant IBS

Defecatory disorders

Idiopathic chronic constipation

Psychosocial

Depression

Low-fiber diet

Sedentary lifestyle

Somatization

GETTING STARTED

- Allow the patient to tell his or her story about the constipation before asking any doctor-centered questions. This will give you diagnostically important data and let the patient feel heard.
- Seek out emotion and address it (see Chapter 4). Patients may be afraid that constipation signals cancer or other serious disease. Responding empathically to emotion helps build a strong doctor-patient relationship[12] and can also allow sensitive or embarrassing psychosocial issues to arise.

Questions	Remember
Tell me about your constipation.	*Avoid interrupting.*
What do you mean when you say that you are constipated?	*Listen for clues of organic illness, psychosocial distress.*
How has this been for you?	*Seek out emotion and use empathy.*
What do you think might be causing your symptoms?	*Learning patient's explanatory model can help allay fears, uncover cultural issues, etc.*

INTERVIEW FRAMEWORK

- Determine whether patient actually has constipation. Range of normal is from 3 bowel movements per week to several per day; patients preoccupied with their bowels may have unreasonable expectation of "regularity."
- Determine whether constipation is acute or chronic (long-standing constipation is less likely to be due to serious disease and more likely to be functional).
- Assess for alarm features.
- Assess for symptoms of other medical conditions causing constipation (eg, hypothyroidism, IBS).
- Obtain a complete medication list, including over-the-counter medications and alternative therapies; assess for constipation as medication side effect.
- If constipation is chronic, determine patient's idea of "normal" bowel function.
- Obtain a dietary history to estimate fiber and fluid intake.

IDENTIFYING ALARM SYMPTOMS

Recent-onset constipation with abdominal pain, weight loss, or rectal bleeding may signal serious organic illness such as colon cancer or stricture. However, abdominal pain is also a prominent feature of IBS, a much more common, benign or functional condition.

Serious Diagnoses

- Colon cancer
- Strictures
- Spinal cord tumors/trauma
- Bowel obstruction or ileus

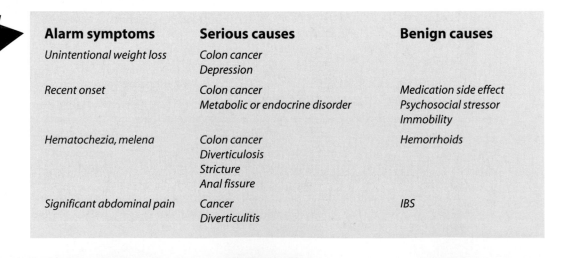

Alarm symptoms	Serious causes	Benign causes
Unintentional weight loss	*Colon cancer* *Depression*	
Recent onset	*Colon cancer* *Metabolic or endocrine disorder*	*Medication side effect* *Psychosocial stressor* *Immobility*
Hematochezia, melena	*Colon cancer* *Diverticulosis* *Stricture* *Anal fissure*	*Hemorrhoids*
Significant abdominal pain	*Cancer* *Diverticulitis*	*IBS*

Change in stool caliber	Colon cancer Stricture Anal fissure	Hemorrhoids IBS
Nausea, vomiting	Bowel obstruction (eg, tumor, stricture)	IBS
Fever	Diverticulitis Cancer	
Back pain, saddle anesthesia, leg weakness/numbness, difficulty urinating	Spinal cord process (eg, cauda equina syndrome)	

FOCUSED QUESTIONS

Questions	Think about
Acute onset of severe constipation	
Do you still pass gas?	Failure to pass gas suggests complete intestinal obstruction
Do you have abdominal pain, cramps?	Intestinal obstruction, eg, cancer, diverticulitis, IBS, ileus
Do you have nausea, vomiting?	Intestinal obstruction
Are you having fecal incontinence?	Fecal impaction
Have you recently started any new medicines?	Medication side effect
Tell me what you've eaten in the last 24 hours, starting with just before coming to the office and working backwards. Does this represent a change in your diet?	Decrease in fiber or liquids can cause constipation
Has your level of activity recently changed?	Bed rest or sedentary state often lead to constipation
What were your bowel habits like before this episode?	Abnormal: chronic condition progressing to complete obstruction. Bouts of constipation alternating with diarrhea: colon cancer, IBS, diabetic autonomic neuropathy, fecal impaction
Have you had abdominal surgery? Radiation?	Strictures Adhesions
Have you suffered a back injury?	Spinal cord trauma
Do you have new weakness in your legs? Numbness around your rectum or genitals? Difficulty passing your urine?	Spinal cord damage from tumor Trauma
Chronic constipation	**Think about**
How often do you have bowel movements? For you, what would normal bowel function be?	Patients with fewer than 2 stools per week are more likely to have slow transit constipation.

(continued)

Chronic constipation	*Think about*
What is the most distressing symptom for you?	*May provide clue to etiology (see next 5 questions for defecatory disorders)*
Do you have difficulty passing even soft stools or enema liquid?	*Defecatory disorder*
Do you ever need to press around your vagina/ rectum with your fingers in order to move your bowels?	*Defecatory disorder*
Do you ever need to evacuate your bowels with your finger?	*Defecatory disorder*
Do you feel like your bowels are blocked?	*Defecatory disorder*
Do you have difficulty letting go or relaxing your muscles to have a bowel movement?	*Defecatory disorder*
Do you have the sensation of incomplete evacuation?	*IBS*
Do you have abdominal pain and bloating that is associated with bowel movements?	*IBS* *Intestinal obstruction*
How often do you experience a call to move your bowels? Do you always heed it?	*Chronic failure to heed may lead to chronic rectal distention, lax muscle tone, slow transit time, and chronic constipation*
What medicines do you take, including over-the-counter and alternative remedies?	*Medication side effect*
What laxatives/enemas/suppositories do you use? What dosage? How often?	*Laxative abuse can lead to chronic constipation. After purging with a laxative or enema, it can take several days for enough stool to accumulate for another bowel movement.*
Are you ever able to have a bowel movement without using a laxative?	*"No" suggests slow transit constipation*
Does increasing your fiber intake improve your constipation?	*Normal transit constipation*
Tell me what you've eaten and drunk in the last 24 hours, starting with just before coming to the office and working backwards.	*Diet low in fiber or liquids can lead to constipation*
Have you had any pregnancies? Deliveries?	*Multiparity is associated with defecatory disorder*
Has your level of activity recently changed?	*Bed rest or sedentary lifestyle can cause constipation*
How is your sleep? Appetite? Mood? Concentration? Interest in things? (See Chapter 60)	*Depression can lead to constipation*
Have you had any weight gain, decreased energy levels, or swelling in your legs?	*Hypothyroidism*
Have you had increased urinary frequency, increased thirst, or even been told that you have diabetes?	*Diabetes and autonomic neuropathy*

In your life, have you been hit, slapped, kicked, or otherwise physically hurt by someone? In your life has anyone ever displayed their genitals to you against your will, inappropriately touched your genitals or forced you to have sexual contact against your will?

Idiopathic chronic constipation and defecatory disorders are often associated with a history of physical or sexual abuse, often unknown to the physician.[10,11] While you may choose not to ask in the initial visit, it is important to consider in patients with refractory constipation.

Quality

Are your stools thin like a pencil or ribbon?

Think about

Narrowing of the distal colon/sigmoid/rectum from colon cancer, strictures.

Do you pass mucus?

IBS

Are your stools watery?

In a debilitated or elderly person, consider fecal impaction (liquid stool passing around the obstructing fecal mass)

Do you have constipation alternating with diarrhea?

IBS
Colorectal cancer

Are your stools mixed with blood?

Colon cancer

Are the outside of your stools streaked with blood?

Anal disorder (hemorrhoids, fissures, ulcers)

Are your stools black?

Bismuth subsalicylate, iron supplements

Time course

When did your constipation begin?

Think about

Postoperative: consider adhesions, ileus. Recent: consider colon cancer, fecal impaction, medication side effect, psychological stress.
Long-standing: consider IBS, chronic idiopathic constipation
Lifelong: consider Hirshsprung disease

Associated symptoms

Do you have abdominal pain or discomfort, which is relieved by a bowel movement? Is the discomfort associated with a change in the number of bowel movements or consistency of your stools?

Think about

IBS

Modifying symptoms

Do you notice any change in your symptoms with stress?

Think about

Increase in symptoms with psychosocial stress suggests IBS

CAVEATS

- Many patients with chronic constipation have idiopathic chronic constipation, a condition that is associated with somatization and occasionally a history of sexual abuse.[9–11]
- New-onset constipation, especially in the elderly, should be taken seriously and evaluated further.
- Constipation associated with abdominal pain or bloating is more likely to be due to mechanical obstruction (eg, colon cancer, strictures, fecal impaction), but these symptoms also commonly occur in IBS, a benign, functional condition. Acute onset of symptoms supports the former; pain relieved with bowel movement suggests the latter.
- After purging with a laxative or enema, it can take several days for enough stool to accumulate for another bowel movement. This delay does not indicate constipation. Patients may need to be educated about this.

- Patients who complain of chronic constipation may do so because of difficulty passing stool rather than because of infrequent bowel movements.
- Most patients with chronic constipation have colorectal motility dysfunction.
- It is not always possible to distinguish organic and functional diagnoses by history alone; further diagnostic evaluation is often needed.
- Data are conflicting about whether it is possible to distinguish slow transit constipation from defecatory disorders by history alone.[3,13,14]

PROGNOSIS

The survival of patients with colon cancer depends on the stage at which the cancer is diagnosed. Advanced disease is more likely when colon cancer presents as acute constipation from obstruction. Strictures usually require surgical intervention. Constipation caused by other conditions (eg, hypothyroidism, medication side effect) usually responds when the underlying disorder is addressed. Chronic idiopathic constipation usually responds incompletely to treatment, but quality of life can be improved, particularly if a history of sexual or physical abuse is uncovered and addressed.

REFERENCES

1. Drossman DA, et al. US householder survey of functional gastrointestinal disorders. Prevalence, sociodemography, and health impact. *Dig Dis Sci.* 1993;38:1569–1580.

2. Locke GR 3rd. The epidemiology of functional gastrointestinal disorders in North America. *Gastroenterol Clin North Am.* 1996;25:1–19.

3. Stewart WF, et al. Epidemiology of constipation (EPOC) study in the United States: relation of clinical subtypes to sociodemographic features. *Am J Gastroenterol.* 1999;94:3530–3540.

4. Sandler RS, Drossman DA. Bowel habits in young adults not seeking health care. *Dig Dis Sci.* 1987;32:841–845.

5. Locke GR 3rd, Pemberton JH, Phillips SF. AGA technical review on constipation. American Gastroenterological Association. *Gastroenterology.* 2000;119:1766–1778.

6. Sonnenberg A, Koch TR. Physician visits in the United States for constipation: 1958 to 1986. *Dig Dis Sci.* 1989; 34:606–611.

7. Arce DA, Ermocilla CA, Costa H. Evaluation of constipation. *Am Fam Physician.* 2002;65:2283–2290.

8. Pare P, et al. An epidemiological survey of constipation in Canada: definitions, rates, demographics, and predictors of health care seeking. *Am J Gastroenterol.* 2001;96:3130–3137.

9. Drossman DA, et al. Sexual and physical abuse in women with functional or organic gastrointestinal disorders. *Ann Intern Med.* 1990;113:828–833.

10. Drossman DA, et al. Sexual and physical abuse and gastrointestinal illness. Review and recommendations [see comments]. *Ann Intern Med.* 1995;123:782–794.

11. Leroi AM, et al. Prevalence of sexual abuse among patients with functional disorders of the lower gastrointestinal tract. *Int J Colorectal Dis.* 1995;10:200–206.

12. Smith RC. *Patient centered interviewing.* 2nd ed. Lippincott Williams & Wilkins; 2002:317.

13. Glia A, et al. Clinical value of symptom assessment in patients with constipation. *Dis Colon Rectum.* 1999;42:1401–1408; discussion, 1408–1410.

14. Rao SS. Constipation: evaluation and treatment. *Gastroenterol Clin North Am.* 2003;32:659–683.

SUGGESTED READING

Lembo A, Camilleri M. Chronic constipation. *N Engl J Med.* 2003;349:1360–1368.

Diagnostic Approach: Constipation

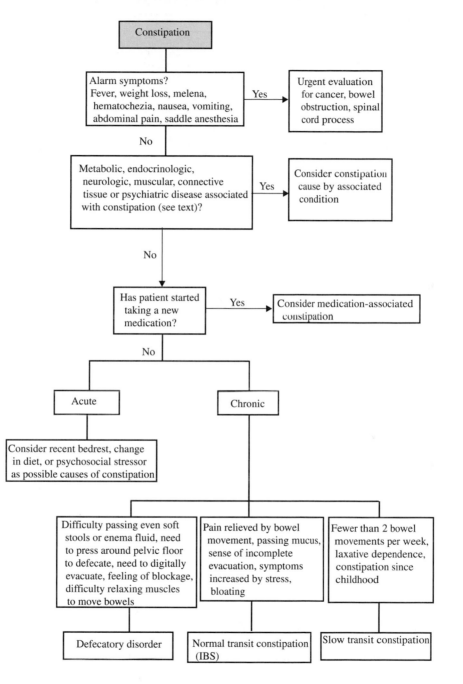

IBS, irritable bowel syndrome.

Diarrhea

Alexander R. Carbo, MD, & Gerald W. Smetana, MD

Diarrhea accounts for up to 28 million office visits and 1.8 million hospital admissions in the United States each year, with up to 200 million total cases per year.[1] The yearly incidence in adult patients has been reported to be 3% to 63% per year, depending on the referral source. In the United States, approximately 6 billion dollars is spent annually on medical care and lost productivity due to diarrhea.[1] Although a strict definition of diarrhea includes stool frequency and stool weight, many patients use the term when they experience increased stool liquidity. This chapter aims to clarify some key components of the history when interviewing a patient with diarrhea.

KEY TERMS

Acute diarrhea	Diarrhea lasting less than 2 weeks.
Chronic diarrhea	Diarrhea lasting at least 4 weeks.
Diarrhea	Increased frequency of stools (> 3 per day) with increased stool weight (> 200 g/d). However, patients may use the term "diarrhea" to describe increased liquidity. In 1 series of patients referred to a gastrointestinal (GI) clinic for diarrhea, only 40% of patients actually had output > 200 g/d.[2]
Dysentery	The passage of bloody stools.
Irritable bowel syndrome (IBS)	A functional disorder characterized by the Rome II criteria, which include "at least 12 weeks, which need not be consecutive, in the preceding 12 months of abdominal discomfort or pain that has 2 of 3 features: relieved with defecation, onset associated with a change in frequency of stool, and/or onset associated with a change in form of stool."[3]
Organic versus functional diarrhea	Diarrhea with a known structural or biochemical explanation (ie, infection, inflammation, neoplasm) versus that without a known underlying cause.[3]
Persistent diarrhea	Diarrhea lasting 2 to 4 weeks. This time frame includes more prolonged and atypical presentations of acute diarrhea. Clinicians should not consider diarrhea to be chronic (and sufficient to evaluate for chronic diarrhea) unless it persists for at least 4 weeks.
Pseudodiarrhea, hyperdefecation	Increased frequency of defecation, but no increase in stool weight or change in stool consistency.
Tenesmus	Spasm of the anal sphincter associated with cramping and ineffective straining at stool.

ETIOLOGY

Since most episodes of diarrhea are self-limited, many patients never seek medical attention. For this reason, prevalence data must be viewed in the proper context: patients referred to specialists are more likely to have chronic diarrhea, and conditions with alarm symptoms may be over-represented. The prevalence of common etiologies of diarrhea in a primary care setting is unknown.

Differential Diagnosis	Prevalence[a]	Prevalence[b]
Functional diarrhea	*45%*	*21%*
Infectious diarrhea	*11%*	
Inflammatory bowel disease (IBD)	*7%*	*3%*
Malabsorption	*5%*	*11%*
Laxative use	*4%*	*2%*
Medication-related (includes caffeine and alcohol)	*4%*	
Postoperative diarrhea	*2.5%*	*20%*
Malignancies	*1%*	
Collagenous colitis		*15%*
Idiopathic		*20%*
Hyperthyroidism		
Ischemic colitis		

[a]Among patients referred to a GI clinic with a complaint of diarrhea[2]; prevalence is unknown when not indicated.
[b]Among patients referred to a tertiary medical center with "undiagnosed or difficult to manage chronic diarrhea"[4]; prevalence is unknown when not indicated.

GETTING STARTED

- Let patients give the history in their own words by saying, for example, "Tell me about the diarrhea."
- Avoid interrupting.
- Assess for related symptoms, beginning with open-ended questions, such as "Are you having any other symptoms?"

INTERVIEW FRAMEWORK

- The most important step in taking the history is to determine duration. The goal is to differentiate between acute and chronic diarrhea, as the respective differential diagnoses differ substantially. Keep in mind that chronic diarrhea will initially present as acute diarrhea that does not resolve over time.
- In acute diarrhea, the initial focus is to determine whether the patient is volume depleted.
- Identify alarm features for both acute and chronic diarrhea.
- Consider comorbidities, accompanying symptoms, and precipitating factors.

IDENTIFYING ALARM SYMPTOMS

Most episodes of acute diarrhea will be self-limited. The astute clinician should look for signs of volume depletion such as thirst, fatigue, or dizziness that may warrant intravenous fluid resuscitation and/or hospitalization. Also look for alarm features, in order to identify serious diagnoses.

In assessing chronic diarrhea, ask about alarm features and symptoms of organic illness that would prompt further evaluation.

Serious Diagnoses

The main goal is to distinguish functional (ie, IBS) and self-limited (ie, gastroenteritis) causes of diarrhea from those due to organic etiologies. Alarm symptoms and features can help differentiate between the 2 groups. Serious diagnoses include neoplasm, IBD (Crohn's disease and ulcerative colitis), infection, intermittent bowel obstruction, systemic disease, and malabsorption.

Alarm features	Serious causes	Benign causes
Weight loss (> 5 pounds)	• With normal appetite: hyperthyroidism, malabsorption • Weight loss precedes diarrhea: neoplasm, diabetes mellitus, tuberculosis, malabsorption.[5]	
Fever	• Invasive pathogens (Salmonella, Shigella, Campylobacter) • Cytotoxic organisms with mucosal inflammation (Clostridium difficile).[6] • IBD	Enteric viruses
Bloody stools (dysentery)	• IBD (ulcerative colitis) • Malignancy • Ischemic colitis • Infection with Salmonella, Shigella, Campylobacter, enterohemorrhagic Escherichia coli (O157:H7), Entamoeba histolytica	• Hemorrhoids • Beet ingestion (may cause red, but not bloody, stool)
Awakening from sleep	Generally associated with organic (not functional) causes, eg, IBD, diabetes mellitus	Self-limited viral syndrome
Family history of colon cancer, IBD, multiple endocrine neoplasia, or celiac sprue	Only useful if positive, since these conditions can develop in patients without a family history.	
Age > 50 with change in symptoms	Organic etiology	
Immunocompromised host	Infection	

FOCUSED QUESTIONS

After making a distinction between acute and chronic diarrhea and assessing for alarm features, focused questions will narrow the differential diagnosis. By asking about the quality and time course of the diarrhea, along with associated symptoms, clinicians can begin to differentiate functional diarrhea (ie, IBS) from other causes. While the history is the first step toward making a diagnosis, further evaluation such as physical examination, stool studies, and imaging techniques may be necessary.

Questions

Quality	*Think about*
Have you had more bowel movements than usual?	Frequent watery voluminous stools usually signify a small bowel etiology. Smaller volumes with lower abdominal pain point toward a large bowel etiology.
Do you have abdominal pain? If so, where is the pain? Can you point to one spot that is bothering you?	
• Periumbilical	Small bowel pathology
• Lower abdominal	Large bowel pathology
	Ulcerative colitis, bacterial dysentery, herpes simplex virus, gonorrhea, Chlamydia, E histolytica[7]
• Tenesmus	Anorectal inflammation such as ulcerative colitis or infectious dysentery
• Generalized	IBS
	Ischemic bowel
	Celiac sprue
Is this pain relieved after a bowel movement?	IBS
Has there been passage of mucus?	IBS
	Ulcerative colitis
Is the stool greasy or oily and difficult to flush?	Steatorrhea due to malabsorption

Time course	*Think about*
Did this begin abruptly?	Viral or bacterial infection; idiopathic secretory diarrhea[4]
Did it come on gradually over time?	IBS
	IBD

Associated symptoms	*Think about*
Do you have abdominal bloating?	IBS
	Lactose intolerance
	Viral enteritis
	Antibiotic administration
	Nonulcer dyspepsia
	Celiac sprue[8]
Have you noticed an increased amount of flatus?	IBS
	Carbohydrate malabsorption
	Viral enteritis
Do you have a feeling of straining, urgency, or incomplete evacuation?	Ulcerative colitis
	IBS
	Proctitis
Do you have nausea or vomiting?	Viral gastroenteritis
	Bowel obstruction

Are there extraintestinal symptoms?

- *Arthritis (joint pain, swelling, redness)*

  Reactive arthritis after infection
  IBD

- *Arthritis, urethritis, or conjunctivitis*

  Reiter syndrome (usually after infection with Salmonella enteritidis or Shigella, Yersinia, Campylobacter)[9]

Modifying symptoms and relevant additional history

Think about

Do milk or dairy products worsen your symptoms? Lactose intolerance

Have you noticed symptoms after eating rye, wheat, or barley? Celiac sprue

Do you chew sugarless gum? *Sorbitol ingestion*

Do your symptoms persist if you stop eating? *Secretory diarrhea*

Have you traveled recently?

- *South or Central America, Mexico, Southeast Asia*

  Various infectious etiologies: enterotoxigenic E coli (most common), Shigella, rotavirus, Salmonella, Campylobacter, Giardia, E histolytica.[6]

- *Russia*

  Cryptosporidium
  Giardia[6]

- *Mountainous areas in United States*

  Giardia[6]

Did you drink any stream water? Giardia

Have you been taking antibiotics? C difficile, *antibiotic-associated diarrhea*

Have you recently begun taking any new medications?

  HMG-CoA reductase inhibitors (statins), proton pump inhibitors, and selective serotonin reuptake inhibitors may cause diarrhea

Have you been hospitalized recently or been to an extended care facility? C difficile, *medication-related*

Have you ever had surgery such as vagotomy, intestinal resection, or cholecystectomy

  Diarrhea occurs due to lack of absorptive surface, decreased transit time, malabsorption of bile acids.[8]

Has anyone else developed these symptoms?
  What did you eat?
  When did you eat it?
  Did you develop other symptoms?

  Food-borne outbreaks[6,7]:
  - *< 6 hours after ingestion:* Staphylococcus aureus *(after mayonnaise, potato/egg salad, custards, poultry),* Bacillus cereus *(classically after fried rice)*
  - *8–14 hours after ingestion:* Clostridium perfringens *(after poorly reheated meats or poultry)*
  - *8–72 hours after eating seafood:* Vibrio species
  - *>14 hours with vomiting: Viral agents*
  - *With dysentery: Enterohemorrhagic* E coli

(continued)

Modifying symptoms and relevant additional history	Think about
	• *With fever or dysentery:* Salmonella, Shigella, Campylobacter
Do you work in a daycare center?	*Rotavirus (sudden, with vomiting)* Shigella Giardia Cryptosporidium[6]
Do you have any pets, such as iguanas, turtles?	Salmonella[7]
Do you engage in anal intercourse?	*Herpes simplex virus, gonorrhea,* Chlamydia *(direct inoculation causing proctitis)* Shigella, Salmonella, Campylobacter, Giardia, E histolytica, Cryptosporidium *(fecal-oral transmission)*[6]
Do you have HIV infection?	Cryptosporidium Microsporidium Isospora Cytomegalovirus Mycobacterium avium complex
Do any diseases run in your family?	*IBD* *Multiple endocrine neoplasia*
Do you use laxatives?	*Laxative abuse*
Are you happy with your body image?	*Laxative abuse*
Have you had associated body flushing?	*Carcinoid syndrome*

CAVEATS

- This review focuses only on adult patients. A different spectrum of disease may apply to infants and children.
- Some patients have > 300 grams of stool per day due to a high fiber diet, but do not complain of diarrhea because their stool consistency is normal.[10]
- Remember to differentiate acute from chronic diarrhea, as failure to do so will lead to consideration of an incorrect differential diagnosis.
- Be sure to review a patient's medications, including over-the-counter medications, as these agents can cause diarrhea.
- Ask about fecal incontinence, the involuntary release of rectal contents, as many patients may confuse this with diarrhea. While diarrhea may lead to incontinence, there are many non-diarrheal causes.
- Laxative abuse is a frequently overlooked cause of chronic diarrhea. Four percent of patients visiting GI clinics and up to 20% of those referred to tertiary centers have laxative abuse as the cause for chronic diarrhea. Many of these patients will deny laxative use.[8]

PROGNOSIS

Most diarrheal episodes are self-limited. However, patients with alarm symptoms and signs of volume depletion at the extremes of age are particularly at risk for mortality. Of the average 3000 annual deaths attributed to diarrhea in the United States, 51% were in those older than 74 years, 78% were in those older than 55 years, and 11% were in those younger than 5 years.[1]

REFERENCES

1. Guerrant RL, Van Gilder T, Steiner TS, et al. Practice guidelines for the management of infectious diarrhea. *Clin Infect Dis.* 2001;32:331–351.

2. Bytzer P, Stokholm M, Andersen I, et al. Aetiology, medical history, and faecal weight in adult patients referred for diarrhoea. A prospective study. *Scand J Gastroenterol.* 1990;25:572–578.

3. Thompson WG, Longstretch GF, Drossman DA, et al. Functional bowel disorders and functional abdominal pain [Rome II: A multinational consensus document on functional gastrointestinal disorders]. *Gut.* 1999;45(S2):II43–II47.

4. Fine, KD, Schiller LR. AGA technical review on the evaluation and management of chronic diarrhea. *Gastroenterology.* 1999;116:1464–1486.

5. Krosner JA, Mertz DC. Evaluation of the adult patient with diarrhea. *Prim Care Clin Office Pract.* 1996;23:629–647.

6. DuPont HL, et al for The Practice Parameters Committee of the American College of Gastroenterology. Guidelines on acute infectious diarrhea in adults. *Am J Gastroenterol.* 1997;92:1962–1975.

7. Hogan DE. The emergency department approach to diarrhea. *Emerg Med Clin North Am.* 1996;14:673–694.

8. Donowitz M, Kokke FT, Saidi R. Evaluation of patients with chronic diarrhea. *N Engl J Med.* 1995;332:725–729.

9. Dworkin MS, Shoemaker PC, Goldoft MJ, et al. Reactive arthritis and Reiter's syndrome following an outbreak of gastroenteritis caused by *Salmonella enteritidis. Clin Infect Dis.* 2001;22:1010–1014.

10. Schiller LR. Diarrhea. *Med Clin North Am.* 2000;84:1259–1274.

SUGGESTED READING

Ilnyckyj A. Clinical evaluation and management of acute infectious diarrhea in adults. *Gastroenterol Clin North Am.* 2001;30:599–609.

Somers SC, Lembo A. Irritable bowel syndrome: evaluation and treatment. *Gastroenterol Clin.* 2003;32:507–529.

Talley NJ, Weaver AL, Zinsmeister AR, et al. Self-reported diarrhea: what does it mean? *Am J Gastroenterol.* 1994;89:1160–1164.

Diagnostic Approach: Diarrhea

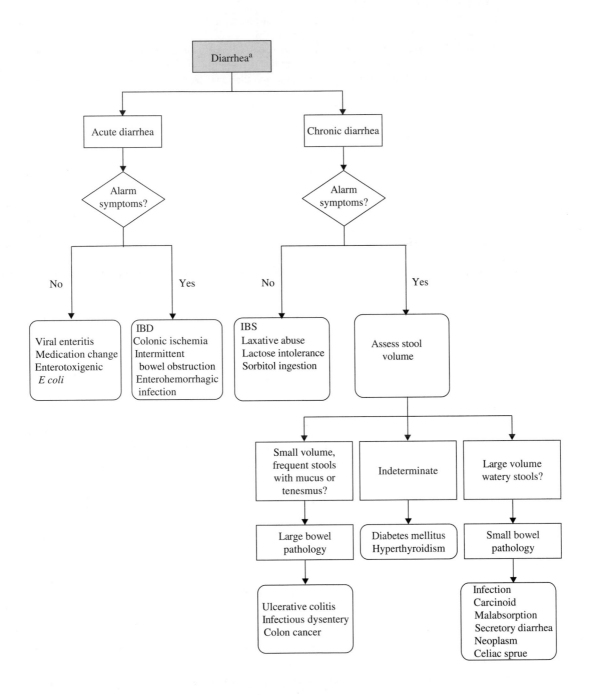

IBD, inflammatory bowel disease; IBS, irritable bowel syndrome.

[a] If hypovolemic, give fluid resuscitation. If patient immunocompromised, consider broader infectious work-up.

Dyspepsia

Sara B. Fazio, MD

Dyspepsia is a general term that refers to symptoms originating from the upper gastrointestinal tract. As such, it may encompass a variety of symptoms. Typically, patients present with a complaint of epigastric pain, but may also complain of heartburn, nausea, vomiting, abdominal distention, heartburn, early satiety and anorexia. The condition occurs in approximately 25% of the population, with a range of 13–40%, though the majority of patients do not seek medical care.[1] Dyspepsia is responsible for 2–5% of visits to a primary care physician,[2] and accounts for 40–70% of gastrointestinal complaints in general practice.[3] An organic cause is found in 40–50% of cases, most often gastric ulcer, gastroesophageal reflux disease, and gastric cancer, but in approximately 50% of cases no cause is found, and the patient is deemed to have functional or "nonulcer" dyspepsia.[2] The approach to a dyspeptic patient should be two-fold: attempting to elicit a symptom complex that may be helpful in diagnosing a specific condition as well as excluding worrisome or "alarm" symptoms.

KEY TERMS

Dysphagia	Difficulty swallowing, food getting stuck.
Flatulence	Passing of gas.
Functional dyspepsia	Symptom without an anatomic correlate for pain; also known as "nonulcer" dyspepsia.
Gastroparesis	Hypoactive bowel activity; often associated with autonomic neuropathy of diabetes. Characterized by abdominal distention, bloating, nausea, and flatulence.
GERD	Gastroesophageal reflux disease.
Irritable bowel syndrome (IBS)	Abdominal pain or discomfort associated with change in stool frequency or consistency and often relieved by defecation.
Negative predictive value	The probability of not having the suspected disease when a particular symptom is absent.
NSAID	Nonsteroidal anti-inflammatory drug.
Organic dyspepsia	Dyspepsia associated with a specific diagnosis.
Positive likelihood ratio	The increase in odds for a particular diagnosis if a symptom or factor is present.
Positive predictive value	The probability of the suspected disease in a patient with a particular symptom.
Regurgitation	Reflux of gastrointestinal contents into the esophagus or mouth, or both.

ETIOLOGY

The cause of dyspepsia proves to be benign in most patients. The most common diagnoses among patients who have undergone endoscopy include functional dyspepsia (prevalence approximating 50–60%), peptic ulcer disease (15–20%), reflux esophagitis (5–15%) and gastric or esophageal cancer (< 2%). The prevalence of a particular condition varies depending on the population being studied. For example, in 1 series, gastric ulcer constituted 30% of dyspepsia diagnoses in persons under the age of 30 but 60% in persons over the age of 60.[4] Similarly, gastric malignancy is much more common in patients over the age of 45 as well as persons of East Asian descent. In addition, it is often difficult to extrapolate data from studies performed in tertiary care centers (ie, gastroenterology clinics) to the general primary care setting, because the incidence of any pathologic finding is likely to be higher in the former.

Differential Diagnosis: Benign Causes	**Prevalence[a]**
Functional dyspepsia	*50–60%[1]*
Peptic ulcer disease (gastric or duodenal ulcer)	*15–25%[1]*
GERD	*5–15%[1]*
Esophagitis	*5–15%[3]*
Gastritis and duodenitis	
Biliary tract disease	
Gastroparesis	
IBS	
Pancreatitis	
Medications (NSAIDs, antibiotics, potassium, iron, alcohol, theophylline, acarbose, alendronate, metformin, corticosteroids, narcotics)	
Celiac disease	
Lactose intolerance	*9%[3]*
Metabolic disturbances (hyperthyroidism, hypothyroidism, diabetes, hyperparathyroidism, adrenal insufficiency)	

[a]Among general population with dyspepsia; prevalence is unknown when not indicated.

GETTING STARTED

Although obtaining a complete history from a patient with dyspepsia is important, the presence of symptoms alone has not been found to be very helpful in establishing a specific diagnosis.[1] Clinicians correctly diagnose only 45–50% of adults on initial presentation.[5] However, certain clusters of symptoms have been found to have a high negative predictive value for organic causes of dyspepsia.[6] In other words, the presence of these features makes a serious cause unlikely. For example, in 1 study, the diagnosis of functional dyspepsia was much more likely if the patient had upper abdominal pain that was not severe and if there was an absence of nocturnal pain, nausea, vomiting or weight loss.[5]

It is important to ask open-ended questions at the beginning of the interview to allow the patient to provide as much of the history as possible without specific prompting. Because clinicians use the term "dyspepsia" to describe a variety of symptoms, it is important to allow the patient to describe the symptoms in detail to avoid coming to a diagnosis prematurely.

INTERVIEW FRAMEWORK

After asking open-ended questions, directed questions should help classify a dyspeptic patient into 1 of 3 categories of benign disease:

1. Ulcer-like dyspepsia. Discomfort is typically well localized and often relieved by food or antacids. Patients often complain of nighttime symptoms.
2. Dysmotility-like dyspepsia. Discomfort is aggravated by meals and associated with bloating or fullness. Nausea, vomiting, and early satiety are frequent complaints.
3. Reflux-like dyspepsia. Patients often complain of a burning sensation that radiates into the chest or throat, associated with a sour taste in the mouth. The symptoms are worse when lying down or after intake of spicy foods, fatty foods, alcohol, chocolate, peppermint, or caffeinated beverages. Patients may complain of regurgitation, or the effortless passage of stomach contents into the mouth. Dysphagia may progressively develop over time, particularly for solids, which often indicates the presence of an esophageal stricture.

Assessment of alarm symptoms, which are suggestive of a more serious disease, is equally important. A paradigm to organize specific questions includes asking about the following:

- Onset
- Duration
- Frequency
- Location
- Character of pain or discomfort
- Radiation
- Associated symptoms
- Exacerbating factors
- Relieving factors

IDENTIFYING ALARM SYMPTOMS

Most serious causes for dyspepsia are rare, with the exception of duodenal or peptic ulcer disease. Duodenal and peptic ulcer disease have been included here because they can cause a gastrointestinal hemorrhage or perforation if left untreated. Gastric or esophageal malignancy, the most feared diagnosis, has a prevalence of < 2% among patients with dyspepsia. Patients with malignancy tend to be older and to seek medical attention earlier (due to severity of symptoms) than persons with a benign disease.[1]

Differential Diagnosis: Serious Causes	**Prevalence[a]**
Gastric or esophageal cancer	*< 2%[1]*
Duodenal ulcer	*25–30%[7]*

(continued)

Differential Diagnosis: Serious Causes	Prevalence[a]
Gastric ulcer	*10–15%*[7]
Infiltrative diseases of the stomach (Crohn's disease, sarcoidosis)	
Ischemic colitis	
Hepatoma	
Pancreatic cancer	
Ischemic heart disease	

[a]Among general population with dyspepsia; prevalence is unknown when not indicated.

Perhaps one of the most important functions of the history for a patient with dyspepsia is the identification of alarm symptoms or features. Definitions of alarm features vary but generally include any of the following: weight loss, bleeding, anemia, dysphagia, severe pain, and protracted vomiting. Age over 45 is often listed as an alarm feature because the incidence of gastric malignancy is higher in this age group. However, it is important to remember that even among this age group, the likelihood of malignancy in a patient with dyspepsia is still less than 3%.[3] Many patients with a diagnosis of malignancy have with 1 or more alarm features. However, these features are not specific for malignancy, as illustrated by a study of 20,000 patients who underwent endoscopy for evaluation of dyspepsia. Only 3% of patients with any of 4 major predictors (age > 45, male sex, anemia, or bleeding) proved to have a malignancy (positive predictive value). However, the negative predictive value was 99% (99% of patients with no significant major predictors had no malignancy).[8] Thus the absence of any alarm features is perhaps the most helpful diagnostic tool.

Alarm features	Serious causes	Positive likelihood ratio (LR+)[a]	Benign causes
Weight loss	*Gastric or esophageal malignancy* *Intra-abdominal malignancy* *Colon cancer* *Ischemic colitis*		*Peptic ulcer disease* *Malabsorption* *Metabolic disturbance*
Bleeding	*Gastric or esophageal malignancy* *Colon cancer* *Peptic or duodenal ulcer* *Ischemic colitis*	*2.90*[8]	
Anemia	*Gastric or esophageal malignancy* *Intra-abdominal malignancy*	*2.28*[8]	*Peptic ulcer disease*
Dysphagia	*Gastric or esophageal malignancy*		*Esophageal stricture* *Esophagitis*
Age > 45	*Gastric or esophageal malignancy* *Intra-abdominal malignancy* *Colon cancer*	*1.72*[8]	*Any etiology*
Male sex	*Gastric or esophageal malignancy*	*1.40*[8]	*Any etiology*

[a]Each LR applies to the adjacent serious cause.

FOCUSED QUESTIONS

After asking open-ended questions and considering alarm symptoms, ask the following questions in order to narrow the differential diagnosis.

Questions	Think about
Do you have a personal history of gastric or duodenal ulcer?	*Peptic ulcer disease is much more common in a person with a prior history.*
Do you have a family history of ulcer disease?	*Peptic ulcer disease*
Do you smoke?	*Peptic ulcer disease* *Reflux esophagitis* *Gastric cancer*
Do you have a history of heavy alcohol use?	*Gastritis* *Reflux esophagitis* *Peptic ulcer disease* *Pancreatitis* *Esophageal cancer*
How often do you take NSAIDs or aspirin?	*NSAID use increases the likelihood of gastrointestinal bleeding in a patient with dyspepsia by a factor of 7 (odds ratio 7.1).[9]*
Are you over the age of 45?	*Age > 45 increases the likelihood of a gastric or esophageal malignancy.*
How long have you had this discomfort?	*More serious diagnoses tend to have a shorter interval until presentation; thus a patient who has had dyspepsia for years with no associated symptoms is more likely to have a benign diagnosis.*

Quality	*Think about*
Is the pain	
• *Burning?*	*Gastritis* *Duodenal ulcer* *Gastric ulcer*
• *Stabbing?*	*Pancreatitis* *Duodenal ulcer* *Gastric ulcer*
• *Severe/unbearable?*	*Acute pancreatitis* *Perforated viscus*
• *Crampy/ colicky?*	*Biliary colic* *IBS* *Intestinal obstruction*
Where is the pain localized?	
• *Epigastric?*	*Gastritis* *Esophagitis* *Duodenal ulcer* *Peptic ulcer* *Pancreatitis* *Gastric or esophageal malignancy* *Pancreatic cancer* *Colon cancer (in transverse colon)* *Functional dyspepsia*

(continued)

Quality	Think about
• Substernal?	Ischemic heart disease Esophagitis
• Right upper quadrant?	Biliary colic IBS Hepatoma
• Periumbilical?	Small bowel disease Small bowel obstruction
• Left upper quadrant?	IBS Lesion in tail of pancreas

Does the pain

• Remain in the same place?	Gastric ulcer
• Radiate from the epigastrium to the back?	Pancreatitis Posterior penetration of peptic ulcer
• Radiate from the epigastrium to the chest or neck?	GERD Ischemic heart disease Esophageal spasm

Is the pain

• Constant?	Gastric malignancy
• Intermittent?	Gastritis Peptic ulcer disease Biliary colic IBS Medication-related dyspepsia

Time course	Think about

Tell me about the onset of the discomfort.

• Abrupt onset?	Acute pancreatitis Perforated viscus Vascular thrombosis
• Gradual increase in intensity?	Peptic ulcer disease Biliary colic

How long does it last?

• Steady for 30 minutes to 2 hours before gradually subsiding	Peptic ulcer disease
• Reaches peak intensity in 15 to 45 minutes and subsides over several hours	Biliary colic

Does the pain wake you from sleep?	Peptic ulcer disease

Associated symptoms	*Think about*
Do you have nausea, or are you vomiting?	Peptic ulcer disease Gastric cancer Biliary colic
Do you have melena?	Peptic ulcer disease Gastric cancer Colon cancer
Do you have chronic cough or hoarseness?	GERD
Is your urine dark? Have you noticed a yellow tone in your skin?	Biliary disease
Are you belching?	Biliary disease IBS GERD
Does your abdomen feel full?	IBS
Do you have heartburn, a bitter taste in your mouth, or regurgitation of food contents?	GERD
Are you passing gas?	IBS Malabsorption Biliary disease
Have you lost weight?	Gastric or esophageal cancer Peptic ulcer disease Colon cancer Intra-abdominal malignancy Malabsorption
Is swallowing difficult?	GERD Esophagitis Esophageal stricture Esophageal cancer
Are you bloated?	IBS
Have you had a change in stool frequency or consistency?	IBS, often associated with "alternating constipation and diarrhea" as well as pencil-thin stools
Are you constipated?	Colon cancer IBS
Is there mucous with passage of stool?	IBS Inflammatory bowel disease
Is bright red blood present with passage of stool?	Colon cancer Diverticulosis Briskly bleeding peptic ulcer Hemorrhoids Inflammatory bowel disease

(continued)

Modifying symptoms	Think about
Worse after eating?	*Gastric ulcer*
	GERD
Worse before eating, relieved by food?	*Duodenal ulcer*
Worse after	
• *Drinking milk?*	*Lactose intolerance*
• *Eating fatty or fried foods?*	*Biliary colic*
	IBS
• *Eating gluten-containing foods (ie, wheat, barley, rye)?*	*Celiac disease*
• *Consuming citrus fruits?*	*Gastritis*
	GERD
• *Drinking alcohol?*	*Gastritis*
	GERD
	Peptic ulcer disease
	Pancreatitis
Worse when lying down?	*GERD*
	Pancreatitis
Relieved by defecation?	*IBS*
Precipitated by stress?	*IBS*
	Gastritis
Related to menstrual cycle?	*Nongastrointestinal etiology. Consider endometriosis, dysfunctional uterine bleeding, ovarian cyst*

DIAGNOSTIC APPROACH

The first step is to determine whether any alarm features are present. If absent, the likelihood of a benign etiology is much higher. If present, immediate evaluation with endoscopy should take place. Among the benign etiologies of dyspepsia, consider 3 subclassifications: ulcer-like dyspepsia, reflux-like dyspepsia, and dysmotility-like dyspepsia. Although distinct from dyspepsia, biliary colic symptoms can often overlap and should also be considered. Certain symptom groupings, if present, will help clarify the diagnosis.

CAVEATS

- Dyspepsia refers to a constellation of symptoms arising from the upper gastrointestinal tract, and as such, has a very broad differential diagnosis.
- Most causes of dyspepsia are benign; the presence of alarm features may help distinguish a patient with a more serious condition. Such patients must be referred for endoscopic evaluation.
- Extensive symptom-overlap occurs between different groups of patients with dyspepsia.[1] The value of the medical history is unfortunately limited as a tool to discriminate between different etiologies. Thus, while history is important, physical examination and diagnostic studies are also important parts of the evaluation.
- Avoid narrowing the differential diagnosis too early. A patient who complains of generalized epigastric discomfort may have a primary cardiac and not gastrointestinal etiology.

- Taking a complete medication history is of paramount importance. Many herbal products and over-the-counter medications can cause dyspepsia, and the patient is unlikely to bring them up unless you ask them directly.
- Gastric malignancies are rare but are more common in patients older than 45 years; in patients with a family history of gastric cancer, gastric surgery, or infection with *Helicobacter pylori;* or in those who have immigrated from an endemic area (eg, Japan, Costa Rica, China, Brazil).[3]

PROGNOSIS

Most patients with dyspepsia have an excellent prognosis, since the most common etiologies are nonulcer dyspepsia, GERD, and peptic ulcer disease. However, dyspepsia can have a significant impact on quality of life, with large societal and individual costs, including multiple physician visits, diagnostic tests, the cost of medications for treatment, and loss of productivity. The symptoms can be quite disabling and distressing. If untreated, peptic ulcer disease can be associated with significant morbidity. Gastric cancer is uncommon, but approximately 95% of symptomatic lesions are discovered at an advanced stage, when the 5-year survival is 10%.[3]

REFERENCES

1. Bazaldua OV, Schneider FD. Evaluation and management of dyspepsia. *Am Fam Physician.* 1999;60:1773–1784.
2. Fisher RS, Parkman HP. Management of nonulcer dyspepsia. *N Engl J Med.* 1998;339:1376–1381.
3. McQuaid K. Dyspepsia. In: Feldman, M, Friedman, LS, Sleisenger, MH, Scharshmidt, BF (editors). *Sleisenger and Fordtran's Gastrointestinal and Liver Disease,* 7th ed. WB Saunders and Company; 2002:102.
4. Richter JE. Dyspepsia: organic causes and differential characteristics from functional dyspepsia. *Scand J Gastroenterol Suppl.* 1991;182:11–16.
5. Talley NJ, McNeil D, Piper DW. Discriminant value of dyspeptic symptoms: a study of the clinical presentation of 221 patients with dyspepsia of unknown cause, peptic ulceration, and cholelithiasis. *Gut.* 1987;28:40–46.
6. Muris JW, Starmans R, Pop P, et al. Discriminant value of symptoms in patients with dyspepsia. *J Fam Pract.* 1994;38:139–143.
7. Zell SC, Budhraja M. An approach to dyspepsia in the ambulatory care setting: evaluation based on risk stratification. *J Gen Intern Med.* 1989;4:144–150.
8. Wallace MB, Durkalski VL, Vaughan J, et al. Age and alarm symptoms do not predict endoscopic findings among patients with dyspepsia: a multicentre database study. *Gut.* 2001;49:29–34.
9. Kurata JH, Nogawa AN, Noritake D. NSAIDs increase risk of gastrointestinal bleeding in primary care patients with dyspepsia. *J Fam Pract.* 1997;45:227–235.

SUGGESTED READING

Talley NJ, Silverstein MD, Agreus L, et al. AGA technical review: evaluation of dyspepsia. American Gastroenterological Association. *Gastroenterology.* 1998;114:582–595.

Bytzer P, Talley NJ. Dyspepsia. *Ann Intern Med.* 2001;134:815–822.

McNamara DA, Buckley M, O'Morain CA. Nonulcer dyspepsia. Current concepts and management. *Gastroenterol Clin North Am.* 2000;29:807–818.

Diagnostic Approach: Dyspepsia

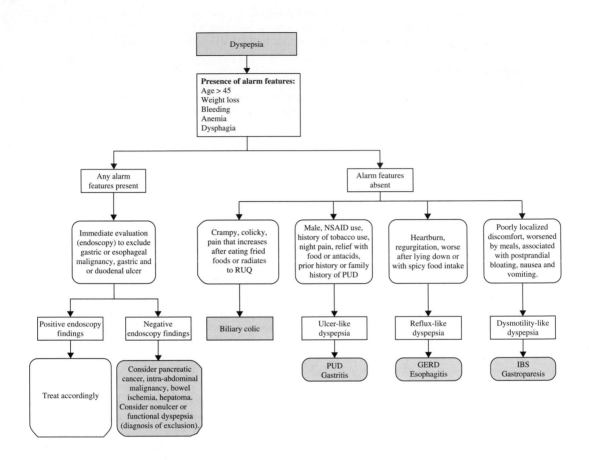

RUQ, right upper quadrant; NSAID, nonsteroidal anti-inflammatory drug; PUD, peptic ulcer disease; GERD, gastroesophageal reflux disease; IBS, irritable bowel syndrome.

Dysphagia

32

Sonal M. Patel, MD, & Anthony Lembo, MD

The word dysphagia derives from the Greek words "dys" (with difficulty) and "phagia" (to eat) and is defined as difficulty in swallowing. It is the sensation of hesitation or delay in passage of food during swallowing. Therefore, dysphagia differs from odynophagia, which refers to pain with swallowing. It is also differs from globus, which is the sensation of a lump or tightness in the throat unrelated to swallowing. The complaint of dysphagia, especially when it is a new symptom, should always be taken seriously since it is the most common presenting symptom of neoplasm of the esophagus.[1]

Two types of dysphagia exist: oropharyngeal and esophageal. They are distinct processes that require different evaluation and management. The history can often distinguish between the 2 types of dysphagia and can correctly identify the cause for the symptoms in 80–85% of cases.[2]

KEY TERMS

Esophageal dysphagia	Difficulty in passage of a bolus from the upper esophagus to the stomach.
Globus	Sensation of lump or tightness in the throat unrelated to swallowing.
Mechanical disorder	Obstruction of the esophageal lumen.
Motor disorder of the esophagus	Discoordination of the esophageal contractions.
Odynophagia	Pain with swallowing.
Oropharyngeal dysphagia	Difficulty initiating the swallowing process (ie, passage of a bolus from the mouth to the proximal esophagus).

ETIOLOGY

The exact prevalence of dysphagia is unknown. Current studies estimate the prevalence as between 16% and 22% among individuals over 50 years of age.[3] In a population survey of persons aged 30–64 years living in the Midwest, the estimated prevalence of dysphagia was 6–9%.[4] In a Swedish survey of the general population, 10% of respondents reported symptoms of dysphagia. Up to 25% of hospitalized patients and 33% of nursing home residents experience dysphagia.[5] Most nursing home residents with dysphagia have oropharyngeal dysphagia.[6] Oropharyngeal dysphagia complicates up to 67% of strokes and places these patients at increased risk for aspiration pneumonia. The 12-month mortality rate in these persons is as high as 45%.[7]

A study at the Mayo Clinic showed that of 499 patients with esophageal dysphagia, 47% had an obstructive lesion in the esophagus, 32% had dysphagia related to disturbed esophageal motility, and 21% had no demonstrable structural or motor abnormalities in the esophagus or oropharynx. Older age, male sex, the presence of weight loss, heartburn, and a history of prior esophageal dilation significantly predicted mechanical causes of dysphagia.[8]

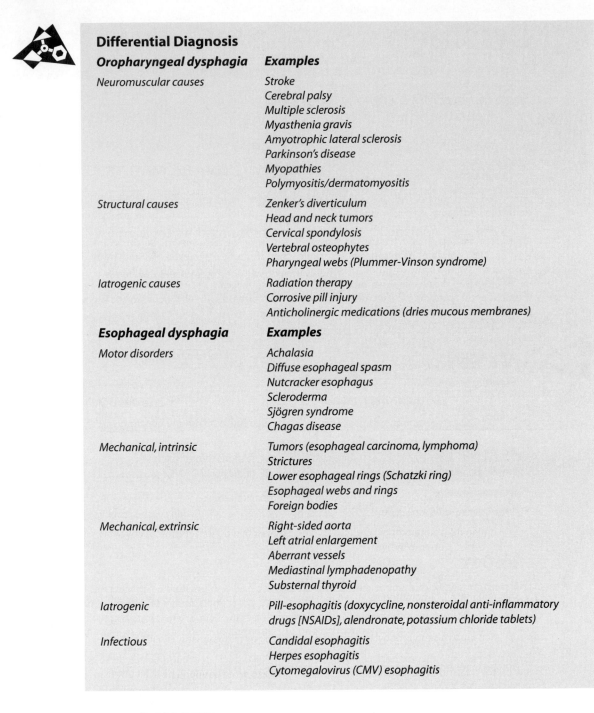

Differential Diagnosis

Oropharyngeal dysphagia	Examples
Neuromuscular causes	Stroke
	Cerebral palsy
	Multiple sclerosis
	Myasthenia gravis
	Amyotrophic lateral sclerosis
	Parkinson's disease
	Myopathies
	Polymyositis/dermatomyositis
Structural causes	Zenker's diverticulum
	Head and neck tumors
	Cervical spondylosis
	Vertebral osteophytes
	Pharyngeal webs (Plummer-Vinson syndrome)
Iatrogenic causes	Radiation therapy
	Corrosive pill injury
	Anticholinergic medications (dries mucous membranes)

Esophageal dysphagia	Examples
Motor disorders	Achalasia
	Diffuse esophageal spasm
	Nutcracker esophagus
	Scleroderma
	Sjögren syndrome
	Chagas disease
Mechanical, intrinsic	Tumors (esophageal carcinoma, lymphoma)
	Strictures
	Lower esophageal rings (Schatzki ring)
	Esophageal webs and rings
	Foreign bodies
Mechanical, extrinsic	Right-sided aorta
	Left atrial enlargement
	Aberrant vessels
	Mediastinal lymphadenopathy
	Substernal thyroid
Iatrogenic	Pill-esophagitis (doxycycline, nonsteroidal anti-inflammatory drugs [NSAIDs], alendronate, potassium chloride tablets)
Infectious	Candidal esophagitis
	Herpes esophagitis
	Cytomegalovirus (CMV) esophagitis

GETTING STARTED

- Ask the patient to describe what happens when he or she swallows.
- Ask open-ended questions.
- Distinguish between oropharyngeal and esophageal dysphagia, remembering that in up to 80% of cases of dysphagia, clinicians may establish the cause based on history alone.

- Determine which types of food result in dysphagia (solids, liquids, or both). Dysphagia to both solids and liquids is suggestive of a motor disorder while dysphagia to solids alone is more likely due to a mechanical obstruction.
- Determine the time course. The new onset of symptoms that progressively worsen requires prompt evaluation because of the concern for malignancy.

Questions	Remember
Tell me what happens when you swallow.	*Avoid interrupting.*
When did you first notice that you were having difficulty swallowing? Are your symptoms getting worse?	*Do not ask focused questions until the patient is done describing his or her symptoms in detail.*
Describe what happens when you try to eat solid foods. *Describe what happens when you drink liquids.*	*Ask the patient to describe these events in detail.*

INTERVIEW FRAMEWORK

- Evaluate the patient's medication list before the interview and consider the potential contribution of the medications in dysphagia.
- Determine whether the patient has symptoms with ingestion of solids only, or both liquids and solids to distinguish between mechanical obstruction and neuromuscular disorders.
- Determine whether symptoms are progressive or intermittent.
- Determine whether the patient has any associated symptoms or comorbid conditions, such as history of stroke, neurologic disorders, tobacco use, or history of reflux disease.
- Assess for additional alarm symptoms (ie, weight loss, bleeding, fevers, hematemesis, advanced age).
- Establish characteristic features of the dysphagia such as onset, duration, frequency, location, and precipitating or alleviating factors. If a patient has not offered this information with your open-ended questioning, be sure to ask directed questions.

IDENTIFYING ALARM SYMPTOMS

- Older patients presenting with progressive dysphagia, particularly those with a past history of alcohol abuse, smoking, obesity, or gastroesophageal reflux, should raise concern about an underlying oropharyngeal or esophageal malignancy.

Serious Causes	Remarks	Prevalence
Oropharyngeal or laryngeal carcinoma	*Associated with tobacco and chronic alcohol use.*	*82% of all patients with oropharyngeal or laryngeal carcinoma experience dysphagia.[9]*
Stroke	*Most common cause of oropharyngeal dysphagia. Onset is often abrupt.*	*45% of all stroke patients experience dysphagia at 3 months.*
Head injury		
Parkinson's disease	*Common cause of oropharyngeal dysphagia.*	*81% of patients with Parkinson's disease have mild dysphagia.*

(continued)

Serious Causes	Remarks	Prevalence
Multiple sclerosis		24–34% of patients with multiple sclerosis have permanent dysphagia.[10]
Amyotrophic lateral sclerosis	Characterized by progressive dysphagia.	
Huntington's chorea		
Myasthenia gravis	Dysphagia becomes progressively worse with repetitive swallows.	67% of patients have dysphagia at the time of diagnosis.
Esophageal carcinoma	Progressive dysphagia to solids, and then to both solids and liquids, is the most common presentation. Squamous cancer of the esophagus is associated with smoking and alcohol use. Adenocarcinoma of the esophagus is associated with gastroesophageal reflux, smoking, and obesity.	6–17% of patients presenting with dysphagia in the primary care setting prove to have carcinoma.
Mediastinal tumors		
Vascular structures (dysphagia lusoria)		
Muscular dystrophies	Can present with dysphagia and ptosis later in life.	

Alarm symptoms	Serious causes	Benign causes
Weight loss	Malignancy	Peptic stricture
Progressive symptoms	Malignancy Neurodegenerative disorders	
Are your symptoms worse with solids than with liquids?	Malignancy	Peptic stricture Esophageal web or ring Foreign bodies
Blood in stools	Malignancy	
Otalgia (ear pain) with dysphagia	Hypopharyngeal lesion (eg, squamous cell cancer or thyroid cancer)	
Hoarseness (dysphonia) or pain with speaking and dysphagia?	Muscular dystrophies	
Dysarthria	Stroke	

FOCUSED QUESTIONS

Questions	Think about
Do you cough, choke, or sense food coming back through your nose after swallowing?	Oropharyngeal dysphagia
Does it feel as if food is getting stuck within the first few seconds of swallowing?	Oropharyngeal dysphagia
Do you have difficulty swallowing liquids, solids, or both?	Liquids and solids = motor disorder Solids progressing to include liquids = mechanical obstruction
Are your symptoms getting worse?	Rapidly progressive symptoms are worrisome for malignancy
Do you always have trouble swallowing or are your symptoms intermittent?	Intermittent, nonprogressive symptoms suggest a distal esophageal web or ring
Have you received radiation therapy in the past?	Radiation esophagitis
Do you take your medications with fluids? Do you take your medications immediately before going to bed?	Pill-esophagitis. Most commonly associated with ingestion of iron supplements, aspirin, potassium, doxycycline, and alendronate.
Do you have a medical condition that suppresses your immune system eg, HIV, chronic steroid use, chemotherapy?	Candidal, herpes simplex virus (HSV), or CMV esophagitis

Quality	*Think about*
Is food sticking or getting stuck after you swallow?	Esophageal dysphagia
Have you experienced nasal regurgitation?	Oropharyngeal dysphagia
Do you have difficulty initiating a swallow?	Oropharyngeal dysphagia
Do you choke or cough when you try to swallow?	Oropharyngeal dysphagia
Have your symptoms remained the same over a long period of time or are they getting worse?	Nonprogressive symptoms indicate benign structural lesions such as Schatzki ring or web

Location	*Think about*
Where exactly does the food stick or hang up?	Oropharyngeal dysphagia: Patients frequently point to their cervical region Esophageal dysphagia: The lesion is at or below the region to which they point

Time course and frequency	*Think about*
Are your symptoms episodic?	Episodic dysphagia to solids over a long period of time suggests a benign disease such as a lower esophageal ring.
How long have you had these symptoms?	Dysphagia of short duration suggests an inflammatory process.

(continued)

Associated symptoms	Think about
Do you hear a gurgling noise when you swallow?	Zenker's diverticulum
Do you feel like you have bad breath?	Halitosis is associated with Zenker's diverticulum
Do you regurgitate old foods?	Distal esophageal obstruction Zenker's diverticulum Achalasia
Is it painful to swallow?	Esophageal mucosal inflammation (ie, esophagitis)
Do you experience chest pain?	Motor disorders of the esophagus (ie, diffuse esophageal spasm, achalasia, and scleroderma)
Do you ever have to bear down or raise your arms over your head to help a food bolus pass?	Motor disorders
Are your symptoms worse with very hot or cold liquids?	Motor disorders
Do you have a long-standing history of heartburn?	Peptic stricture
Are your symptoms relieved by repeated swallows?	Motor disorders
Have you ever experienced the sudden onset of dysphagia after swallowing pieces of meat?	Esophageal ring "Steak house syndrome" (Recurrent episodes of obstruction in distal esophagus often after eating a piece of steak or bread. The obstruction is the result of a lower esophageal ring and is usually relieved by drinking large amounts of water.)
Are your symptoms worse when you swallow cold foods?	Motor disorders

CAVEATS

- Dysphagia should always be taken seriously and should prompt further evaluation. Dysphagia should never be perceived as functional and always mandates a careful evaluation. The duration and frequency of a patient's dysphagia provide useful clues and can help make the diagnosis.
- Distinguish between oropharyngeal and esophageal dysphagia at the beginning of the interview.
- Dysphagia related to esophageal disease, such as a peptic stricture, may sometimes be felt in the suprasternal notch.
- A history of dry mouth or eyes may indicate inadequate salivary production. In such cases, it is particularly important to obtain a detailed review of medications. Anticholinergics, antihistamines, and certain antihypertensives can reduce salivary flow. Sjögren syndrome should also be considered.
- If a patient describes food getting stuck and that the only way to relieve this is by regurgitation, the patient probably has a mechanical obstruction. On the other hand, if certain physical maneuvers assist the passage of food, then the patient likely has a motility disorder.

REFERENCES

1. Cohen S. Parkman H. Diseases of the Esophagus. In: Goldman, editor. *Cecil's Textbook of Medicine.* WB Saunders and Company; 2000.
2. Spieker M. Evaluating dysphagia. *Am Fam Physician.* 2000;61:3639–3648.
3. Lind C. Dysphagia: evaluation and treatment. *Gastroenterol Clin.* 2003;32:553–575.

4. Talley N, Weaver A, Zinmeister A, Melton L. Onset and disappearance of gastrointestinal symptoms and functional gastrointestinal disorders. *Am J Epidemiol.* 1992;136:65–77.

5. Layne KA, Losinski DS, Zenner PM, Ament JA. Using the Fleming index of dysphagia to establish prevalence. *Dysphagia.* 1989;4:39–42.

6. Lynn R. Dysphagia. In: Edmundowicz S, editor. *20 Common Problems in Gastroenterology.* McGraw-Hill; 2002.

7. Croghan JM, Burke EM, Caplan S, Denman S. Pilot study of 12-month outcomes of nursing home patients with aspiration on videofluoroscopy. *Dysphagia.* 1994;9:141–146.

8. Kim C, Weaver A, Hsu J, et al. Discriminate Value of Esophageal Symptoms: A Study of the Initial Clinical findings in 499 Patients With Dysphagia of Various Causes. *Mayo Clin Proceedings.* 1993;68:948–954.

9. Chua KS, Reddy SK, Lee MC, Patt RB. Pain and loss of function in head and neck cancer survivors. *J Pain Symptom Manage.* 1999;18:193–202.

10. De Pauw A, Dejaeger E, et al. Dysphagia in multiple sclerosis. *Clin Neurol Neurosurg.* 2003;104:345–351.

SUGGESTED READING

Goyal R. Dysphagia. In: Fauci A, editor. *Harrison's Principles of Internal Medicine.* McGraw Hill; 1998.

Koch W. Swallowing Disorders. Diagnosis and Therapy. *Med Clin North Am.* 1993;77:571.

Richter J. Dysphagia, Odynophagia, Heartburn and other Esophageal Symptoms. In: *Sleisenger's and Fordtram's Gastrointestinal and Liver Disease.* Elsevier; 2002.

Diagnostic Approach: Dysphagia

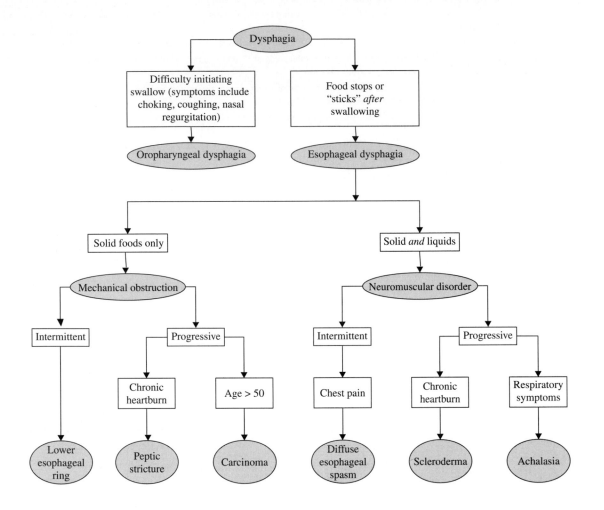

Acute Gastrointestinal Bleeding | 33

Liana Vesga, MD, & Kenneth R. McQuaid, MD

Gastrointestinal (GI) bleeding is a common medical condition. Occasionally, patients are seen in the office setting, but most patients with bleeding go to the emergency department or bleeding develops while they are hospitalized for another reason. The annual incidence of acute upper GI bleeding is 100–200 cases and of lower GI bleeding is 20–27 cases per 100,000 population.[1–5] Distinguishing between upper and lower GI bleeding is paramount because the differential diagnosis and management vary. The causes of GI bleeding are myriad, ranging from trivial to life-threatening.

Patients with GI bleeding require rapid evaluation and treatment. The initial history and physical examination provide information about the severity, duration, location, and possible etiology of GI bleeding. This initial assessment guides initial fluid resuscitation, triage within the hospital, and timing of diagnostic procedures and therapy.

KEY TERMS

Hematemesis	*Vomiting of bright red (fresh) blood or old "coffee ground" material.*
Hematochezia	*Bright red blood, maroon blood, or clots per rectum.*
Hemodynamic instability	*Systolic blood pressure < 100 mm Hg and/or pulse > 100 beats per minute. Indicates significant intravascular volume loss.*
Lower gastrointestinal bleeding (LGIB)	*Bleeding that originates distal to the ligament of Treitz (ie, small intestine [5%] or colon [95%]). Manifested by hematochezia.*
Upper gastrointestinal bleeding (UGIB)	*Bleeding that originates proximal to the ligament of Treitz (ie, esophagus, stomach, or duodenum). Manifests in 3 ways: (1) hematemesis, (2) melena, or (3) hematochezia.*
Melena	*Black, tarry, foul-smelling stools.*
Positive nasogastric aspirate	*The presence of bright red blood, clots, or coffee grounds aspirated from nasogastric tube; confirms an UGIB. Red blood suggests active bleeding.*

ETIOLOGY

UGIB originates from sources above the ligament of Treitz. Lack of hematemesis does not exclude UGIB because bleeding may be intermittent or arising from the distal duodenum. LGIB originates from sources beyond the ligament of Treitz. Melena usually indicates UGIB; however bleeding from the small intestine or proximal colon with slow transit time may also cause melena. Hematochezia usually indicates LGIB, although 10% of episodes are caused by brisk UGIB.

Differential Diagnosis

Common Causes of UGIB[2,8]		Frequency
Peptic ulcers	Ulcerations > 3 mm in size caused by Helicobacter pylori or nonsteroidal anti-inflammatory drugs (NSAIDs)	50%
Gastroesophageal varices	Dilated veins in the esophagus or stomach caused by portal hypertension, usually secondary to cirrhosis	10–20%
Erosions	Small mucosal breaks (< 3 mm) commonly caused by NSAIDs or severe physiologic stress ("stress gastritis")	5–10%
Mallory-Weiss tear	Mucosal laceration at the gastroesophageal junction, commonly occurring after retching	5–8%
Uncommon Causes of UGIB		
Angiodysplasia or vascular ectasias	Congenital or acquired abnormal dilation of submucosal veins and capillaries.	2–5%
Gastric antral vascular ectasia	Diffuse vascular ectasias of antrum ("watermelon stomach")	2–5%
Portal hypertensive gastropathy	Dilated submucosal veins caused by portal hypertension.	< 5%
Tumors	Adenocarcinoma, lymphoma, or stromal tumors	1–5%
Dieulafoy lesion	Rupture of a large, tortuous artery in the proximal stomach.	1–5%
Erosive esophagitis	Seldom a cause of overt UGIB	< 1%
Aortoenteric fistula	Fistula between aorta and duodenum, most commonly in patients with prior abdominal aortic aneurysm surgery.	< 1%
Hemobilia	Bleeding from liver lesion into bile duct.	< 1%
Hemosuccus pancreaticus	Bleeding from pancreatic lesion into pancreatic duct.	< 1%
Colonic Sources of LGIB[4]		**Account for > 95% of LGIB**
Diverticulosis	Herniations of the mucosa through intestinal wall at sites of penetrating arteries. Bleeding occurs in < 5% of patients and stops spontaneously in 75% of episodes.	40–55%
Angiodysplasia or vascular ectasia.	Most commonly found in the cecum or ascending colon.	3–8%

Colorectal malignancy	Usually manifests with occult bleeding or blood mixed with stool. Seldomly presents with severe bleeding.	5–10%
Ischemic colitis	Impaired colonic blood supply caused by reduced cardiac output or occlusion of mesenteric arteries. Bleeding usually is self-limited.	5–8%
Infectious colitis	Manifested by dysentery (ie, blood mixed with stool and pus). Causes include infection with Shigella, Campylobacter, Salmonella, and Escherichia coli O157:H7	5%
Postpolypectomy hemorrhage	Bleeding occurs in 1 of 300 patients after colonoscopic removal of polyps. > 70% stop spontaneously.	2–8%
Inflammatory bowel disease	Bloody diarrhea is common with ulcerative colitis, but major bleeding is uncommon.	2%
Stercoral ulcers	Rectal ulcerations caused by chronic constipation.	1–2%
Radiation proctitis	Occurs months to years after pelvic radiation.	1–2%
Hemorrhoids	The most common cause of minor hematochezia; usually characterized by blood streaking stool and dripping into toilet during defecation. Uncommonly cause serious LGIB.	< 5%
Small Intestine Sources		**Account for < 5% of LGIB**
Angiodysplasias or vascular ectasias	Commonly cause chronic, occult bleeding leading to anemia; but may cause acute, severe bleeding.	3–5%
Meckel's diverticulum	Vitelline duct remnant located in terminal ileum. Most common cause of small bowel bleeding in patients younger than 25 years.	
Crohn's disease	Most common in terminal ileum or proximal colon.	< 1%
NSAID-induced ulcers	Erosions, ulcers, or webs occur throughout the small intestine, but clinically significant bleeding is uncommon.	1–2%
Tumors	Adenocarcinoma, lymphoma, carcinoid, stromal tumors	< 1%

GETTING STARTED

The first step in evaluating patients with acute GI bleeding is to assess the severity of the bleeding to determine whether hemodynamic resuscitation is necessary. The provider should initially obtain the patient's vital signs (pulse and blood pressure), perform a focused history, and insert intravenous catheters for fluid replacement. Based on this initial evaluation, the clinician is able to make a preliminary assessment of the severity of bleeding, whether the bleeding is likely from an upper or lower source, and whether it is ongoing.

- Determine whether the patient has lost substantial volumes of blood.
- Seek clues as to whether the bleeding is ongoing or may have stopped.
- Determine whether the bleeding is likely originating from the upper or lower gastrointestinal tract.

Questions	Remember
Describe what you saw in the toilet bowl.	*Melena suggests UGIB or slow LGIB. Hematochezia suggests either LGIB or massive UGIB. Blood mixed with or coating stool suggests a hemodynamically insignificant bleed from an anorectal source.*
Have you had vomiting? If so, describe what it looks like.	*Hematemesis indicates an UGIB. Coffee-ground emesis suggests that the bleeding has slowed or stopped. Bright red emesis indicates recent or ongoing bleeding.*
When did you first notice the bleeding?	*Bleeding that began more than 4–6 hours earlier may have led to significant blood loss.*
How many times have you had hematochezia or vomiting?	*Repeated episodes suggest significant blood loss.*
Have you been passing or vomiting cups of blood or only streaks or small clots?	*Although patient estimations of blood loss are of questionable reliability, bloody streaks or small clots mixed with emesis or stool suggest minor blood loss.*
When was the last time you passed a black or bloody stool?	*Blood in the GI tract is a potent cathartic. If no melena or hematochezia has occurred in the last 4–6 hours, bleeding may have slowed or stopped.*
Do you have any dizziness?	*Dizziness suggests significant intravascular volume loss.*
Obtain the patient's vital signs (blood pressure and pulse) while supine. If normal, obtain vital signs after patient assumes a sitting or standing position.	*See below.*

INTERVIEW FRAMEWORK

After the initial assessment has been performed and appropriate fluid resuscitation has been initiated, a more complete history and physical examination is obtained. Most causes of bleeding can be ascertained from the patient's presenting symptoms and past medical history. Information obtained about the current bleeding episode, prior bleeding episodes, recent GI symptoms, past medical history, medications, and social history will provide clues to the most likely bleeding source and guide decisions about admission to an intensive care unit or regular hospital unit.

- A past history of GI bleeding or other GI disorders may suggest potential causes of the current bleeding.
- Aspirin and NSAIDs may cause or potentiate UGIB or LGIB due to their ulcerogenic and antiplatelet effects. Other antiplatelet agents (clopidrogel) and anticoagulants (heparin, warfarin) may exacerbate but do not cause GI bleeding.

IDENTIFYING ALARM SIGNS AND SYMPTOMS

The sight of GI bleeding is frightening to patients and providers alike. Certain symptoms and signs suggest massive GI bleeding or raise concern that the patient is at increased risk for morbidity and mortality. Such patients usually warrant admission to the intensive care unit.

- Reassure and calm the patient, who may be anxious and frightened.
- Vital signs: Supine systolic blood pressure < 100 mm Hg or pulse > 100 beats per minute indicates significant (> 20%) intravascular volume loss and the need for immediate fluid resuscitation. Orthostatic hypotension or tachycardia indicates intravascular volume loss of 10–20%.

- Hematochezia with hematemesis or a positive nasogastric lavage indicates active, life-threatening UGIB and should prompt urgent evaluation and therapy.
- Elderly patients may have concomitant cardiovascular disease, placing them at increased risk for adverse events from bleeding, hypotension, or anemia.
- Dizziness and lightheadedness suggest significant intravascular volume depletion.
- Patients with chronic liver disease may have severe bleeding due to portal hypertension and coagulopathy, and are at increased risk for complications.
- GI bleeding in hospitalized patients carries increased risk of morbidity and mortality compared with bleeding that begins in outpatients, irrespective of the cause.

Alarm symptoms	Serious causes	Benign causes
Ongoing hematemesis, bright red blood per nasogastric tube with hematochezia, or unstable vital signs	Massive UGIB due to esophageal or gastric varices Peptic ulcer disease (PUD) Aortoenteric fistula	
Ongoing hematemesis, or bright red blood from nasogastric tube with melena	Esophageal or gastric varices Peptic ulcer with arterial bleed Dieulafoy lesion Aortoenteric fistula	Mallory-Weiss tear Erosive esophagitis Erosive gastritis Portal hypertensive gastropathy
Ongoing, brisk hematochezia with no blood from nasogastric lavage	LGIB due to diverticulosis, vascular ectasia, or NSAID-ulcers If vital signs unstable, also consider UGIB from duodenal ulcer or aortoenteric fistula (without blood refluxing into stomach)	Radiation proctitis Stercoral ulcers Inflammatory bowel disease Hemorrhoids
Weight loss	Neoplasm	Peptic ulcer with gastric outlet obstruction
Acute onset of lower or mid-abdominal pain followed by bleeding	Mesenteric or colonic ischemia	Ulcerative colitis Crohn's disease Cramps from cathartic effects blood
Prior aortic repair	Aortoenteric fistula	
Shortness of breath, chest pain, lightheadedness	Cardiac ischemia secondary to significant blood loss	Anxiety
UGIB that begins in hospitalized, critically ill patient	Stress-related erosions or ulcers of stomach or duodenum	Esophagitis NSAID-induced gastric erosions

FOCUSED QUESTIONS

After obtaining the initial history, vital signs, and assessing for alarm symptoms, perform a more complete history focusing on associated GI symptoms, past medical history, medications, and social history.

Questions

Associated symptoms

Have you had

- *Vomiting, retching?*

- *Heartburn?*

- *Odynophagia (pain on swallowing)?*

- *Dysphagia?*

- *Dyspepsia (epigastric discomfort or pain)?*

- *Evidence of chronic liver disease (jaundice, scleral icterus, ascites, spider telangiectasias, palmar erythema, gynecomastia, hepatosplenomegaly)?*

- *Bloody diarrhea (dysentery)?*

- *Straining with defecation, constipation?*

Think about

Mallory-Weiss tear (< 50% have a history of vomiting or retching)

Erosive esophagitis

Pill-induced esophageal ulceration
Infections (cytomegalovirus [CMV], Candida, herpesvirus)

Esophageal neoplasm
Gastroesphageal reflux with esophageal stricture

PUD or erosive gastritis; however, patients with bleeding from PUD may be asymptomatic.

Esophageal or gastric varices
Portal hypertensive gastropathy.

Infectious diarrhea or inflammatory bowel disease (ulcerative colitis, less likely Crohn's disease). Symptoms present for > 2 weeks suggest inflammatory bowel disease.

Distal colonic or rectal neoplasm
Hemorrhoids
Stercoral ulcer

Past medical history

Do you have

- *History of peptic ulcer?*

- *History of gastric surgery or gastric bypass?*

- *History of immunodeficiency (HIV disease with low CD4 count, immunosuppression, chemotherapy)?*

- *History of esophageal, gastric, or colonic neoplasm?*

- *History of diverticulosis?*

- *History of inflammatory bowel disease?*

- *History of radiation therapy?*

- *History of coronary artery disease or peripheral artery disease?*

- *Chronic renal disease?*

Think about

Ulcer recurrence

Ulcer at anastomosis between intestine and stomach

CMV ulcers
Fungal infections
Kaposi sarcoma

Recurrence of neoplasm

Bleeding occurs in < 5% of patients with diverticulosis

Ulcerative colitis is a more common cause of bleeding, usually presenting with bloody diarrhea. Crohn's disease uncommonly presents with acute hemorrhage from ulceration.

Postradiation esophagitis, proctitis

Increased risk of ischemic bowel disease. Also, likely use of antiplatelet agents and/or anticoagulants.

Increased risk of angiodysplasias. Potential for worsened bleeding from any cause due to uremic-induced platelet dysfunction.

- *Osteoarthritis?* | *Likely use of NSAIDs*
- *History of hepatitis or known chronic liver disease?* | *Increased risk of bleeding from varices or portal hypertensive gastropathy*
- *Have you had an endoscopy or colonoscopy with biopsy, sphincterotomy, or polypectomy within prior 2 weeks?* | *Bleeding from biopsy or polypectomy site*

Medications | ### Think about

What medications are you taking?

- *Aspirin, NSAIDs* | *Erosions or peptic ulcer in stomach, duodenum, small bowel, or proximal colon. Due to antiplatelet effects, may potentiate bleeding from upper or lower GI tract source.*
- *Anticoagulants (eg, warfarin, heparin, enoxaparin, clopidrogel)* | *Do not directly cause GI bleeding, but potentiate bleeding from preexisting lesions within GI tract.*
- *Immunosuppressants (chemotherapy, prednisone, antirejection drugs)* | *Opportunistic infections (CMV, herpes simplex virus, Candida)*
- *Recent use of antibiotics?* | *Clostridium difficile colitis*
- *Bisphosphonates (alendronate), potassium, quinidine, iron, antibiotics* | *Pill-induced esophageal ulcer (usually not a cause of significant bleeding)*

Social history | ### Think about

Is the patient

- *An immigrant from a developing country (Mexico, Central America, Africa, Asia)* | *In a patient with UGIB, peptic ulcer may be due to chronic infection with H pylori.*
In a patient > 40 years of age, also consider H pylori-associated gastric cancer or lymphoma.
- *A US resident from lower socioeconomic background (especially blacks and Hispanics)* | *In a patient with UGIB, peptic ulcer may be due to chronic infection with H pylori.*
In a patient > 40 years of age, also consider H pylori-associated gastric cancer or lymphoma.

Do you drink alcohol? How much? Do you have a history of drinking alcohol? | *Gastroesophageal varices or portal hypertensive gastropathy secondary to alcoholic cirrhosis.*

Have you traveled recently? If so, where? | *Infectious diarrhea*

Do you have a history of sexual activity leading to increased risk of anal-oral contamination? | *Infectious diarrhea*

CAVEATS

- UGIB and LGIB cause overlapping symptoms and share broad differential diagnoses.
- Nasopharyngeal and pulmonary disorders cause epistaxis or hemoptysis, which may be misinterpreted as hematemesis.
- Bleeding in the duodenum may not always reflux into the stomach. Hence, lesions in the duodenum do not always cause hematemesis or positive nasogastric lavage.

PROGNOSIS

The overall mortality rate from UGIB is < 10% and from LGIB is < 5%. Approximately 80% of GI bleeding stops spontaneously. Persistent or recurrent bleeding markedly increases the risk of morbidity and mortality. The 2 most important prognostic factors are the cause of bleeding and the presence of comorbid illnesses.[6,7,9] Bleeding originating from gastroesophageal varices, ulcers with visible blood vessels, or advanced malignancies have an increased risk of adverse outcome. Patients with serious comorbid illnesses, especially coronary ischemia or heart failure, advanced liver disease, renal failure, or disseminated malignancy have increased rates of rebleeding and mortality. Other independent risk factors for mortality from GI bleeding include age and the presence of shock (systolic blood pressure < 100 mm Hg) on admission.[6,7,9] For both upper and lower GI bleeding, endoscopy may help localize the source of bleeding, determine the risk of rebleeding, and allow therapy if indicated. If adequate visualization cannot be achieved or if there is hemodynamic instability, angiography with attempted embolization of the bleeding lesion should be considered. Surgery may be required for treatment of persistent or recurrent bleeding that cannot be treated with endoscopy or embolization.

REFERENCES

1. Rockall TA, Logan RFA, Devlin HB, Northfield TC. Incidence of and mortality from acute upper gastrointestinal haemorrhage in the United Kingdom. *BMJ.* 1995;311:222–226.

2. Longstreth GF. Epidemiology of hospitalization for acute upper gastrointestinal hemorrhage: a population-based study. *Am J Gastroenterol.* 1995;90:206–210.

3. Zuckerman GR, Prakash C. Acute lower intestinal bleeding: Part II: Etiology, therapy, and outcomes. *Gastointest Endosc.* 1999;49:228–238.

4. Longstreth GF. Epidemiology and outcome of patients hospitalized with acute lower gastrointestinal hemorrhage: a population-based study. *Am J Gastroenterol.* 1997;92:419–424.

5. Blatchford O et al. Acute upper gastrointestinal hemorrhage in west of Scotland: case ascertainment study. *BMJ.* 1997; 315:510–514.

6. Rockall TA et al. Risk assessment after acute upper gastrointestinal haemorrhage. *Gut.* 1996;38:316–321.

7. Blatchford O et al. A risk score to predict need for treatment for upper gastrointestinal haemorrhage. *Lancet.* 2000;356: 1318–1321.

8. Gupta PK et al. Nonvariceal upper gastrointestinal bleeding. *Med Clin North Am.* 1993;77:973–992.

9. Barkun A et al. Consensus recommendations for managing patients with nonvariceal upper gastrointestinal bleeding. *Ann Intern Med.* 2003;139:843–857.

SUGGESTED READING

Bounds BC et al. Lower gastrointestinal bleeding. *Gastroenterol Clin North Am.* 2003;32:1107–1125.

Fallah M et al. Acute gastrointestinal bleeding. *Med Clin North Am.* 2000;84:1183–1208.

Huang CS, Lichtenstein DR. Nonvariceal upper gastrointestinal bleeding. *Gastroenterol Clin North Am.* 2003;32:1053–1078.

Sharara AI et al. Gastroesophageal variceal hemorrhage. *N Engl J Med.* 2001;345:669–681.

Diagnostic Approach: Upper Gastrointestinal Bleeding

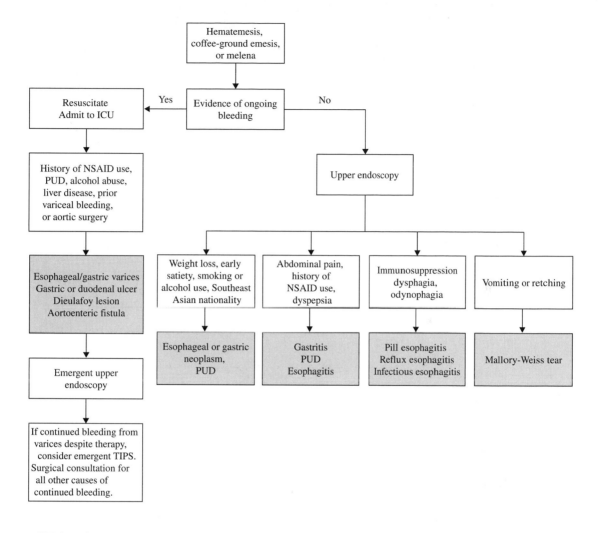

ICU, intensive care unit; NSAID, nonsteroidal anti-inflammatory drug; PUD, peptic ulcer disease; TIPS, transvenous intrahepatic portosystemic shunt.

Diagnostic Approach: Lower Gastrointestinal Bleeding

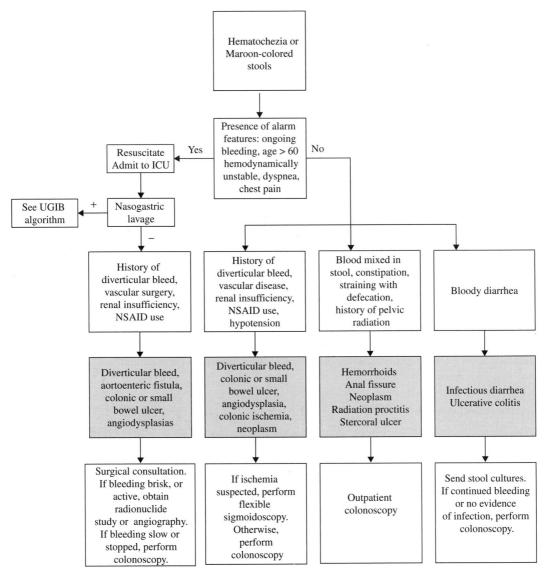

ICU, intensive care unit; NSAID, nonsteroidal anti-inflammatory drug; UGIB, upper gastrointestinal bleeding.

Jaundice

Thomas E. Baudendistel, MD, FACP, & Estella M. Geraghty, MD, MS

Jaundice is a yellow discoloration of body tissues due to an excess of bilirubin, a pigment produced during the metabolism of heme. Normally, serum bilirubin should never exceed 1–1.5 mg/dL. Levels above 2 mg/dL result in detectable jaundice, first in the sclerae, next under the tongue and along the tympanic membranes, and finally in the skin. Thus, cutaneous jaundice implies higher levels of bilirubin than isolated scleral icterus.

A thorough dietary and medication history can exclude the yellow skin discoloration of carotenemia, isotretinoin, or rifampin overdose, all of which spare the sclerae. Once these mimickers are excluded, jaundice must be recognized as a manifestation of advanced underlying liver disease, biliary duct obstruction, or less commonly hemolysis or abnormal bilirubin metabolism. The history should proceed in 2 parallel routes: (1) arrive rapidly at a likely diagnosis and (2) identify alarm features that may necessitate urgent intervention.

KEY TERMS

Budd-Chiari syndrome	Hepatic vein obstruction, often due to an underlying hypercoagulable state (eg, oral contraceptives, polycythemia vera, paroxysmal nocturnal hemoglobinuria, antiphospholipid antibody syndrome); the acute form classically presents with tender hepatomegaly, jaundice, and ascites.
Cholestasis	Retention of bile in the liver.
Conjugated bilirubin	Formed in the liver when unconjugated bilirubin is metabolized, then released into bile; may be filtered by the glomerulus and appear in the urine.
Fulminant hepatic failure	Onset of hepatic encephalopathy within 8 weeks of liver injury, often accompanied by coagulopathy. Common causes include acute viral hepatitis, ingestions (eg, acetaminophen or Amanita mushrooms), and hepatic ischemia. Less common causes include Wilson's disease, autoimmune hepatitis, acute Budd-Chiari syndrome, other infections, and malignancy.
Hepatocellular jaundice	Accumulation of conjugated bilirubin in the serum due to hepatocyte dysfunction.
Hyperbilirubinemia	Elevated serum levels of bilirubin (> 1.2 mg/dL).
Icterus	Synonymous with jaundice.
Infiltrative liver disease	Subset of liver disease marked by cholestasis due to diffuse involvement within the liver including granulomatous disease (sarcoidosis, Wegener's granulomatosis, fungal and mycobacterial infections), amyloidosis, Wilson's disease, hemochromatosis, lymphoma, and metastatic cancer.

(continued)

KEY TERMS

Jaundice	*Yellow pigmentation of the skin and sclerae.*
Nonalcoholic fatty liver disease (NAFLD)	*Also referred to as nonalcoholic steatohepatitis (NASH); parenchymal liver disease common in obese diabetics.*
Obstructive jaundice	*Excess conjugated bilirubin in the serum due to impaired bile flow in the intrahepatic or extrahepatic bile ducts.*
Unconjugated bilirubin	*The main circulating form of bilirubin, produced upon heme breakdown and delivered to the liver for further metabolism.*

ETIOLOGY

The numerous causes of jaundice can be divided into 4 broad categories (see Figure, Causes of Jaundice Based on Mechanism of Bilirubin Accumulation):

1. Impaired bilirubin metabolism
   a. Excess bilirubin production
   b. Impaired bilirubin uptake
   c. Impaired conjugation of bilirubin
2. Impaired secretion of bile into bile canaliculi
3. Liver disease
4. Obstruction of the bile ducts.

Most disorders in the first category cause unconjugated hyperbilirubinemia, and—with the exceptions of sepsis and acute hemolytic reactions—are milder. Predominantly conjugated hyperbilirubinemia is more common and generally implies a more serious condition. In adults, most jaundice results from gallstone disease, cancer (pancreatic and hepatobiliary), and cirrhosis (due to alcohol abuse, chronic viral hepatitis, or NAFLD).

Differential Diagnosis	Prevalence[a,1–3]
Gallstones	*20%*
• Biliary colic	*20% of patients with gallstones*
• Choledocholithiasis	*15% of patients with gallstones*
Alcoholic cirrhosis	
NAFLD	
Gilbert syndrome	*4% (10% among whites)*
Hepatitis A	*38% seroprevalence*
Hepatitis B	*0.1–2% carrier prevalence*
Hepatitis C	*1.4–1.8% antibody (+)*
Wilson's disease	*1 in 30,000*
Hemochromatosis	*0.5% in whites*
Primary biliary cirrhosis	*4.5 per 100,000 women 0.7 per 100,000 men*

Primary sclerosing cholangitis	
Pancreatic cancer	7.9 per 100,000 women
	12.8 per 100,000 men
Hepatocellular carcinoma	3–5% annual risk in patients with cirrhosis
Cholangiocarcinoma	0.01–0.46%

[a]Among general population in the United States; prevalence is unknown when not indicated.

GETTING STARTED

Jaundice seldom occurs as an isolated event and is often a late manifestation of a chronic illness. However, the patient may not immediately relate jaundice—a skin or eye complaint—to other symptoms. Therefore, allow the patient time to disclose other key etiologic information.

Open-ended questions

Tell me how you were feeling when you first noticed the color change.

What other symptoms have accompanied this color change?

When did you last feel your health was normal?

Tips for effective interviewing

- Be nonjudgmental so patients can feel safe revealing details of high-risk behaviors (eg, alcohol intake, illicit drug use, suicide attempts)
- Begin to formulate and rank items on your differential diagnosis

INTERVIEW FRAMEWORK

- Determine the acuity of onset, which will dictate the pace of the diagnostic evaluation. Slow progression of jaundice over months may not warrant an urgent evaluation, whereas rapid onset over days should prompt immediate investigation.
- Early questioning should focus on risk factors and symptoms associated with biliary duct obstruction and hepatocellular disease.

The Most Common Causes of Acute and Subacute Jaundice

Risk factors and symptoms of obstructive etiology

- Older age
- Prior biliary tract surgery
- History of gallstones
- More severe pain
- Weight loss

Risk factors and symptoms of hepatocellular disease

- Viral prodrome (anorexia, malaise, fatigue)
- Risk factors for viral hepatitis: injection drug use, sexual promiscuity, blood transfusion prior to 1990
- Hepatotoxin exposure: alcohol, acetaminophen, new medications or herbal supplements, Amanita mushrooms
- Local outbreak of hepatitis

IDENTIFYING ALARM SYMPTOMS

Jaundice usually indicates a serious illness, although there are a few benign causes (eg, Gilbert syndrome, hematoma). Medical emergencies include ascending cholangitis, fulminant hepatic failure, and severe/massive hemolysis (eg, transfusion reaction, disseminated intravascular coagulation, thrombotic thrombocytopenic purpura, *Clostridium perfringens* sepsis, or falciparum malaria). Painless jaundice classically suggests pancreas or bile duct cancer. The presence of fever or abdominal pain suggests complications from gallstones, sepsis, or acute viral or alcoholic hepatitis. Encephalopathy with jaundice implies either hypotension or fulminant hepatic failure; the latter concern should prompt immediate consideration of liver transplantation.

Serious Diagnoses	Prevalence[a]
Pancreatic or biliary carcinoma	20–35%
Gallstone disease	13%
Alcoholic cirrhosis	10–21%
Sepsis or shock	22%
Drug or toxin-mediated hepatitis (most commonly acetaminophen)	5.8%
Acute viral hepatitis	1.7%
Autoimmune hepatitis	1.7%

[a]Among patients with jaundice.[4,5]

Alarm features	Serious causes	Benign causes
Fever[a]	Cholangitis Gallstone disease Acute hepatitis (viral, toxin/alcohol, medication-induced) Sepsis	
Right upper quadrant pain[a]	Cholangitis Gallstone disease Acute hepatitis Budd-Chiari syndrome Right-sided heart failure	Varicella zoster Right lower lobe pneumonia Right-sided pleural effusion Peptic ulcer disease Atypical renal colic Musculoskeletal pain
Confusion or altered mentation[a]	Cholangitis Hepatic encephalopathy Sepsis Intracranial bleed due to coagulopathy Hypoglycemia Seizure	Delirium of any cause

Gum bleeding or epistaxis	Thrombocytopenia due to fulminant hepatic failure Disseminated intravascular coagulation Thrombotic thrombocytopenic purpura Evans syndrome Falciparum malaria Hypersplenism due to portal hypertension	Minor gum or nasal trauma
Back pain	Acute hemolysis	Musculoskeletal pain
Pregnancy	Hyperemesis gravidarum Acute fatty liver of pregnancy Eclampsia HELLP syndrome Intrahepatic cholestasis of pregnancy	
Dark urine	Hemoglobinuria from acute hemolysis Bilirubinuria (due to any cause of conjugated hyperbilirubinemia) Porphyria (port-wine color or red urine) Myoglobinuria due to rhabdomyolysis Gross hematuria	Dehydration, medications (rifampin—orange urine), beets (red urine)
Involuntary weight loss	Pancreatic or hepatobiliary cancer	

HELLP: hemolysis, elevated liver enzymes, and low platelet count.

[a]**Charcot's triad** refers to jaundice, fever, and right upper quadrant pain, classically associated with cholangitis and present in 22–75% of cases of cholangitis. The addition of altered mentation and hypotension comprise **Reynold's pentad,** a surgical or endoscopic emergency.[6,7]

FOCUSED QUESTIONS

If answered in the affirmative	Think about
Have you had previous biliary surgery?	Retained stones after cholecystectomy Biliary stricture Obstruction from recurrent malignancy
Have you recently ingested any acetaminophen, new medications, herbal supplements, or wild mushrooms?	Fulminant hepatic failure from numerous medications (eg, acetaminophen, isoniazid, anticonvulsants) or Amanita mushrooms

(continued)

If answered in the affirmative	Think about
Do you drink alcohol?	*Acute alcoholic hepatitis, chronic alcoholic cirrhosis, and "therapeutic misadventure"—liver injury at therapeutic doses of acetaminophen in an alcoholic*
Have you ever used injection drugs?	*Hepatitis C: 65% prevalence among injection drug users[8]*
Are you younger than age 20?	*Familial disorders of bilirubin metabolism (Gilbert, Crigler-Najjar, Dubin-Johnson, and Rotor syndromes)*
Are you between the ages of 15 and 40?	*Wilson's disease* *Autoimmune hepatitis (especially in women)* *Primary sclerosing cholangitis (especially in men)*
Are you older than 40?	*Increased risk of primary biliary cirrhosis (especially in women)* *Hemochromatosis* *Cancer of the pancreas or bile ducts*
Have you been recently exposed to anyone with hepatitis?	*Hepatitis A is a common cause of food-borne outbreaks of hepatitis* *Hepatitis B can be transmitted through sexual activity (hepatitis C to a much lesser extent)*
Have you received any blood transfusions?	*Acute transfusion reaction may rarely cause massive hemolysis. Past blood transfusions may increase the risk for hepatitis B and C; this risk is low today, but transfusions prior to 1990 were not routinely tested for hepatitis C*
Does anyone in your family have hepatitis or a history of jaundice?	*Hepatitis B transmitted vertically from mother to child at the time of birth may remain asymptomatic for years; familial causes include hemochromatosis, Wilson's disease; and Gilbert, Crigler-Najjar, Dubin-Johnson, and Rotor syndromes*
Have you become jaundiced with prior illnesses?	*Gilbert syndrome, present in 10% of whites, often coincides with a viral illness*
Are you diabetic?	*Diabetes (and obesity) are risk factors for NAFLD; diabetes may also be a manifestation of hemochromatosis*
Do you have sickle cell disease?	*Sickle cell patients have 2 reasons for jaundice: chronic hemolysis due to sickled hemoglobin, and predisposition to pigment gallstone formation (resulting in biliary colic).*
Do you have a history of ulcerative colitis?	*Primary sclerosing cholangitis develops in 1–4% of patients with ulcerative colitis; whereas 67% of patients with primary sclerosing cholangitis have ulcerative colitis*
Do you have a history of heart failure?	*Decompensated heart failure* *Constrictive pericarditis*
Have you or anyone in your family ever had blood clots?	*Hypercoagulable states may result in Budd-Chiari syndrome*
Time course	***Think about***
Was onset abrupt?	*Choledocholithiasis* *Cholangitis* *Acute hepatitis*

	Acute Budd-Chiari syndrome
	Hemolysis
	Sepsis
Was onset over weeks to months?	*Pancreatic and hepatobiliary cancers*
	Any cause of chronic cirrhosis
	Infiltrative liver disease
	Heart failure
Are episodes recurrent and self-limited?	*Biliary colic and familial disorders of bilirubin metabolism (eg, Gilbert syndrome)*

Associated symptoms

Do you have

Think about

• *Epigastric pain?*	*Pancreatitis*
	Pancreatic cancer
• *Nausea, vomiting?*	*Choledocholithiasis*
	Cholangitis
	Acute hepatitis (viral, toxin/alcohol, medication-induced)
	Budd-Chiari syndrome
	Sepsis
• *Prodrome of malaise, fatigue, anorexia?*	*Viral hepatitis*
	Pancreatic or hepatobiliary cancer
• *Clay-colored stools?*	*Biliary duct obstruction*
• *Silver stool?*	*Cancer at the head of the pancreas causing melena without bile (tumor obstructs bile duct and may bleed into intestinal lumen)*
• *Hematuria or flank pain?*	*Renal cell carcinoma with associated paraneoplastic reversible hepatic dysfunction (Stauffer syndrome)*
• *Increased abdominal girth?*	*Suggests either ascites (due to decompensated chronic liver disease or Budd-Chiari syndrome) or abdominal mass (hepatoma, pancreatic cancer, lymphoma)*
• *Pruritus?*	*Subacute or chronic cholestatic process such as primary biliary cirrhosis, medication injury (estrogens, oral contraceptives, anabolic steroids, erythromycin, parenteral nutrition), benign recurrent intrahepatic cholestasis, intrahepatic cholestasis of pregnancy*
• *Increased or easy bruisability?*	*Coagulopathy due to impaired clotting factor synthesis from cirrhosis*
• *Missed menses?*	*Pregnancy*
• *Arthralgias?*	*Prodrome of viral hepatitis; also seen in hemochromatosis*

Modifying symptoms

| | **Think about** |
| *Worsening coincides with viral illness or reduced oral intake?* | *Gilbert syndrome* |

CAVEATS

- Most patients will not complain of "jaundice" per se but rather of discolored eyes or skin, or of the accompanying symptoms that may be more concerning to the patient.
- Prevalence data must be interpreted with caution: the main outpatient causes of jaundice are biliary obstruction and decompensated alcoholic liver disease. Sepsis and hepatic ischemia emerge as common causes in the inpatient setting.[5] The literature likely underestimates the prevalence of acute and chronic viral hepatitis among etiologies of jaundice.
- Life-threatening causes of jaundice fall under 1 of 2 broad categories: liver injury or biliary tract obstruction. Unfortunately, the history alone is limited in its ability to reliably discriminate between the two, and combined history and physical are only 80% accurate.[9] Depending on the urgency of the situation, physical examination, laboratory evaluation, and often abdominal imaging may be needed to arrive at an accurate diagnosis.
- A complete ingestion history is vital, including acetaminophen and other medications, toxins (eg, alcohol), foods (eg, *Amanita* mushrooms), and herbal remedies. Even medications taken at therapeutic doses can result in fulminant hepatic failure. Combinations of medications or hepatotoxins can provoke a toxic reaction at lower doses, such as seen with concomitant alcoholic liver disease and acetaminophen use.

PROGNOSIS

The mortality rate among hospitalized patients with jaundice was 32% in 1 study[5] but varied by underlying cause. Highest mortality rates were seen with sepsis or hypotensive liver injury, followed closely by malignancy and cirrhosis; whereas gallstone disease had a more favorable prognosis. Fulminant hepatic failure of any cause warrants immediate evaluation for liver transplantation.

Pancreatic cancer has a dismal overall prognosis, with 5-year survival rates between 2% and 5%. Select patients with smaller tumors involving the pancreas head may reach survival rates of 20–40%.[1]

Among patients infected with hepatitis C virus, chronic disease will develop in 80% and 20% will progress to cirrhosis over 20 years. For an immunocompetent adult infected with hepatitis B, chronic infection will develop in less than 5%. Only the small subset of chronically infected hepatitis B patients with actively replicating virus is at risk for progressing to cirrhosis. Once hepatitis B or C results in cirrhosis, the annual risk of developing hepatocellular carcinoma is 3–5%.[1]

REFERENCES

1. Friedman LS. Liver, biliary tract, & pancreas. In: Tierney Jr., LM, McPhee SJ, Papadakis MA (editors). *Current Medical Diagnosis and Treatment,* 43rd ed. McGraw Hill; 2004:656–697.

2. Lidofsky SD. Jaundice. In: Feldman M, Friedman LS, Sleisenger MS (editors). *Sleisenger & Fordtran's Gastrointestinal and Liver Disease: Pathophysiology/Diagnosis/Management,* 7th ed, volume1. WB Saunders; 2002:249–262.

3. Chowdhury NR, Chowdhury JR. Diagnostic approach to the patient with jaundice or asymptomatic hyperbilirubinemia. UpToDate,Version 11.3, 2004; accessed February 2, 2004. Topic last changed 10/22/1999.

4. Reisman Y, Gips CH, Lavelle SM, Wilson JH. Clinical presentation of (subclinical) jaundice—the Euricterus Project in The Netherlands. United Dutch Hospitals and Euricterus Project Management Group. *Hepatogastroenterology.* 1996;43: 1190–1195.

5. Whitehead MW, Kingham JGC. The causes of obvious jaundice in South West Wales: perceptions versus reality. *Gut.* 2001; 48:409–413.

6. Csendes A, Diaz JC, Burdiles P, et al. Risk factors and classification of acute suppurative cholangitis. *Br J Surg.* 1992; 79:655–658.

7. Saik RP, Greenburg AG, Farris JM, Peskin GW. Spectrum of cholangitis. *Am J Surg.* 1975;130:143–150.

8. Garfein RS, Vlahov D, Galai N, et al. Viral infections in short-term injection drug users: the prevalence of the hepatitis C, hepatitis B, human immunodeficiency, and human T-lymphotropic viruses. *Am J Public Health.* 1996;86:655–661.

9. Reisman Y, van Dam GM, Gips CH, et al. Physicians' working diagnosis compared to the Eiricterus Real Life Date Diagnostic Tool in three jaundice databases: Euricterus Dutch, independent prospective, and independent retrospective. *Hepatogastroenterology.* 1997;44:1367–1375.

SUGGESTED READING

O'Grady JG, Alexander GJM, Hayllar KM, Williams R. Early indicators of prognosis in fulminant hepatic failure. *Gastroenterology.* 1989;97:439–445.

Causes of Jaundice Based on Mechanism of Bilirubin Accumulation

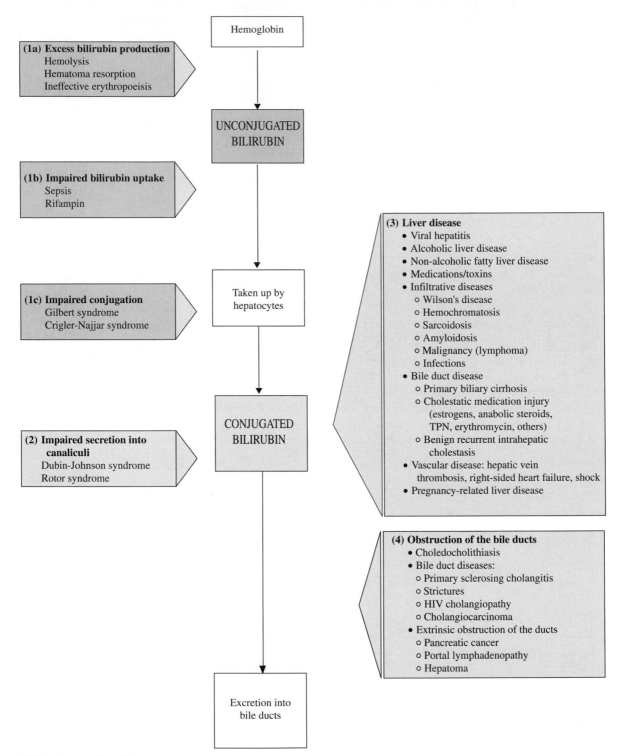

Hemoglobin

(1a) Excess bilirubin production
Hemolysis
Hematoma resorption
Ineffective erythropoeisis

UNCONJUGATED BILIRUBIN

(1b) Impaired bilirubin uptake
Sepsis
Rifampin

Taken up by hepatocytes

(1c) Impaired conjugation
Gilbert syndrome
Crigler-Najjar syndrome

(3) Liver disease
- Viral hepatitis
- Alcoholic liver disease
- Non-alcoholic fatty liver disease
- Medications/toxins
- Infiltrative diseases
  - Wilson's disease
  - Hemochromatosis
  - Sarcoidosis
  - Amyloidosis
  - Malignancy (lymphoma)
  - Infections
- Bile duct disease
  - Primary biliary cirrhosis
  - Cholestatic medication injury
    (estrogens, anabolic steroids,
    TPN, erythromycin, others)
  - Benign recurrent intrahepatic
    cholestasis
- Vascular disease: hepatic vein
  thrombosis, right-sided heart failure, shock
- Pregnancy-related liver disease

(2) Impaired secretion into canaliculi
Dubin-Johnson syndrome
Rotor syndrome

CONJUGATED BILIRUBIN

(4) Obstruction of the bile ducts
- Choledocholithiasis
- Bile duct diseases:
  - Primary sclerosing cholangitis
  - Strictures
  - HIV cholangiopathy
  - Cholangiocarcinoma
- Extrinsic obstruction of the ducts
  - Pancreatic cancer
  - Portal lymphadenopathy
  - Hepatoma

Excretion into bile ducts

TPN, total parental nutrition.

Key: Darker shading reflects predominantly unconjugated hyperbilirubinemia; lighter shading indicates conjugated hyperbilirubinemia.

Diagnostic Approach: Jaundice

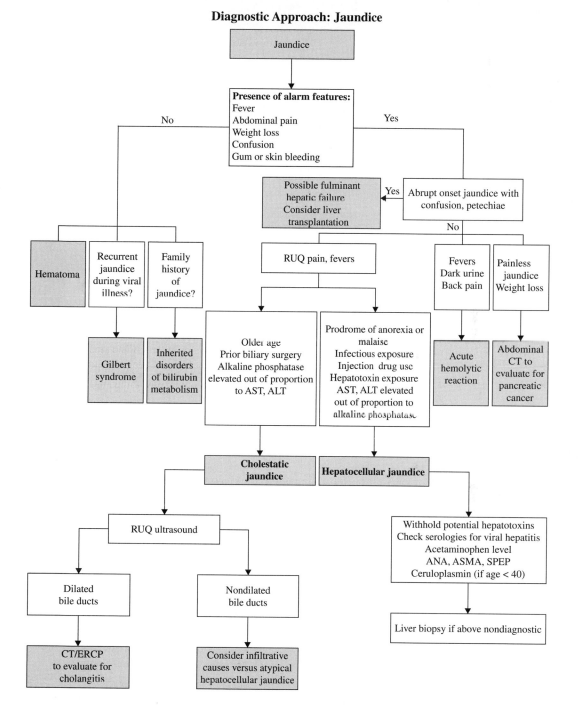

RUQ, right upper quandrant; AST, aspartate aminotransferase; ALT, alanine aminotransferase; CT, computed tomography; ERCP, endoscopic retrograde cholangiopancreatography; ANA, antinuclear anitbody; ASMA, anti-smooth muscle antibody; SPEP, serum protein electrophosresis.

Nausea and Vomiting

35

Randall E. Lee, MD

Nausea and vomiting are symptoms experienced by both the young and the elderly. While they are often manifestations of minor self-limited illnesses, these symptoms may also be harbingers of life-threatening disease. Nausea and vomiting cause significant worldwide reductions in worker productivity and increases in healthcare costs, particularly among pregnant women, patients who are receiving cancer chemotherapy, and those who are recovering from surgery. Nausea frequently, but not always, is associated with vomiting.[1]

KEY TERMS[1]

Chronic nausea and vomiting	*The persistence of the symptoms for more than 1 month.*
Early satiety	*The sensation of feeling full after eating an unusually small amount of food.*
Nausea	*The unpleasant sensation of the imminent need to vomit that may or may not ultimately lead to the act of vomiting.*
Post-chemotherapy nausea and vomiting (PCNV)	*3 types: acute, within 24 hours; delayed, more than 24 hours later; and anticipatory, just before the next chemotherapy dose.*
Recurrent vomiting	*3 or more episodes*
Regurgitation	*The passive retrograde flow of esophageal contents into the mouth without the muscular activity associated with vomiting, and without antecedent nausea.*
Retching	*The "dry heaves." Spasmodic respiratory movements against a closed glottis with contractions of the abdominal musculature without expulsion of any gastric contents. Retching often immediately precedes vomiting.*
Rumination	*Chewing and swallowing of regurgitated food that has come back into the mouth through a voluntary increase in intraabdominal pressure within minutes of eating or during eating.*
Vomiting	*The forceful oral expulsion of gastric contents associated with contraction of the abdominal and chest wall musculature.*

ETIOLOGY

The initial differential diagnosis of nausea and vomiting is broad but may be narrowed significantly by the clinical context.

The evaluation of an infant or young child who has acute vomiting merits special consideration. For instance, the possibility of a toxic ingestion is much more likely in a child than an adult. Despite a declining incidence, Reye's syndrome remains a consideration in an acutely vomiting child who has had a viral infection.

Similarly, the differential diagnosis for a recurrently vomiting infant or young child should be expanded to include congenital abnormalities (eg, malrotation, pyloric stenosis, and esophageal atresia), inherited metabolic disorders (eg, urea cycle enzyme deficiencies), and neurogastrointestinal disorders (eg, cyclic vomiting syndrome). Remember, what is reported as vomiting may simply be regurgitation due to physiologic gastroesophageal reflux.

Differential Diagnosis	Percentage of patients with specific diagnosis who have nausea and vomiting[a]
Acute nausea and vomiting	
Gastrointestinal infections and toxins (gastroenteritis, hepatitis, food poisoning)	
Medications (chemotherapeutics, antibiotics, analgesics, etc.)	Cancer patients receiving narcotics for pain control: 40–70%[1] Patients receiving cisplatinum chemotherapy: 90%[1] Post–general anesthesia: 37% nausea, 23% vomiting[1]
Visceral pain (pancreatitis, appendicitis, biliary colic, acute small bowel obstruction, renal colic, intestinal ischemia, myocardial infarction)	
Conditions affecting central nervous system (CNS) (eg, labyrinthitis, motion/space sickness, head trauma, stroke, Reye's syndrome, meningitis, increased intracranial pressure)	Skull fracture: 28% adults, 33% children[2]
Metabolic (pregnancy, ketoacidosis, uremia)	First trimester of pregnancy: 70%[1]
Radiation	Radiation therapy to abdomen: 80%[1]
Chronic nausea and vomiting	
Gastric (mechanical obstruction or functional dysmotility, ie, gastroparesis, dyspepsia)	
Small intestinal dysmotility (pseudo-obstruction, scleroderma)	
Metabolic (pregnancy, hyperthyroidism, adrenal insufficiency)	
CNS (increased intracranial pressure due to tumor, pseudotumor cerebri)	
Psychogenic (eating disorder)	
Cyclic vomiting syndrome	

[a]Prevalence is unknown when not indicated.

GETTING STARTED

- The approach to a patient with nausea and vomiting begins by clearly defining the symptoms and characterizing their duration, severity, and associated factors.

- Assess the patient for alarm symptoms that require immediate intervention.
- Distinguish between acute and chronic symptoms to narrow the broad differential diagnosis.
- Finally, ask focused questions to further refine the differential diagnosis.

Open-ended questions

Tell me about your nausea and vomiting.

Tell me about the first time this happened.

What do you think is the cause of your nausea and vomiting?

Think about your most recent episode of nausea and vomiting. What did you do that day, starting from when you woke up in the morning?

Tips for effective interviewing

- *Allow the patient to tell the story without interruption.*
- *When the patient pauses, prompt for more information by asking "what else?"*

INTERVIEW FRAMEWORK

- Define the patient's symptoms based upon the above definitions or key terms. For instance, is the patient truly experiencing vomiting, or is it regurgitation?
- Assess the patient for alarm symptoms.
- Determine the following symptom characteristics:
  –Duration of the nausea and vomiting (acute or chronic?)
  –Frequency of the symptoms
  –Severity of the nausea and vomiting
  –Relationship of the vomiting to meals and medications
  –Quality and quantity of vomitus
- Determine associated symptoms.
- Determine modifying symptoms.

IDENTIFYING ALARM SYMPTOMS

Serious Diagnoses	Prevalence[a]
Hyperemesis gravidarum	*0.3–1.0%[3]*
Acute fatty liver of pregnancy (AFLP)	*0.008%[3]*
HELLP syndrome (hemolytic anemia, elevated liver enzymes, low platelet count)	*0.1% in pregnant women (4–12% of women with preeclampsia)[3]*
Intra-abdominal emergency (obstruction, perforation, peritonitis)	
Acute myocardial infarction	
CNS disorder (skull fracture, infection, increased intracranial pressure, bleed)	
Toxic ingestion	
Upper gastrointestinal bleeding	

[a]Prevalence is unknown when not indicated.

Alarm symptoms	Serious causes	Likelihood ratio (LR+)	Benign causes
Large volume hematemesis (grossly bloody or black, like coffee-grounds)	Major upper gastrointestinal bleeding from peptic ulcer, varices, or Mallory-Weiss tear		
History of head trauma	Skull fracture	Adult, LR+ 4.17 Child, LR+ 2.82[2]	
Headache	Intracranial bleed, mass, or infection	Jolt accentuation of headache LR+ 2.4 for meningitis[4]	Migraine headache
Neck stiffness	Meningitis		
Altered mental state	Intracranial bleed, mass or infection		
Right lower quadrant pain	Acute appendicitis	LR+ 8.0[5]	
Migration of periumbilical pain to right lower quadrant	Acute appendicitis	LR+ 3.1[5]	
Abdominal pain before vomiting	Acute appendicitis	LR+ 2.76[5]	
Abdominal pain that worsens with jolting movements, such as going down stairs (peritoneal pain)	Peritonitis		
Upper abdominal pain: steady pain > 30 minutes (biliary colic)	Acute cholecystitis		
Acute chest pain	Acute myocardial infarction	Pain radiation to left arm LR+ 2.3 Pain radiation to both left and right arms LR+ 7.1[6]	Gastroesophageal reflux disease
Postural symptoms, lethargy, unable to retain oral liquids for > 8 hours in a child (12 hours in an adult)	Hypovolemia and/or electrolyte imbalances requiring immediate treatment		

FOCUSED QUESTIONS

Questions	Think about
Do you also have diarrhea? Do others in your community (family, day care, cruise ship, summer camp) also have vomiting and diarrhea?	Viral gastroenteritis Food poisoning
Do you have any symptoms of pregnancy: late menstrual period; breast swelling, tingling, or tenderness?	Early pregnancy (LR + 2.70)[7]
Are you pregnant (first trimester)?	Hyperemesis gravidarum
Are you pregnant (second or third trimester)?	AFLP or HELLP syndrome
Does the room feel like it is moving? (vertigo)	Labyrinthitis (see Chapter 6)
Have you been receiving chemotherapy for cancer?	PCNV
Has your weight gone up and down (30–40 lbs) this past year? Do you always vomit into the toilet, never on the floor or in public? Do you make yourself vomit?	Eating disorder[8] (see Chapter 15)
Do you have a history of kidney disease or failure?	Uremia
Do you have a history of peptic ulcer? Do you feel full after eating just a small amount of food (early satiety)?	Gastric outlet obstruction
Do you have a history of heart disease?	Acute myocardial infarction, digoxin toxicity
Have you had previous abdominal surgery?	Intestinal obstruction due to adhesions
Is anyone else who ate or drank the same thing also having nausea and vomiting?	Food poisoning
Did the symptoms occur within a few hours after eating or drinking something?	Food poisoning due to Staphylococcus aureus or Bacillus cereus toxin
Did you drink liquids that were stored in a metal container? Do you also have a metallic taste?	Heavy metal ingestion (zinc, copper, tin, iron, cadmium)
Did you eat raw fish?	Anisakiasis
Did you eat home canned or preserved food?	Botulism[9]
Did the bumps in the car ride make your abdominal pain worse?	Peritonitis
Do you have diabetes?	Diabetic ketoacidosis or gastroparesis
Does the child's ear hurt? Is the child rubbing or pulling on the ear?	Acute otitis media LR+ 3 to 7.3[10] (see Chapter 16)
Did the child recently have the flu or a cold? Did the child receive aspirin?	Reye's syndrome

Quality	*Think about*
Is the vomitus grossly bloody?	Peptic ulcer Esophageal varices Mallory-Weiss tear
Does the vomitus contain partially digested food?	Gastroparesis Gastric outlet obstruction

(continued)

Quality	**Think about**
Is the vomitus bilious (containing green bile)?	Small bowel obstruction
Is it feculent?	Bowel obstruction
Does it contain undigested food regurgitated (not truly vomited)?	Achalasia
	Zenker diverticulum
	Esophageal stenosis
Do you have nausea without vomiting?	Pregnancy
Is it projectile?	Pyloric stenosis
	Increased intracranial pressure

Time course	**Think about**
Do you vomit	
• In the morning before breakfast?	Pregnancy
	Increased intracranial pressure
• ≥ 1 hour after eating?	Gastroparesis
	Gastric outlet obstruction
• During or soon after a meal?	Gastric ulcer
	Eating disorder
• Soon after taking medications?	Medication side-effect
• Recurrent, but intermittent pattern	Cyclic vomiting syndrome

Associated symptoms	**Think about**
Do you have	
• Diarrhea, headache, myalgia, fever?	Viral gastroenteritis
• Headache, neck stiffness, altered mentation, photophobia?	Meningitis
• Low weight, weight loss?	Eating disorder
	Gastrointestinal malignancy
• Lack of concern regarding weight loss or vomiting?	Eating disorder
• Jaundice, dark urine, light stools?	Hepatitis
	Choledocholithiasis
• Chest pain, cold sweats (diaphoresis)?	Myocardial infarction
• Crampy, colicky abdominal pain?	Bowel obstruction
• Upper abdominal pain (biliary colic)?	Cholecystitis
• Epigastric abdominal pain radiating to the back?	Pancreatitis
• Abdominal pain that worsens with jolting movements?	Bowel perforation
	Peritonitis
• Migraine headaches?	Cyclic vomiting syndrome
• Vertigo?	Labyrinthitis

Modifying symptoms	**Think about**
Do you get sick	
• Only as a passenger in a vehicle?	Motion sickness/sea sickness/space sickness
• Only during periods of stress?	Psychogenic

DIAGNOSTIC APPROACH

The diagnostic approach to the patient with nausea and vomiting has 2 basic goals: (1) determine the need for immediate intervention, and (2) identify the specific cause of the symptoms. The comprehensive history and subsequent physical examination directs the selection of diagnostic tests such as esophagogastroduodenoscopy, computed tomography scans, abdominal ultrasonography, and barium radiographs.

CAVEATS

- By itself, a clinical history of nausea and vomiting has only 30% sensitivity and 60% specificity for the diagnosis of acute meningitis in adults.[4]
- No single clinical finding has sufficient diagnostic power to establish or exclude a diagnosis of acute cholecystitis in a patient with upper abdominal pain without further testing, such as abdominal ultrasonography.[11]

PROGNOSIS

The prognosis depends on the underlying cause of the nausea and vomiting. In general, a careful history and physical examination readily yields the etiology and subsequent therapy of acute nausea and vomiting. In contrast, the cause of chronic nausea and vomiting may be more elusive, and the management of chronic symptoms more challenging.

REFERENCES

1. American Gastroenterological Association Clinical Practice and Practice Economics Committee. AGA Technical Review on Nausea and Vomiting. *Gastroenterology.* 2001;120:263–286.
2. Nee PA, Hadfield JM, Yates DW, Faragher EB. Significance of vomiting after head injury. *J Neurol Neurosurg Psychiatry.* 1999;66:470–473.
3. Knox T, Olans L. Liver disease in pregnancy. *N Engl J Med.* 1996;335:569–576.
4. Attia J, Hatala R, Cook DJ, Wong JG. The rational clinical examination. Does this adult patient have acute meningitis? *JAMA.* 1999;282:175–181.
5. Wagner J, McKinney W, Carpenter J. The rational clinical examination. Does this patient have appendicitis? *JAMA.* 1996;276:1589–1594.
6. Panju A, Hemmelgarn B, Guyatt G, Simel D. The rational clinical examination. Is this patient having a myocardial infarction? *JAMA.* 1998;280:1256–1263.
7. Bastian L, Piscitelli J. The rational clinical examination. Is this patient pregnant? *JAMA.* 1997;278:586–591.
8. Woodside DB. Eating disorders. *Clin Perspect Gastroenterol.* 2001;4:333–339.
9. Bishai W, Sears C. Food poisoning syndromes. *Gastroenterol Clin North Am.* 1993;22:579–608.
10. Rothman R, Owens T, Simel D. The rational clinical examination. Does this child have acute otitis media? *JAMA.* 2003;290:1633–1640.
11. Trowbridge R, Rutkowski N, Shojania K. The rational clinical examination. Does this patient have acute cholecystitis? *JAMA.* 2003;289:80–86.

SUGGESTED READING

American Gastroenterological Association Clinical Practice and Practice Economics Committee. American Gastroenterological Association Medical Position Statement: Nausea and Vomiting. *Gastroenterology.* 2001;120:261–262.

Lee M. Nausea and Vomiting. In: Feldman M, Friedman L, Sleisenger M ed. *Gastrointestinal and Liver Disease,* 7th ed. 2002: 119–130.

Li B, Misiewicz L. Cyclic vomiting syndrome: a brain-gut disorder. *Gastroenterol Clin North Am.* 2003;32:997–1019.

Diagnostic Approach: Nausea and Vomiting

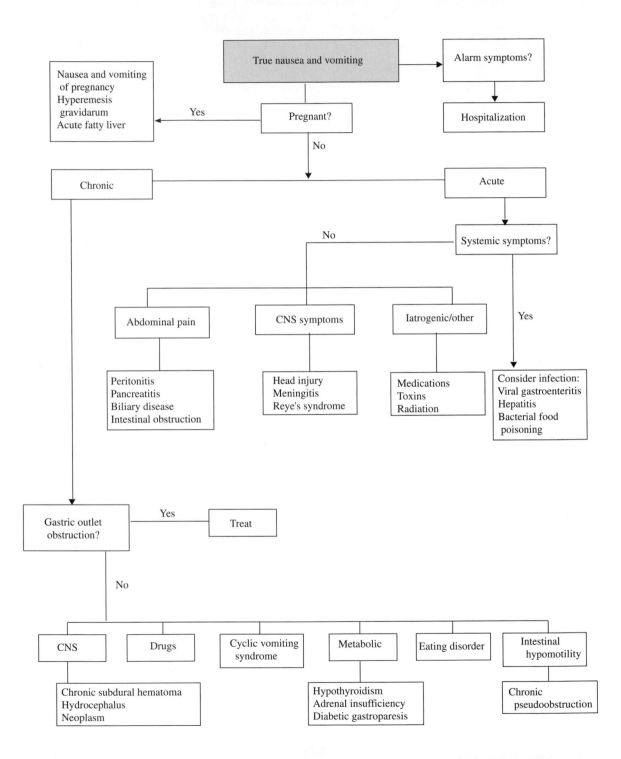

Anorectal Pain

36

David S. Fefferman, MD, & Ciaran P. Kelly, MD

Symptoms of anorectal disease are common. However, due to the reluctance of both patients and clinicians to discuss these symptoms in detail, problems may be attributed hastily to internal hemorrhoids and not investigated adequately. In many cases, a thorough history will point to a specific diagnosis, or at least help target the physical examination and indicate the appropriate special tests. No matter how clear the history seems to be, a perianal inspection and digital anorectal examination is mandatory unless the anal canal is too tender or too stenotic to allow a digital examination. Anoscopy is an important adjunct to the physical examination in patients with anorectal symptoms. Through the combination of a detailed history, physical examination, and anoscopy, further or more invasive diagnostic testing may become unnecessary.

KEY TERMS

Anal fissure	A cut or tear of the anal mucosa.
Coccydynia	Referred pain from injured, inflamed, or hypersensitive coccyx.
Defecatory dysfunction or anismus	Dysfunction, weakness, or faulty coordination of the muscles that effect defecation.
Fecal impaction	Obstruction of the anal outlet with stool.
Fistula	Abnormal tunnel of infection or inflammation into the perianal skin, usually originating from an anal gland.
Foreign body	An item placed within the rectum for therapeutic or recreational purposes can cause rectal irritation, obstruction (if retained), or trauma including tearing of the anal mucosa and a painful anal fissure.
Hemorrhoid	Dilation of the superior or inferior hemorrhoidal venous plexus (cushions) resulting in internal or external hemorrhoids, respectively.
Levator ani syndrome	Idiopathic dull ache possibly resulting from dysmotility of the muscles supporting the anus.
Perianal abscess	Collection of infection within or adjacent to the perianal space.
Proctalgia fugax	Idiopathic recurrent sharp pain lasting seconds that is unrelated to bowel movements.
Proctitis	Inflammation, infection, or ischemia of the rectum.
Prostatitis	Infection or inflammation of prostate gland.
Pruritus ani	This is not an etiology of anorectal pain but rather a symptom of itching in the skin of the anal canal or perianal region. It has a variety of causes including many of those listed above in addition to local irrita-

(continued)

KEY TERMS

tion of the perianal skin from fecal soilage, infection (bacterial, fungal, viral, parasitic), inflammation, and dermatologic abnormalities. It may also be idiopathic.

Sacral nerve compression   *Referred pain from compression or inflammation of sacral nerve.*

ETIOLOGY

The pathophysiology of pain from the anorectum varies greatly depending on the disorder. However, useful groupings include: local causes, referred causes, and functional disorders (for which no known pathophysiologic mechanism has been demonstrated). Because of the varied mechanisms, it is difficult by history alone, to differentiate between them without performing a physical examination. Basic knowledge of the different innervations of the anal mucosa and rectal mucosa, which are separated anatomically by the dentate line, may help localize the lesion. The anal mucosa is innervated by pain sensory nerve fibers which, when irritated or inflamed, produce sharp well-localized symptoms. Conversely, lesions of the rectum, which contain only stretch fibers, result in poorly localized pressure sensations.

Differential Diagnosis

There have been no published studies summarizing the prevalence of disease or predictive value of symptoms in patients presenting with anorectal pain. Population surveys have found that 80% of people with anorectal symptoms do not seek medical attention.[1] Since many symptoms are falsely attributed to hemorrhoids, the relative prevalence of other anorectal disorders may be underestimated. The relative prevalence of the different etiologies for anorectal pain in the general population are outlined below. Although anal or rectal carcinoma presenting with anorectal pain is quite rare, this serious diagnosis should be considered in every patient.

Local causes	*Frequency*
Anal fissure	*Very common*
Thrombosed external hemorrhoid	*Very common*
Perianal abscess	*Common*
Thrombosed/prolapsed internal hemorrhoid	*Common*
Defecatory dysfunction or anismus	*Common*
Fistula	*Infrequent*
Proctitis	*Infrequent*
Fecal impaction	*Infrequent*
Anal or rectal neoplasm (benign or malignant tumors of the anal canal or rectum)	*Rare*
Referred pain	*Frequency*
Coccydynia	*Rare*
Sacral nerve compression	*Rare*
Prostatitis	*Rare*
Uterine disease	*Rare*

• Referred pain from inflamed or enlarged uterus
• Direct compression or invasion of rectum

Pelvic inflammatory disease	Rare
Referred pain from inflamed reproductive organs	
Functional syndromes	**Frequency**
Proctalgia fugax	Common
Levator ani syndrome	Rare

GETTING STARTED

Ask open-ended questions initially. Determine the onset of symptoms, frequency, and association with bowel movements. Obtain a detailed history of bowel movements including frequency, consistency, urgency, episodes of fecal incontinence, the presence of blood in the stool, bleeding after defecation, or the presence of a palpable swelling in the anal area during or after defecation. Next, ask targeted follow-up questions to obtain a complete and detailed history. Obtaining a past medical history, including complete surgical and gynecologic histories, is imperative. Assess the family history specifically for gastrointestinal malignancies and inflammatory bowel disease (IBD). Inquire about medication use including the use of enemas or suppositories. Ask specifically about anal instrumentation or trauma (including the insertion of digits or participation in receptive anal intercourse) that is temporally related to the onset or alteration of anorectal symptoms.

Questions	**Remember**
Tell me about the symptoms you are experiencing.	• *Let patients use their own words*
What were the events surrounding the first time you experienced the symptoms?	• *Refrain from using the word pain; the patient may be experiencing other sensations, such as a dull ache, a poorly defined sense of discomfort, or even pruritus.*
Under what circumstances do your symptoms typically occur?	
What do you think may be causing your symptoms?	

INTERVIEW FRAMEWORK

Characterize the type, onset, duration, frequency, and severity of pain or discomfort.
Assess for the following:

- The temporal association of symptoms with bowel movements.
- The presence of blood with or after bowel movements.
- The presence or absence of a palpable mass, lump, or bulge.
- If a palpable mass, lump, or bulge is present, determine whether it develops only when straining during defecation and resolves spontaneously or following manual reduction.
- The presence of alarm symptoms.

IDENTIFYING ALARM SYMPTOMS

Although a rare cause of anorectal pain, neoplasia should be considered in every patient. Even though a change in bowel habits, presence of blood in the stool or constitutional symptoms (weight loss, fatigue, fever) may be attributed to benign conditions, they should trigger a suspicion for a more serious process that may warrant colonoscopic and/or radiologic evaluation. Similarly, acute onset of pain with fever or abdominal pain and tenderness, especially with a history of IBD, should raise concern for serious inflammatory or infectious conditions including intra-abdominal or perirectal abscess.

Serious Diagnoses

- Anorectal cancer
- Perirectal or pelvic abscess
- Intraperitoneal infection
- IBD

Alarm symptoms	Serious causes	Benign causes
Weight loss, fatigue	Cancer Infection IBD	
Chronic anemia	Cancer IBD Infection	
Blood in the stool	Cancer IBD Infection	Hemorrhoidal bleeding Anal fissure
Dark blood or blood mixed in with the stool	Suggests a bleeding source more proximal than the anorectum	
Fevers	Infection IBD Cancer	
Abdominal pain	Abscess Infection IBD	Fecal obstruction Levator ani syndrome Coccydynia Uterine disease
Gradual increase in pain over days	Abscess	Fecal obstruction
Loss of sensation or muscle weakness	Neoplasm or infection affecting the spinal cord, nerve roots, or peripheral nerves	
Change in bowel habits in patients older than 50 years	Colon cancer	

FOCUSED QUESTIONS

Pain related to bowel movements	Possible etiology
Was the onset of pain associated with moving your bowels?	Anal fissure Thrombosed or prolapsed internal hemorrhoid
Did sharp pain develop with the passage of a large hard bowel movement?	Anal fissure
With the passage of stool, does the pain feel like being cut by glass?	Anal fissure
With the passage of stool, is there painful passage or scant amounts of red blood on the toilet paper?	Anal fissure

Did a dull pain or sensation of rectal fullness start after prolonged straining?	Thrombosed or prolapsed internal hemorrhoid Rectal prolapse
Was there a sudden onset of severe sharp pain associated with the development of a tender perianal swelling?	Thrombosed external hemorrhoid
Is there a sensation of rectal pressure with a recurrent urge to defecate and passage of small amounts of feces or mucus?	Proctitis

Pain not related to bowel movements

Possible etiology

Is there pain regardless of bowel movements with a full, tender area lateral to the anus or on the buttock?	Perianal abscess or fistula
Is there pain regardless of bowel movement with a small amount of bloody or purulent discharge from an area lateral to the anus?	Perianal fistula
Is the pain associated with the onset of vesicles, blisters, or ulcerations in the perianal region?	Perianal infection (herpes simplex virus [HSV], chancroid) or inflammation
Are the symptoms temporally related to the onset of menses?	Endometriosis
Is there deep pelvic pain with intercourse?	Endometriosis Pelvic inflammatory disease Uterine pathology
Does the pain come on suddenly, lasting only seconds to minutes?	Proctalgia fugax
Does the pain come on episodically at night?	Proctalgia fugax
Did the pain start after a fall or other trauma to the tailbone?	Coccydynia
Is there tenderness of the sacrum or coccyx?	Coccydynia
Is the pain made worse by movement of the legs or back?	Sacral nerve lesion

Pain characteristics

Possible etiology

Is the pain sharp? *Does it localize to the anal canal (below the dentate line on the anal mucosa)?*	Anal fissure Thrombosed external hemorrhoid Perirectal abscess or fistula
Is the pain dull? *Is the pain poorly localized inside the rectum (above the dentate line on the rectal mucosa)?*	Proctitis Fecal impaction Defecatory dysfunction Thrombosed/prolapsed internal hemorrhoid Prostatitis Uterine disease Rectal cancer Referred pain

(continued)

Pain characteristics	**Possible etiology**
Was the pain mild initially but then gradually increased in intensity over several days?	Perianal infection or abscess Obstruction

Associated symptoms and history	**Possible etiology**
Do you painlessly pass drips of blood into the toilet after a bowel movement?	Bleeding from internal hemorrhoid
Does rectal bleeding occur with the onset of menses?	Colonic endometriosis
Does purulent material drain from an area adjacent to the anus?	Perianal fistula
Is there a lump, bulge, or a mass?	Thrombosed external hemorrhoid Prolapsed internal hemorrhoid Rectal prolapse Infection IBD Cancer
Did a new tender perianal lump develop suddenly with the onset of pain?	Thrombosed external hemorrhoid
Is there a soft painless lump that develops while straining at stool and is reducible?	Prolapsed internal hemorrhoid Rectal prolapse
Is there a soft painless lump that develops while straining during defecation, is reducible, and at times drips bright red blood?	Prolapsed, bleeding internal hemorrhoid
Is there a history of constipation or difficulty passing a bowel movement?	Anal fissure Internal hemorrhoid Fecal impaction Trauma during attempted digital disimpaction or administration of an enema
Is there a history of recent anorectal instrumentation or receptive anal intercourse?	Anorectal trauma Infection Retained foreign body
Personal history or family history of colon carcinoma of early onset (age younger than 50 years)	Colonic neoplasia
Is there a personal or family history of IBD?	Ulcerative colitis Ulcerative proctitis Crohn's proctocolitis or perianal Crohn's disease
Are there vesicles, blisters, or ulcerations in the perianal region?	Perianal infection (HSV, chancroid) or inflammation

CAVEATS

- Anorectal pain is common and often caused by anal fissures, thrombosed external hemorrhoids and perirectal abscesses. Despite a clear history suggesting a benign cause and the rarity of anorectal cancers presenting with pain, cancer must be considered in every patient, especially the elderly.

- Due to the reluctance of both patients and clinicians to discuss anorectal symptoms and function in detail, problems may be hastily attributed to hemorrhoids and not investigated adequately.
- Every patient should be screened with a thorough history, review of symptoms, and physical examination including perianal and digital rectal examinations. When applicable, anoscopy should also be performed. A detailed history and examination will frequently lead to a specific clinical diagnosis. In a young patient without alarm symptoms and no risk factors for infectious or neoplastic disease, an initial management plan can be instituted without further testing. However, further investigations such as stool testing, colonoscopy, or abdominal imaging are indicated in patients of advanced age and in those with alarm symptoms or evident risk factors for infection or neoplasia.
- When obtaining a history ask the patient exactly what they mean by pain in the rectal area because the patient may be experiencing a different sensation, such as a dull ache, a poorly defined sense of discomfort, rectal fullness, tenesmus or even pruritus.
- Sharp, well-localized anorectal pain usually originates in the anal canal.
- Diffuse, poorly localized anorectal discomfort often originates in the rectum or is referred from other structures.
- An anal fissure usually presents with the sudden onset of anal pain while passing a hard bowel movement and is often associated with sharp pain (cutting like glass) and bleeding with subsequent bowel movements.
- A thrombosed external hemorrhoid presents with the sudden onset of severe perianal pain associated with the development of a tender perianal swelling.
- Proctalgia fugax is characterized by recurrent brief episodes of rectal pain without other significant symptoms or signs.
- Coccydynia frequently follows a fall or other trauma and is associated with tenderness of the coccyx.
- No matter how clear the diagnosis seems to be by history, a perianal inspection and digital anorectal examination is mandatory unless the anal canal is too tender or too stenotic.

REFERENCES

1. Nelson RL, Abcarian H, Davis FG, Persky V. Prevalence of benign anorectal disease in a randomly selected population. *Dis Colon Rectum.* 1995;38:341–344.

SUGGESTED READING

Gopal DV. Diseases of the rectum and anus: a clinical approach to common disorders. *Clin Cornerstone.* 2002;4:34–48.

Hull T. Examination and Diseases of the Anorectum. In: Feldman M, Friedman LS, Sleisenger MH, editors. *Sleisenger & Fordtran's Gastrointestinal and Liver Disease,* 7th ed. WB Saunders Co; 2002:2277–2293.

Pfenninger JL, Zainea GG. Common anorectal conditions: Part I. Symptoms and complaints. *Am Fam Physician.* 2001;15;63:2391–2398.

Pfenninger JL, Zainea GG. Common anorectal conditions: Part II. Lesions. *Am Fam Physician.* 2001;64:77–88.

Diagnostic Approach: Anorectal Pain with Defecation

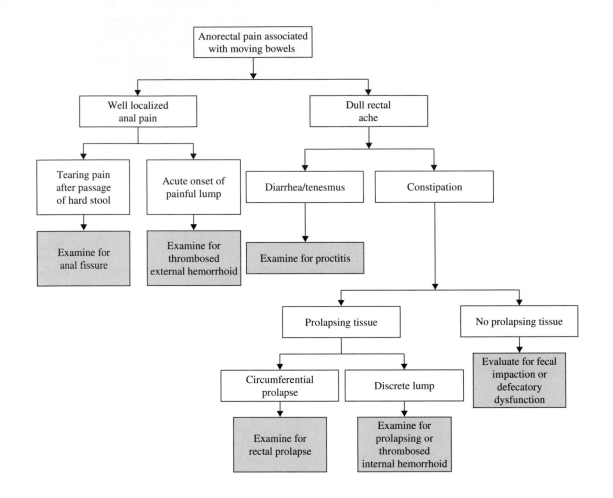

Diagnostic Approach: Anorectal Pain without Defecation

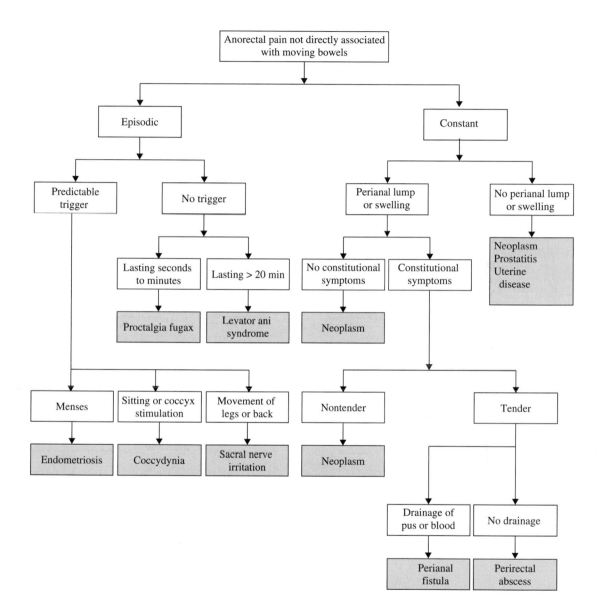

SECTION VIII
Genitourinary System

Dysuria

Paul L. Fine, MD, & Sanjay Saint, MD, MPH

Dysuria is defined as pain, burning, or discomfort experienced during or immediately after urination. Though it has a broad differential diagnosis, dysuria most often results from inflammation or infection of the bladder and/or the urethra.[1]

KEY TERMS

Frequency	*Voiding at abnormally brief intervals.*
Urgency	*An intensely exaggerated sense of needing to urinate immediately.*
Urinary tract infection (UTI)	*An infection of the urethra, bladder, prostate, or kidney. Lower UTI implies infection of the bladder (ie, cystitis). Upper UTI usually indicates infection of the kidney (ie, pyelonephritis).*

ETIOLOGY

Infection of the urinary tract (including the urethra, bladder, or prostate) is by far the most common cause of dysuria; data concerning the relative prevalence of other causes of dysuria have not been published. Women are affected much more often than men; almost 25% of adult women experience an acute episode of dysuria each year.[2] The complaint is more common in younger, sexually active women. Among men, the incidence of UTI increases with age.[1] In women with dysuria and vaginal discharge, vulvovaginitis is much more common than a UTI. On the other hand, in women with dysuria without vaginal symptoms, UTI is far more common.[3]

Differential Diagnosis[1]

Infection

Cystitis

Urethritis

Prostatitis

Cervicitis

Vulvovaginitis

Pyelonephritis

Malformation

Bladder neck obstruction (eg, benign prostatic hyperplasia)

Urethral strictures or diverticuli

Neoplasm

Cancers of the bladder, prostate, vagina, or penis

(continued)

Differential Diagnosis[1]

Inflammation	***Trauma***
Urethral or vesicular calculi	*Urinary catheter insertion*
Behçet syndrome	***Hormonal conditions***
Reiter syndrome	*Endometriosis*
Interstitial cystitis	*Atrophic vaginitis*
Drug side effects	
Psychogenic conditions	
Somatization disorder	
Depression	

GETTING STARTED

- UTIs tend to recur in many patients, especially young, sexually active women. Therefore, for some patients, the interview may be streamlined by the recognition that the patient has had similar symptoms previously.
- In such situations, it is always useful to compare the most recent symptoms with the patient's past experiences. When symptoms recur in a woman who has had cystitis previously, an infection is identified in about 90% of patients.[4]

Questions

Have you been treated previously by a physician for a UTI?

If so, how would you compare your current symptoms to those you had at that time?

Have these symptoms ever failed to improve with antibiotics?

Remember

- If the patient's symptoms match those of a prior, successfully treated infection, it is very likely that a recurrent UTI is present.
- If the patient's current symptoms differ from those of previous infections, further investigation will be necessary.

INTERVIEW FRAMEWORK

Efficiency is important when taking a history from a patient with dysuria. Since most patients have an infectious etiology, try to confirm the presence of a UTI expediently without extending the interview unnecessarily. It is reasonable to begin with the hypothesis that there is an infection, which is supported by the presence of the following characteristic features: recent-onset dysuria, mild suprapubic pain, urinary urgency and frequency, and cloudy urine.

IDENTIFYING ALARM SYMPTOMS[5]

Although most patients with dysuria have a lower UTI, clinicians must keep an open mind regarding alternative diagnoses so that serious diagnoses can be ruled out. Although alarm symptoms are unusual in patients with dysuria, it is important to consider them, especially when an aspect of the history is atypical for infection.

Serious Diagnoses	Think about
Infection	Pyelonephritis Urethritis Cervicitis
Neoplasm	Cancers of the bladder, prostate, vagina, or penis
Inflammation	Behçet syndrome Reiter syndrome

Alarm symptoms	Consider
Have you had vaginal bleeding or discharge? Have you had urethral discharge?	Chlamydia or gonococcal infection
Have you had joint aches, mouth ulcers, or eye symptoms?	Behçet syndrome Reiter syndrome
Have you had a gradual onset of your symptoms over weeks, blood in the urine, or unintentional weight loss?	Renal cell carcinoma Bladder cancer
Have you had fever, chills, flank pain, or nausea and vomiting?	Pyelonephritis

FOCUSED QUESTIONS

After a patient notes the presence of dysuria, one can begin to assess the likelihood of the various possible diagnoses by asking questions regarding the quality of the dysuria, its time course, associated symptoms, and modifying symptoms.

Questions

Quality	*Think about*
When urinating, do you experience a burning sensation, as if the urine were hot?	Dysuria is usually related to inflammation of the lower urinary tract, as outlined in the introduction. The full differential diagnosis is listed above.

Time course	*Think about*
How long has painful urination been present?	
• 1–2 days?	Bacterial cystitis
• 2–7 days?	Urethral syndrome
• > 14 days?	Chlamydia infection or interstitial cystitis
Was the onset	
• Sudden?	Bacterial cystitis
• Gradual?	Chlamydia infection or interstitial cystitis

(continued)

Associated symptoms	**Think about**
Do you urinate more frequently than usual during the day?	*Daytime urinary frequency suggests increased urine production (polyuria), decreased bladder capacity (seen with bladder inflammation or infection), or incomplete bladder emptying (common in benign prostatic hyperplasia)*
Is the amount passed with each void less than usual?	*Bladder inflammation* *Incomplete bladder emptying*
Is the amount passed with each void more than usual?	*Diabetes mellitus* *Diabetes insipidus* *Diuretics* *Excessive water intake*
Do you have an exaggerated sense of needing to urinate immediately?	*Urgency results from irritability of the inflamed bladder and decreased bladder compliance. It is common in cystitis, bladder cancer, radiation damage, and neurogenic bladder dysfunction.*
Is the urge to void sometimes so immediate that you urinate involuntarily?	*Acute cystitis* *Upper motor neuron lesions* *Detrusor muscle instability* *Bladder tumors*
(For men) Do you have pain with urination without frequency or urgency?	*Urethritis*
Has the appearance of your urine changed?	*Cloudy urine suggests infection; bloody urine (hematuria) may be seen with cystitis, benign prostatic hypertrophy, urologic and renal malignancy, and nephrolithiasis*
Does your urine smell of ammonia?	*UTI with urea-splitting Proteus species*
(For men) Do you have a urethral discharge?	*Gonococcal or chlamydial urethritis*
(For women) Do you have vaginal discharge or vulvar itching?	*Vaginitis*
(For women) Is sexual intercourse painful?	*Dyspareunia (especially during initial penetration) suggests vulvovaginitis or urethritis*
Do you have flank pain?	*Pyelonephritis or nephrolithiasis*
Do you have an uncomfortable fullness in the perineal and/or rectal areas?	*Cystitis or prostatitis*
Do you have fevers and/or chills?	*Pyelonephritis*
Modifying symptoms	**Think about**
Is the discomfort worse at the beginning of the stream?	*Urethritis*
Is the discomfort worse at the end of the stream?	*Cystitis or prostatitis*

CAVEATS

- Certain symptoms in combination are particularly useful in suggesting the diagnosis of cystitis. For example, for women, the presence of dysuria and frequency without vaginal discharge or irritation raises the probability of cystitis to more than 90%.[4]
- Conversely, vaginal irritation or discharge reduces the likelihood of cystitis by about 20%.[4]
- There is increasing evidence that telephone-based management of selected women with acute uncomplicated UTI is safe and economically efficient.[6,7]

PROGNOSIS

Most conditions associated with dysuria can be treated successfully. In particular, the infectious etiologies, such as cystitis and urethritis, respond well to appropriate antibiotic therapy.

REFERENCES

1. Bremnor JD, Sadovsky R. Evaluation of dysuria in adults. *Am Fam Physician.* 2002;65:1589–1596.
2. Hooton TM, Stamm WE. Diagnosis and treatment of uncomplicated urinary tract infection. *Infect Dis Clin North Am.* 1997;11:551.
3. Bent S, Nallamothu BK, Simel D, Fihn SD, Saint S. Does this woman have an acute uncomplicated urinary tract infection? *JAMA.* 2002;287:2701–2710.
4. Fihn SD. Acute uncomplicated urinary tract infection in women. *N Engl J Med.* 2003;349:259–266.
5. Roberts RG, Hartlaub PP. Evaluation of dysuria in men. *Am Fam Physician.* 1999;60:865–872.
6. Saint S, Scholes D, Fihn SD, Farrell RG, Stamm WE. The effectiveness of a clinical practice guideline for the management of presumed uncomplicated urinary tract infection in women. *Am J Med.* 1999;106:636–641.
7. Barry HC, Hickner J, Ebell MH, Ettenhofer T. A randomized controlled trial of telephone management of suspected urinary tract infections in women. *J Fam Pract.* 2001;50:589–594.

SUGGESTED READING

Gupta K, Hooton TM, Roberts PL, Stamm WE. Patient-initiated treatment of uncomplicated recurrent urinary tract infections in young women. *Ann Intern Med.* 2001;135:9–16.

Diagnostic Approach: Dysuria

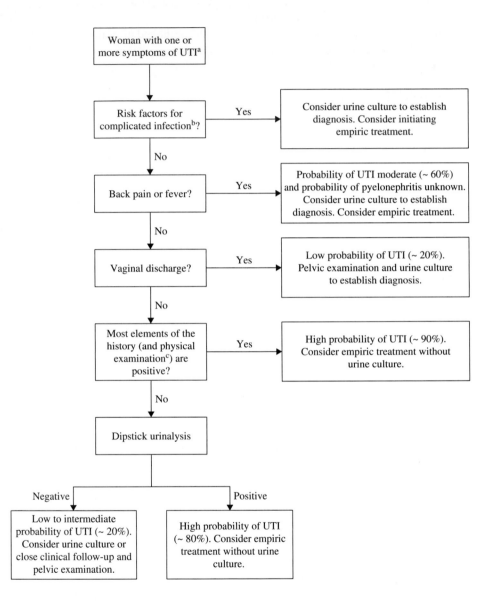

UTI, urinary tract infection.

[a] In women who have risk factors for sexually transmitted diseases, consider testing for chlamydia. The US
Preventive Services Task Force recommends chlamydia screening of all women age 25 or younger and
women of any age with more than 1 sexual partner, a prior history of sexually transmitted disease, or inconsistent
use of condoms.

[b] "Complicated" refers to a UTI in a person with a functional or anatomic abnormality of the urinary tract (including
a history of polycystic renal disease, nephrolithiasis, neurogenic bladder, diabetes mellitus, immunosuppression,
pregnancy, indwelling urinary catheter, or recent urinary tract instrumentation).

[c] The only physical examination finding that increases the likelihood of UTI is costovertebral angle tenderness, and
clinicians may consider not performing this test in patients with typical symptoms of acute, uncomplicated UTI
(as in telephone management).

Hematuria

Virginia U. Collier, MD, FACP

Few symptoms are more alarming to patients than grossly red or brown urine. The first priority is to determine whether the discoloration is due to blood in the urine or another cause. The diagnosis of gross hematuria, or visible blood in the urine, must be confirmed by centrifuging the urine specimen (see Figure, Diagnostic Approach: Gross Hematuria).

Microscopic hematuria is usually not noticed by the patient, but rather diagnosed on routine urinalysis during screening for insurance or employment purposes. Neither the US Preventive Health Services Task Force nor the Canadian Task Force on Periodic Health recommends routine screening for microscopic hematuria. They note that microscopic hematuria has a low predictive value for bladder cancer, even in high-risk elderly patients, and that there is currently no evidence that early detection improves prognosis.[1,2]

For purposes of the ensuing discussion, it is assumed that the diagnosis of true gross or microscopic hematuria has already been established. Although the prevalence of serious disease (eg, malignancy) is higher in patients with gross hematuria, microscopic hematuria may also indicate significant genitourinary pathology.[3,4] A careful history is essential in the evaluation of the patient with either condition.

KEY TERMS

Hematuria	*Bleeding from the urinary tract.*
Gross hematuria	*The presence of blood in the urine in sufficient quantity to be visible to the naked eye. A recent study indicates that more than 95% of clinicians will only recognize gross hematuria when > 3500 red blood cells per high power field are present.[5]*
Microscopic hematuria	*2–3 red blood cells per high power field on urine microscopy. A lower cutoff results in more false-positive results (decreased specificity), a higher cutoff in more missed disease (decreased sensitivity).*

ETIOLOGY

Prevalence of Microscopic Hematuria

In 5 studies examining prevalence, the percentage of patients with asymptomatic microscopic hematuria varied from 0.19% to 16.1%.[6] Some studies indicate the prevalence is higher in older people and higher among women than among men.[1]

Common Causes of Microscopic and Gross Hematuria[3]

	Hematuria, No. (%) of Patients	
	Microscopic (n=1689)	Gross (n=1200)
Urologic cancer	**86 (5.1)**	**270 (22.5)**
Bladder	63 (4.0)	178 (15.0)
Renal	9 (0.5)	45 (3.6)
Prostate	8 (0.5)	29 (2.4)
Ureteral	3 (0.2)	10 (0.8)
Other	3 (0.2)	8 (0.6)
Other significant lesions		
Nephrolithiasis	84 (5.0)	130 (11.0)
Renal disease	37 (2.2)	
Urinary tract infection	73 (4.3)	394 (33.0)
Prostatic hyperplasia	217 (13.0)	153 (13.0)
No source found	**717 (43.0)**	**101 (8.4)**

When considering a more exhaustive list of etiologies, it is useful to divide hematuria into nonglomerular or glomerular causes (see Figure, Diagnostic Approach: Microscopic Hematuria). Since renal biopsy is not routinely done to evaluate patients with hematuria, it is difficult to determine what percentage of patients has a glomerular source.[1] Estimates range from 0.1[7] to 14%.[8]

Nonglomerular and Glomerular Causes

Nonglomerular	Think
Lower urinary tract source	Urethritis, prostatitis
	Benign prostatic hypertrophy
	Cystitis
	Bladder carcinoma[a]
	Prostate carcinoma[a]
	Exercise induced
Upper urinary tract source	Ureteral calculus[a]
	Renal calculus
	Hydronephrosis[a]
	Pyelonephritis
	Polycystic kidney disease
	Hypercalciuria, hyperuricosuria, without stones
	Renal trauma
	Papillary necrosis
	Interstitial nephritis (drug-induced)[a]
	Sickle cell trait or disease
	Renal infarct (embolic eg, secondary to subacute bacterial endocarditis or atherosclerosis)[a]
	Renal tuberculosis
	Renal vein thrombosis

Glomerular	Think
Primary glomerulonephritis	IgA nephropathy
	Postinfectious
	Idiopathic (eg, focal glomerulosclerosis, etc.)
Secondary glomerulonephritis	Systemic lupus erythematosus[a]
	Wegener's granulomatosis[a]
	Other vasculitides[a]
Familial	Thin basement membrane disease (benign familial hematuria)
	Hereditary nephritis (Alport syndrome)
Other	
Factitious	

[a]Etiologies of hematuria classified as highly significant (could pose a clear threat to the patient's life or require a major surgical procedure)[9,10] and for which alarm symptoms should be sought (see below).

Prevalence of Serious Disease in Patients with Hematuria

Multiple studies have demonstrated that patients with gross hematuria have a higher likelihood (up to 4 to 7 times greater) of malignancy than those with microscopic hematuria.[3,4]

The prevalence of serious disease in patients with microscopic hematuria depends on the population studied. A general population has a lower prevalence when compared with patients who have been referred to urologists or nephrologists. In addition, older men with known risk factors (see Alarm Symptoms) have a higher prevalence of serious disease than younger men or those with no risk factors.[1] In multiple studies, urologic malignancy has been identified in approximately 9% of men older than 50 years with asymptomatic microscopic hematuria.[4,11] By contrast, in a study of 636 young Israeli men, only 0.1% had neoplasia.[9] In a prospective study of 177 women ranging from 22 to 87 years old with microscopic hematuria,[12] no bladder malignancies were diagnosed, and only 2 patients had highly significant disease. In a population study of patients of all ages with microscopic hematuria in Rochester, Minnesota, 0.5% had highly significant disease.[10]

GETTING STARTED

Determine whether the patient is seeking medical attention because of an abnormal urinalysis without symptoms (asymptomatic microscopic hematuria) or if the patient has gross hematuria (see Figure, Diagnostic Approach: Gross Hematuria).

Questions	Remember
Have you ever been told that there was blood in your urine?	• A patient with microscopic hematuria may be asymptomatic.
Describe an episode of seeing blood in your urine.	• If the patient has gross hematuria, allow him or her to discuss the presentation and associated symptoms with minimal interruption.
	• Remember that the presence of blood in the urine is frightening to most patients. Demonstrate concern and understanding, but do not reassure the patient until you have excluded "alarm features" (see p. 358).

INTERVIEW FRAMEWORK

- First, the examiner should determine whether there are predisposing factors suggesting a transient cause:
  - –Presence of menses
  - –History of trauma (to flank or abdomen)
  - –Recent genitourinary infection or instrumentation, including insertion of Foley catheter
  - –Recent extreme exercise (eg, running a marathon)
- Next, look for alarm symptoms or aspects of the family history and personal and social history suggesting the possibility of serious disease.
- Finally, ask specific questions about accompanying symptoms and the characteristics of the hematuria, which may pinpoint the lesion within the urinary tract.

IDENTIFYING ALARM SYMPTOMS AND FEATURES

- Increased age (particularly older than 40–50 years) and male sex are associated with an increased incidence of neoplasm.
- Constitutional symptoms (weight loss, appetite loss, chronic malaise or fatigue) suggest malignancy or chronic infection.
- A variety of factors in the personal and social history may result in an increased likelihood of a malignancy or other significant disease including exposure to aniline dyes in leather, tire, or rubber manufacturing industries; previous treatment with cyclophosphamide or pelvic irradiation; ingestion of herbal weight loss preparations containing aristolochic acid.
- A positive family history of deafness or renal disease suggests familial disease.

Alarm symptoms	Serious causes	Benign causes
Increased age (> 40)	*Cancer*	
Male sex	*Cancer*	
Weight loss, chronic malaise	*Cancer* *Chronic infection*	
Appetite loss	*Cancer* *Chronic infection*	
Fever	*Cancer (renal cell carcinoma), infection*	*Acute pyelonephritis*
Flank, back, or abdominal pain	*Renal infarct* *Ureteral calculus* *Embolus from bacterial endocarditis* *Cyst rupture* *Neoplasm*	*Renal calculus* *Acute pyelonephritis*
Recent sore throat, acute upper respiratory tract infection	*Acute glomerulonephritis*	
Swelling of eyelids and feet	*Acute glomerulonephritis*	

Nausea, vomiting	Uremia secondary to acute or chronic glomerulonephritis	Symptoms associated with renal calculus or pyelonephritis
Deafness	Alport disease (hereditary nephritis)	
Hemoptysis	Wegener's granulomatosis Goodpasture's syndrome	
Recurrent sinusitis	Wegener's granulomatosis	
Joint pain or skin rash	Acute glomerulonephritis secondary to an underlying connective tissue disease (systemic lupus erythematosus, polyarteritis nodosa)	
Easy bruising, bleeding from gums	Bleeding disorder (eg, thrombocytopenia or excessive anticoagulation)	

Alarm features in past medical history, family history, and personal and social history

Use of herbal weight loss preparations (containing aristolochic acid)	Genitourinary neoplasm
Prior treatment with cyclophosphamide	Bladder cancer
History of pelvic irradiation	Bladder cancer
Prior treatment with analgesics containing phenacetin	Bladder cancer
Medications including aspirin, antibiotics, non-steroidal anti-inflammatory drugs (NSAIDs)	Interstitial nephritis
History of irregular heart beat	Renal embolus from atrial fibrillation
History of nephrotic syndrome	Renal vein thrombosis
Family history of renal disease	Hereditary nephritis Polycystic kidney disease
Occupation in the leather, dye, rubber or tire manu-facturing industries	Bladder cancer
Cigarette smoking	Bladder cancer

FOCUSED QUESTIONS

After allowing the patient to describe the episode(s) of hematuria and asking about alarm symptoms or features, ask a more focused series of questions to narrow the differential diagnosis. First, consider whether the episode was isolated or episodic, and then ask about the character of the urine. Finally, look for associated symptoms and other aspects of the medical history that suggest a more benign cause of hematuria.

Questions	Think about
Time course	
Is this the first episode of blood in your urine?	Transient or self-limited disease
Did you exercise vigorously prior to the hematuria?	Exercise-induced hematuria
Have you had a recent injury to your abdomen, back, or flank?	Trauma
Are you having your menstrual period?	Vaginal source or endometriosis
Have you recently had a urinary catheter in place, a urologic procedure, or a urinary tract infection?	Iatrogenic trauma or recurrent urinary tract infection
Have you had multiple episodes over months to years?	IgA nephropathy
When did the episodes first start?	IgA nephropathy is often seen in young adults
Does anything seem to precipitate an episode?	IgA nephropathy is often preceded by a sore throat or upper respiratory infection symptoms
Quality	**Think about**
Does the urine contain clots?	Nonglomerular source
Do the clots look like pipes?	Bleeding from ureter
Are the clots bulky and look like balls?	Bleeding from bladder
Is blood present	
• At the beginning of the urine stream?	A lesion in the urethra or a location distal to the bladder neck
• At the end of voiding?	A lesion in the posterior urethra, bladder neck, prostate, or bladder trigone
• Throughout urination?	Hemorrhagic cystitis Renal or ureteral source
Associated symptoms	**Think about**
Had you had fevers or felt feverish?	Acute pyelonephritis Acute prostatitis Prostatic abscess
Do you have pain or burning on urination?	Urinary tract infection Hemorrhagic cystitis Passage of renal calculus Acute prostatitis
Do you have sharp pain in your lower abdomen above the groin?	Renal calculus
Do you have suprapubic pain?	Cystitis
Do you have flank pain or back pain?	Acute pyelonephritis Renal calculus Papillary necrosis

Do you have to urinate frequently at night or have you noticed a decreased force of your urine stream?	*Benign prostatic hypertrophy*
Pertinent medical history	**Think about**
Are you currently taking	
• A blood thinner (eg, warfarin)?	*Anticoagulation, especially excessive anticoagulation, may unmask an underlying genitourinary lesion.*
• Cyclophosphamide?	*Hemorrhagic cystitis. Occurs in a dose-dependent fashion in patients receiving intravenous (greater than oral) cyclophosphamide.*
Have you ever had kidney stones?	*Urinary calculus*
Have you ever had gout?	*Uric acid stones*
Do you have sickle cell anemia?	*Hematuria from sickling of red blood cells*

DIAGNOSTIC APPROACH

All patients with even a single episode of gross hematuria should receive a thorough history and physical examination followed by urologic or nephrologic evaluation unless self-limited, transient causes can be identified (trauma, infection, menses, exercise induced). Even in patients who have transient causes, if there are significant risk factors for malignancy, further evaluation should be considered.

A careful history should also be performed in all patients with microscopic hematuria. Most experts recommend further evaluation only if one or more repeated urinalyses confirm microscopic hematuria.[1,13] However, there is no evidence to suggest that an isolated episode is less serious than recurrent episodes.[1] Thus, some authors recommend that unless a self-limited cause is found, a complete evaluation should be undertaken, especially in men over the age of 40 and those with risk factors for significant disease.[5,6,14]

CAVEATS

- Hematuria in patients receiving anticoagulation therapy should not be attributed solely to the anticoagulant.[15]
- Blood in the urine can be an irritant and may cause dysuria, even in the absence of urinary tract infection or kidney stone disease.

PROGNOSIS

The prognosis of hematuria depends on the etiology. Advanced (metastatic) genitourinary malignancy results in death in most patients. Localized malignancy is curable in a significant percentage of patients, with the cure rate dependent on the site of the malignancy. An acute progressive glomerulonephritis occurs in approximately 10% of patients with IgA nephropathy, the most common cause of microscopic hematuria. In 20–30%, chronic renal failure develops over 1 or 2 decades. The remaining patients continue to have gross or microscopic hematuria but significant renal dysfunction does not develop. The majority of cases of acute postinfectious glomerulonephritis resolve in weeks to months, whereas other forms of acute glomerulonephritis (rapidly progressive, membranoproliferative) can progress rapidly to irreversible renal failure despite treatment with immunosuppressive agents.

REFERENCES

1. Cohen RA, Brown RS. Microscopic hematuria. *N Engl J Med.* 2003;348:2330–2338.

2. Preventive Services Task Force. Guide to clinical preventive services: report of the US Preventive Services Task Force. 2nd ed. Williams & Wilkins; 1996.

3. Sutton JM. Evaluation of hematuria in adults. *JAMA*. 1990;263:2475–2480.

4. Khadra MH, Pickard RS, Charlton M, et al. A prospective analysis of 1930 patients with hemtauria to evaluate current diagnostic practice. *J Urol*. 2000;163:524–527.

5. Peacock PR, Souto HL, Benner GE et al. What is gross hematuria? Correlation of subjective and objective assessment. *J Trauma*. 2001;50:1060–1062.

6. Woolhandler S, Pels RJ, Bor DH, et al. Dipstick urinalysis screening of asymptomatic adults for urinary tract disorders. I. Hematuria and proteinuria. *JAMA*. 1989;262:1215–1224.

7. Froom P, Ribak J, Benbassat J. Significance of microhematuria in young adults. *BMJ*. 1984;288:20–22.

8. Mohr DN, Offord KP, Melton LJ III. A symptomatic microhematuria and urologic disease. A population-based study. *JAMA*. 1986;256:224–229.

9. Carson CC, Segura JW, Greene LF. Clinical importance of microhematuria. *JAMA*. 1979;241:149–150.

10. Greene LF, O'Shaughnessey JEJ, Hendricks ED. Study of five hundred patients with asymptomatic microscopic hematuria. *JAMA*. 1956;161:610–613.

11. Messing EM, Young TB, Hunr VB, et al. Home screening for hematuria: results of a multi-clinic study. *J Urol*. 1992; 148:289–292.

12. Bard RH. The significance of asymptomatic microhematuria and proteinuria in adult primary care. *CMAJ*. 2002;166: 348–353.

13. House AA, Cattran DC. Nephrology 2. Evaluation of asymptomatic hematuria and proteinuria in adult primary care. *CMAJ*. 2002;166:348–353.

14. Ritchie CD, Bevan EA, Collier SJ. Importance of occult hematuria found at screening. *BMJ*. 1986;292:681–683.

15. Van Savage JG, Fried FA. Anticoagulant associated hematuria: a prospective study. *J Urol*. 1995;153:1594–1596.

Diagnostic Approach: Gross Hematuria

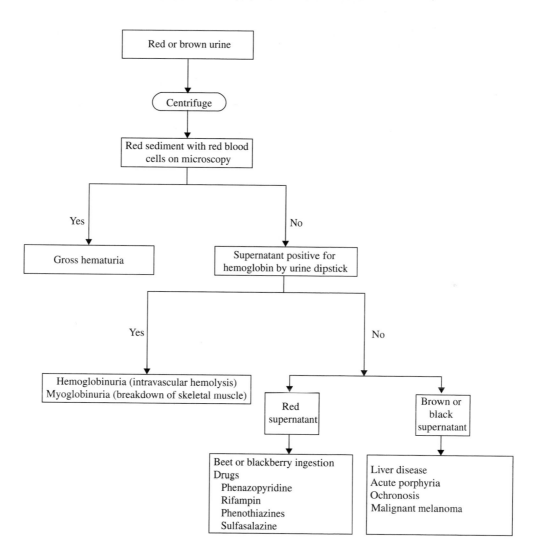

Diagnostic Approach: Microscopic Hematuria

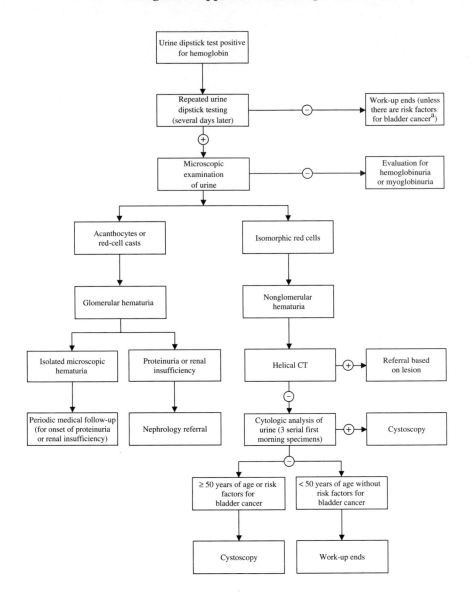

CT, computed tomography.

(Adapted with permission from Cohen RA, Brown RS. *N Engl J Med.* 2003; 348:2330-2338.)

[a]Risk factors for bladder cancer include cigarette smoking, occupational exposure to chemicals used in certain
industries (leather, dye, and rubber or tire manufacturing), heavy phenacetin use, past treatment with high
doses of cyclophosphamide, and ingestion of aristolochic acid found in some herbal weight-loss preparations.

Flank Pain

39

Paul Aronowitz, MD

Flank pain refers to pain occurring just below the 12th rib, encompassing the costovertebral angle and area lateral to that angle. Patients often describe flank pain as unilateral upper back pain. The initial differential diagnosis depends on a patient's age, gender, and comorbidities. However nephrolithiasis, pyelonephritis, and musculoskeletal strain account for the vast majority of cases.

A careful history often suggests one of these possibilities or raises suspicion for a less common cause. For example, a history of chronic atrial fibrillation increases the likelihood of a renal vascular embolus. Splenic infarct as a cause of left flank pain is unusual, but should be considered in patients with suspected endocarditis. If "red flags" arise in the history, life-threatening diagnoses (eg, rupturing abdominal aortic aneurysm [AAA] or retroperitoneal hemorrhage) must also be considered.

KEY TERMS

Dysuria	*Difficulty urinating or pain with urination.*
Gross hematuria	*Bloody urine visible to the patient.*
Renal colic	*Pain caused by obstruction of the ureter. This pain is caused by increased hydrostatic pressure proximal to the obstruction and is considered to be one of the most painful conditions experienced by patients, just short of labor or childbirth.*

ETIOLOGY

Unfortunately there is little data on prevalence of the various causes of flank pain. Furthermore, patients rarely say to a health care provider "I have flank pain"; most complain of back pain.

Flank pain is often caused by sudden obstruction of a ureter by a renal calculus or renal colic. The pain of renal colic tends to be sudden, severe, and debilitating. As the offending calculus descends through the collecting system, pain may also occur in the lower abdominal quadrants and genitalia. Dysuria, frequency, urgency, and hematuria may also accompany nephrolithiasis.

Pyelonephritis commonly causes flank pain, particularly in women. Because women have shorter urethras than men, women have a greater incidence of lower urinary tract infections; pyelonephritis may develop as infection ascends to one or both kidneys. Pain is caused by inflammation of the kidney with stretching of the renal capsule; it may be less severe and more insidious than renal colic. A history of fever or dysuria suggests pyelonephritis, although dysuria may not occur in patients with indwelling urinary catheters. Occasionally, a kidney stone may obstruct the flow of urine, leading to the development of pyelonephritis. Such patients have *both* pyelonephritis and nephrolithiasis, the 2 most common causes of flank pain.

Musculoskeletal causes of flank pain are often clinically obvious. The patient usually describes a precipitating event, such as swinging a baseball bat or lifting a heavy object.

It is helpful to think about the most common diagnoses first and then consider the less common or rare causes.

Differential Diagnosis	Frequency[a]
Nephrolithiasis	Common
Pyelonephritis	Common
Musculoskeletal (muscle strain)	Common
Herpes zoster	Common
Papillary necrosis	Uncommon
Renal abscess	Uncommon
Renal infarct (cardioembolic)	Uncommon (except with atrial fibrillation)
Renal vein thrombosis	Uncommon
Adult polycystic kidney disease (APKD) • Infected renal cyst • Rupturing renal cyst • Hemorrhage into renal cyst	Common in patients with APKD
Renal tuberculosis	Rare in the United States but more common in developing world
Retroperitoneal fibrosis	Rare
AAA	Uncommon
Retroperitoneal hemorrhage	Uncommon; consider in patients receiving anticoagulants
Bacterial endocarditis with splenic infarct	Rare
Pulmonary embolism	Uncommon
Pneumonia (lower lobe)	Uncommon
Pleural effusion	Uncommon
Subphrenic abscess	Uncommon
Biliary tract (gallbladder) disease	Uncommon
Psoas abscess	Uncommon
Diverticulitis	Rare
Appendicitis	Rare
Vertebral compression fracture	Uncommon
Retroperitoneal malignancy (lymphoma, pancreatic cancer, metastatic cancer)	Uncommon
Malingering	Uncommon

[a]Among patients with flank pain.

GETTING STARTED

Open-ended questions

Tell me about the pain you are having.

Did the pain come on suddenly or gradually?

Where in your body did you first notice the pain?

Tips for effective interviewing

• *Listen.*
• *Don't interrupt.*
• *Don't jump to conclusions.*
• *Be empathic—the patient will often be in pain throughout the initial history.*

INTERVIEW FRAMEWORK

• Characterize the onset, location, duration, quality, and associated features of the pain.
• Determine whether the patient has ever had similar pain before.
• Keep in mind the myriad medical conditions that predispose to renal stone formation—from hyperparathyroidism to myeloproliferative disorders to renal tubular acidosis.
• Obtain a careful occupational history and substance use or abuse history (eg, an intern on duty for long periods may not drink adequate fluids, putting her at higher risk for a kidney stone).

IDENTIFYING ALARM SYMPTOMS

• Flank pain associated with unusual features such as pleuritic chest pain, cough, or drenching night sweats, requires urgent attention.
• Flank pain with a normal urinalysis should prompt consideration of pathology outside the kidney.
• Be extremely cautious in patients whose history suggests hypotension, ie, dizziness, fainting, or confusion. A rupturing AAA or retroperitoneal hemorrhage can cause flank pain and hypotension. The mortality is quite high for patients with AAA presenting with shock, even if the diagnosis is made early.

Serious Diagnoses

Serious causes of flank pain tend to be rare or uncommon. Fortunately, the urinalysis rapidly narrows the initial differential diagnosis.

Alarm symptoms	Serious causes	Benign causes
Confusion and fever	*Pyelonephritis with sepsis (urosepsis)* *Cholecystitis* *Pneumonia*	
Orthostatic dizziness	*Shock from rupturing AAA or hemorrhage*	*Volume depletion from poor oral intake (easily corrects with intravenous fluids)*
Concurrent use of anticoagulants	*Retroperitoneal hemorrhage*	
Pleuritic chest pain	*Pulmonary embolism* *Pneumonia* *Subphrenic abscess*	*Pleurisy or muscle strain*
Associated abdominal pain	*AAA* *Subphrenic abscess* *Pancreatitis*	

(continued)

Alarm symptoms	Serious causes	Benign causes
Weight loss	*Malignancy*	
Slow onset and failure to resolve	*Malignancy* *Abscess*	
Prolonged fever with sudden onset flank pain	*Endocarditis with septic emboli*	*Viral syndrome*
Pain associated with eating	*Cholecystitis* *Bowel obstruction* *Pancreatitis*	
Sudden onset of flank pain	*AAA* *Nephrolithiasis* *Retroperitoneal hemorrhage* *Pulmonary embolism* *Renal infarct*	

FOCUSED QUESTIONS

After letting the patient tell the story, focus on alarm symptoms or features suggestive of causes other than nephrolithiasis, pyelonephritis or musculoskeletal disease.

General questions	Think about
Have you ever had a problem with your blood calcium?	Nephrolithiasis
Have you ever had kidney stones?	Nephrolithiasis
Have you had any problems urinating recently?	Pyelonephritis
Have you been urinating more frequently than usual or urinating small amounts?	Pyelonephritis
Do you recall exactly when the pain began?	Nephrolithiasis (if sudden) Pyelonephritis if more insidious
Have you had fevers?	Pyelonephritis
Do you consume large amounts of rhubarb?	Nephrolithiasis (calcium oxalate stones)
Do you use injection drugs?	Endocarditis with subphrenic abscess or splenic infarct

Quality	*Think about*
Is the flank pain	
• *Coming and going? ("colicky")*	Nephrolithiasis
• *Severe and the worst pain you've ever had?*	Nephrolithiasis
• *10 out of 10 in severity?*	Nephrolithiasis
• *A dull ache that has gradually worsened?*	Pyelonephritis or other causes
• *Sudden onset with little change?*	Renal embolus Retroperitoneal hemorrhage
• *Burning*	Herpes zoster

Time course	***Think about***
Did the pain	
• *Come on suddenly?*	*Nephrolithiasis*
	AAA
	Retroperitoneal hemorrhage
	Pulmonary embolism
	Renal embolus
• *Come on during physical activity?*	*Musculoskeletal strain*
• *Present at right flank and come on after eating, especially a high-fat meal?*	*Cholecystitis*
Has the pain been present for weeks to months?	*Malignancy*

Associated symptoms	***Think about***
Do you have	
• *Pain radiating to other places: penis, vagina, groin, or lower quadrants of abdomen?*	*Nephrolithiasis*
• *Bloody urine?*	*Nephrolithiasis*
• *Intermittent bloody diarrhea or a history of Crohn's disease?*	*Nephrolithiasis*
• *Nausea or vomiting?*	*Nephrolithiasis*
	Pyelonephritis
	Cholecystitis
	Pancreatitis
• *Dysuria, urgency, frequency?*	*Pyelonephritis*
	Nephrolithiasis
• *Fever?*	*Pyelonephritis*
	Cholecystitis
	Pneumonia
	Nephrolithiasis with pyelonephritis
• *Unilateral midabdominal pain?*	*Nephrolithiasis*
	Pyelonephritis
• *Diffuse abdominal pain?*	*AAA*
	Bowel obstruction
• *Constipation?*	*AAA*
	Bowel obstruction
• *Palpitations?*	*Cardioembolic renal infarct from atrial fibrillation*
• *Pain increased with touching skin on flank?*	*Herpes zoster*
• *Rash in region of pain?*	*Herpes zoster*
• *Frequent cough?*	*Pneumonia*
• *Cough productive of sputum?*	*Pneumonia*

(continued)

Associated symptoms	**Think about**
Is the pain worse with deep inspiration?	Pneumonia
	Subphrenic abscess
	Pulmonary embolism
Modifying symptoms	**Think about**
Does the pain improve with rest?	Musculoskeletal strain
Has it occurred in past and resolved on own without medical attention?	Nephrolithiasis

CAVEATS

- Age is important in establishing the initial differential diagnosis of flank pain. A young woman with flank pain is highly unlikely to have an AAA, but AAA must be considered in an older man with peripheral vascular disease even if he has flank pain, fever, and dysuria.
- Kidney stones may recur; often the patient will tell you the diagnosis since this pain tends to be unforgettable.
- Always consider a rupturing AAA—an uncommon but potentially life-saving diagnosis if made early enough.
- Injection drug abuse is a "red flag" in all patients with flank pain; such patients require a more careful evaluation.
- Attempt to differentiate pyelonephritis from nephrolithiasis because the latter usually requires a computed tomographic scan or intravenous pyelogram.
- Listen to the patient's story—it will save time and prevent unnecessary testing.
- Remember that other common diseases (pneumonia, cholecystitis) can present in an uncommon fashion—namely, with flank pain.

PROGNOSIS

Prognosis depends on the underlying diagnosis. Patients with pyelonephritis generally do well with antibiotics. Patients with nephrolithiasis may do well with conservative management or sometimes need urologic intervention (eg, lithotripsy), depending on the size and location of the kidney stone. Patients presenting with an enlarging AAA without shock have a much better prognosis than those with shock (22% versus 88% mortality, respectively), highlighting the need for early diagnosis.

SUGGESTED READING

Heptinstall RH. Urinary Tract Infection and Clinical Features of Pyelonephritis. In: *Pathology of the Kidney.* 4th ed. Little, Brown; 1992;v.3:1433–1488.

Lederle FA, Parenti CM, Chute EP. Ruptured abdominal aortic aneurysm: the internist as diagnostician. *Am J Med.* 1994; 96:163–167.

Sobel JD, Kaye D. Urinary Tract Infections. In: *Principles and Practice of Infectious Disease.* 5th ed. Churchill Livingstone; 2000; v. 1:773–805.

Tambyah PA, Maki DG. Catheter-associated urinary tract infection is rarely symptomatic. *Arch Intern Med.* 2000;160:678–682.

Teichman JMH. Acute renal colic from ureteral calculus. *N Engl J Med.* 2004;350:684–693.

Diagnostic Approach: Flank Pain

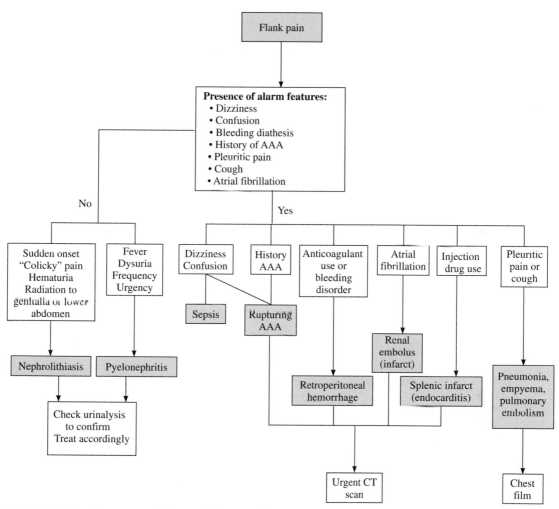

AAA, abdominal aortic aneurysm; CT, computed tomography.

Erectile Dysfunction

40

Mary O'Keefe, MD, & David Gutknecht, MD

Erectile dysfunction (ED) is the inability to attain and sustain an erection of sufficient rigidity for sexual activity. It affects 30 million men in the United States, most commonly those over age 50.[1] The prevalence is 52% in men ages 40–70, and doubles each decade over age 50.[2] ED is a marker for several important diseases and may be the presenting symptom.

KEY TERMS

Impotence	*An outdated and potentially disparaging label for what we now call ED.*
Loss of libido	*Loss of sexual interest.*
Premature ejaculation	*A sexual problem characterized by loss of an adequate erection through early involuntary climax, sometimes confused with ED. More common than ED in patients younger than 50 years.*

ETIOLOGY AND PATHOPHYSIOLOGY

α-Adrenergic sympathetic tone limits blood flow to the penis and maintains the flaccid state. Erection occurs when erotic stimuli inhibit sympathetic tone and release nitric oxide and other transmitters from nerve endings and endothelial cells in the penile arterioles. The cavernosal sinusoids become engorged with blood and erection ensues. This is aided by a passive inhibition of venous outflow as the subtunical venous plexus is compressed between the expanding sinusoids and the unyielding tunica albuginea. Forcible compression of the base of the penis by the ischiocavernous muscles then further increases the intracavernous pressure. Any derangement in these events can cause ED. ED in men over 40 is usually due to a physical (organic) disorder, although concurrent psychological problems, such as depression, are common.[3]

Differential Diagnosis	Approximate Frequency
Psychogenic	*20%[1,4,5]*
Vascular	*Variable* *Although not proven to be the cause, 70% of patients over 60 with ED have vascular disease.[6]*
Drug-induced	*Over 25%[4,7]*
Hormonal	
• Thyroid, pituitary, gonadal disease	*Variable reports, perhaps 3–19% excluding diabetes[4,8]*
• Diabetes	*5–9%[4,9]*

(continued)

Differential Diagnosis	Approximate Frequency
Neurogenic	*7%[4]*
Other	*Urologic 6%[4]*
	Renal disease
	Sickle cell disease
	Sleep disorder[10]
	Liver disease

GETTING STARTED

ED is a sensitive but very important topic, affecting the patient's sexual activity and self-image, as well as the patient's partner. You must specifically ask about ED or you will miss many cases. Routinely incorporate questions about ED in your review of systems. Differentiate ED from loss of libido, lack of orgasm, or premature ejaculation.

Questions	Remember
Many men have occasional problems getting or maintaining an erection. Has this happened to you?	• *Use nonjudgmental, professional language.*
I always ask my patients some very personal questions related to their health. Do you ever have any problems with sexual intercourse? With erections?	• *Teach small bits of information (it's common, it's treatable, it's an appropriate topic to broach with your doctor) interspersed with questions.*
I'm glad you feel comfortable telling me about this. I'd like to ask you some specific questions about sexual function to figure out what we should do.	• *Overcome patient hesitance by asking direct questions first, later returning to open questions.*

INTERVIEW FRAMEWORK

- Determine the patient's agenda. For example, some patients want a prescription for a "cure-all" and others need only an explanation.
- Differentiate psychogenic from physical (organic) causes of ED but remember that patients often have a combination of both.
- When considering physical (organic) causes, differentiate between vascular, hormonal, neurologic, drug-induced, and other causes. It is common for patients to have more than one cause.
- Find unrecognized contributory diseases (see Focused Questions section).

IDENTIFYING ALARM SYMPTOMS

In patients with ED, systemic diseases such as diabetes, alcoholism, depression, or vascular diseases are often self-evident but may not be recognized without directed questioning. Serious diagnoses are rare.

Alarm symptoms	Serious causes	Less serious causes
Concurrent hip and buttock cramps with walking	*Abdominal aortic aneurysm*	*Intermittent claudication*
Leg weakness, numbness, perineal numbness	*Spinal cord compression or pelvic mass*	*Nerve root compression Peripheral neuropathy*

Bowel or bladder incontinence	Spinal cord compression or pelvic mass	Bladder infection
Fecal impaction
Many others
Galactorrhea (milk flow from the breast)	Pituitary tumor	
Abnormal secondary sexual characteristics (loss of beard or body hair and female body habitus)	Pituitary tumor	Normal variant, primary testicular failure
Visual field cuts (loss of portions of vision)	Pituitary tumor	Other eye disorders

FOCUSED QUESTIONS

If answered in the affirmative	**Think about**
Do you have	
• *History of depression, schizophrenia, or bipolar disorder?*	*Psychogenic*
• *Loss of interest, trouble concentrating, trouble with memory, feel sad, etc?*	*Psychogenic (depression)*
• *Difficulties with relationship with partner?*	*Psychogenic*
• *Performance anxiety?*	*Psychogenic*
Are you a smoker?	*Vascular*
Do you have high cholesterol, hypertension, chest pain, and/or leg claudication?	*Vascular*
Do you have a history of coronary artery disease? Do any members of your family? Is there any history of peripheral vascular disease?	*Vascular*
Is there a past history of pelvic or spinal trauma, radiation, or surgery?	*Neurologic (injury)*
Have you had perineal numbness, bowel or bladder incontinence?	*Neurologic (spinal cord or pelvic plexus)*
Have you felt any foot or leg numbness, weakness?	*Neurologic (diabetes; spinal cord, brain or pelvic plexus lesion)*
Are you taking medications known to cause ED (eg, antihypertensives, antidepressants, antiandrogenics, antihistamines, corticosteroids, digitalis)	*Drug-induced*
Do you ever drive under the influence?
Ever tried to cut down, get angry when others ask about alcohol use, feel guilty, drink a morning eye-opener? (CAGE questions)	*Alcoholism*

(continued)

If answered in the affirmative	Think about
Alcohol, marijuana and other drug use?	*Drug-induced* *Depression or other psychogenic cause*
Do you have	
• *History of thyroid disease*	*Hormonal (thyroid disease)*
• *Heat/cold intolerance*	*Hormonal (thyroid disease)*
• *Constipation/diarrhea*	*Hormonal (thyroid disease)*
• *Weight gain/loss*	*Hormonal (thyroid disease)*
• *Tremor*	*Hormonal (thyroid disease)*
• *History of gonadal disease*	*Hormonal (gonadal disease)*
• *Gynecomastia, loss of body hair, thinning of beard, decreased testicular size.*	*Hormonal (pituitary or gonadal)*
• *History of pituitary disease*	*Hormonal (pituitary)*
• *Visual field cuts, headache*	*Hormonal (pituitary mass)*
• *Decreased libido*	*Hormonal (gonadal or pituitary) or psychogenic*
• *A personal or family history of diabetes?*	*Diabetes*
• *Polyphagia, polyuria, polydipsia?*	*Diabetes*
• *History of renal disease?*	*Renal disease*
• *Priapism, bone pains?*	*Sickle cell disease*
Do you snore or not feel refreshed on awakening? *Do you have daytime somnolence?*	*Sleep disorder[10]*
Jaundice, pruritus, nausea?	*Liver disease*
Quality	***Think about***
Do erections take longer to achieve, have shorter duration and less rigidity?	*Physical (organic) etiology.*
Is the problem severe, preventing sexual activity, or of a more minor annoyance?	*Impacts on patient's desire for treatment*
Time course	***Think about***
Was the onset	
• *Sudden?*	*Drug induced (if concurrent with medication start) or psychogenic*
• *Gradual?*	*Physical (organic) etiology*
• *Intermittent?*	*Psychogenic*
Do you achieve normal erection but lose it too early?	*Psychogenic*
Triggering psychological event (ie, discord with partner)?	*Psychogenic*
Associated symptoms	***Think about***
Painful bending of penis with erection?	*Peyronie disease (Fibrous plaque, usually on dorsum of penis, which does not*

	distend as normal skin does. With erection, failure to distend causes penis to bend towards side of plaque, causing pain and loss of erection.)
Difficulty retracting foreskin?	Phimosis
Modifying symptoms	**Think about**
Better with different partner?	Psychogenic
Better with masturbation or visual stimuli?	Psychogenic
Better with nocturnal erections?	Psychogenic

CAVEATS

- Normal morning erections with ED almost always indicates a psychogenic cause.
- Sudden onset of ED suggests a drug or a psychogenic cause.
- Specific therapy is available for ED due to a drug, a hormonal problem other than diabetes, or a psychogenic cause. Be sure to look for these causes.
- ED may be the presenting symptom of an underlying serious, treatable disorder.

PROGNOSIS

If ED is drug-induced, discontinuation of the medication should be effective. Psychiatric therapy for psychogenic ED leads to improvement in 50–80%. Testosterone replacement usually improves severely hypogonadal patients. Identifying drugs, sleep disorders, endocrinopathies, or psychiatric disorders may allow specific treatment options. Medications and devices may assist with erection in appropriately selected patients. Sildenafil is effective in 70% of unselected patients with ED.

REFERENCES

1. NIH consensus Conference on Impotence. NIH Consensus Development Panel on Impotence. *JAMA.* 1993;270:83–90.
2. Johannes CB, Araugo AB, Feldman HA, et al. Incidence of erectile dysfunction in men ages 40–69: longitudinal results from the Massachusetts male aging study. *J Urol.* 2000;163:460–463.
3. Cohan P, Korenman SG. Erectile dysfunction. *J Clin Endocrinol Metab.* 2001;86:2391–2394.
4. Slag MF, Mosley JE, Elson MK, et al. Impotence in medical clinic outpatients. *JAMA.* 1983;249:1736–1740.
5. Kaiser FE, Viosca SP. Impotence and aging: clinical and hormonal factors. *J Am Geriatr Soc.* 1988;36:511–519.
6. Benet AE, Sharaby JG, Melman A. Male erectile dysfunction—assessment and treatment options. *Comp Ther.* 1994;20:669–673.
7. Feldman HA, Goldstein I, Hatzichristou GH, et al. Impotence and its medical and psychosocial correlates: results of the Massachusetts male aging study. *J Urol.* 1994;151:54–61.
8. Johnson AR, Jarow JP. Is routine endocrine testing of impotent men necessary? *J Urol.* 1992;147:1542–1543.
9. Sairam K, Kulinskaya GB, Hanbury DC, McNicholas TA. Prevalence of undiagnosed diabetes mellitus in male erectile dysfunction. *BJU Int.* 2001;88:68–71.
10. Seftel AD, Strohl KP, Loye TL, et al. Erectile dysfunction and symptoms of sleep disorders. *Sleep.* 2002;25:643–647.
11. O'Keefe M, Hunt DK. Assessment and treatment of impotence. *Med Clin North Am.* 1995;79:415–434.

SUGGESTED READING

Lue TF. Erectile dysfunction. *N Engl J Med.* 2000;342:1802–1813.
Ralph D, McNicholas T. UK management guidelines for erectile dysfunction. *BMJ.* 2000;321:499–503.

Diagnostic Approach: Erectile Dysfunction

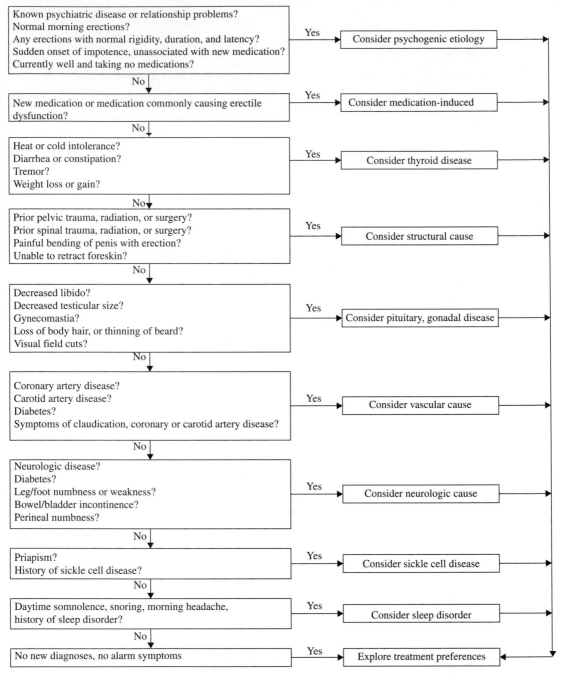

Adapted from O'Keefe M, Hunk DK. Assessment and treatment of impotence. *Med Clin North Am.* 1995;79:415–434.

Urinary Incontinence

41

Calvin H. Hirsch, MD

Occasional involuntary leakage of urine is common in men and women, affecting approximately 5% of men and 30% of women younger than 64 years, and over 15% of men and 50% of women older than 64 years. When urinary incontinence (UI) is severe, it can result in social isolation, depression, and even institutionalization. In the United States, the annual direct cost of UI (in 2000 dollars) has been estimated at $3.0 billion for men and $11.2 billion for women.[1]

KEY TERMS

Detrussor hyperactivity with impaired contractility (DHIC)	*Found mainly in debilitated older persons. Despite an overactive bladder, detrussor contractions are ineffective, resulting in bladder distention and overflow incontinence. (See definition of **Overflow incontinence** below.)*
Detrussor disinhibition	*Spontaneous triggering of the spinal reflex voiding mechanism when the bladder reaches a threshold volume and there is inadequate inhibition of bladder contractions by the central nervous system. Urine loss may occur with or without warning. Also called neurogenic detrussor overactivity.*
Detrussor-sphincter dyssynergy	*Failure to synchronize bladder contractions with release of sphincter, due to multiple sclerosis or other conditions causing supra-sacral spinal cord lesions. (See definition of **Overflow incontinence** below.)*
Functional incontinence	*Incontinence despite a normally functioning bladder due to the inability to reach a toilet in time.*
Idiopathic overactive bladder	*Involuntary detrussor contractions that occur before the bladder is full, creating a sensation of urgently needing to void. May occur with or without incontinence.*
Incontinence	*The involuntary leakage of urine. There are several types: urge, detrussor disinhibition, stress, overflow (includes detrussor hyperactivity with impaired contractility and detrussor-sphincter dyssynergy), functional, and mixed.*
Mixed incontinence	*Incontinence from multiple etiologies, most commonly stress and urge.*

(continued)

KEY TERMS

Overflow incontinence	*Due to urinary retention, pressure in the bladder exceeds outlet (sphincter) resistance, causing leakage until the bladder pressure drops below outlet resistance; examples include DHIC and detrussor-sphincter dyssynergy.*
Stress incontinence	*Leakage caused by an increase in intra-abdominal pressure, as produced by a cough, sneeze, laughing, standing up, or heavy lifting (Figure 41–1). Also called sphincter incompetence.*
Urge incontinence	*Involuntary detrussor contractions cause an urgent need to void. After a variable period of time (seconds to minutes), the contractions exceed bladder outlet resistance (normally produced by the internal sphincter), resulting in incontinence (see Figure 41–2). Also called detrussor hyperreflexia and idiopathic detrussor overactivity with incontinence.*

ETIOLOGY

The prevalence of the incontinence types varies across age groups and by gender. An overactive bladder—with or without incontinence—has a similar prevalence in men and women, rising from about 5% among those aged 25 to 34 to approximately 30% after age 74. However, the prevalence of UI resulting from an overactive bladder increases more rapidly with age in women than in men; by age 75, twice as many women experience urge incontinence.[2] Stress incontinence occurs predominantly in women because of pelvic floor laxity; however, it may occur in men who have damage to the internal sphincter resulting from instrumentation or prostate surgery. Incontinence in older women is more likely to have an urge component, compared with younger women. However, in a survey of 647 currently incontinent women aged 48 to 79 years, over 80% described symptoms suggesting a mixed etiology that included urgency and stress.[3]

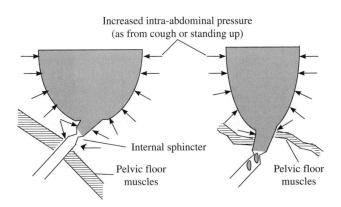

A. Normal bladder outlet

B. Hypermobile urethra with internal sphincter outside abdominal cavity

Figure 41–1. **A:** With a normal bladder outlet, increased intra-abdominal pressure is applied equally to outside of bladder and sphincter, keeping the bladder pressure-sphincter pressure ratio unchanged. **B:** When the sphincter drops below the pelvic diaphragm, all the increased intra–abdominal pressure is applied above the sphincter, causing the bladder pressure to exceed the sphincter pressure, resulting in leakage. (Adapted from Kane et al, 1994.)

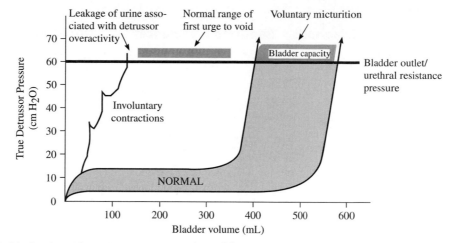

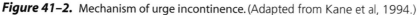

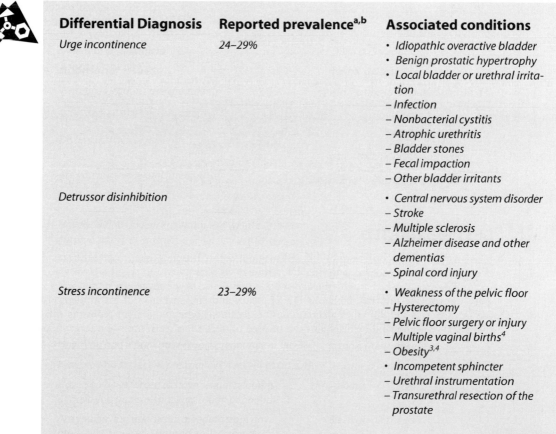

Figure 41–2. Mechanism of urge incontinence. (Adapted from Kane et al, 1994.)

Differential Diagnosis	Reported prevalence[a,b]	Associated conditions
Urge incontinence	*24–29%*	• *Idiopathic overactive bladder* • *Benign prostatic hypertrophy* • *Local bladder or urethral irritation* – *Infection* – *Nonbacterial cystitis* – *Atrophic urethritis* – *Bladder stones* – *Fecal impaction* – *Other bladder irritants*
Detrussor disinhibition		• *Central nervous system disorder* – *Stroke* – *Multiple sclerosis* – *Alzheimer disease and other dementias* – *Spinal cord injury*
Stress incontinence	*23–29%*	• *Weakness of the pelvic floor* – *Hysterectomy* – *Pelvic floor surgery or injury* – *Multiple vaginal births[4]* – *Obesity[3,4]* • *Incompetent sphincter* – *Urethral instrumentation* – *Transurethral resection of the prostate*

(continued)

Differential Diagnosis	Reported prevalence[a,b]	Associated conditions
Overflow incontinence	*5–10%*	• *Bladder outlet obstruction* – *Benign prostatic hypertrophy* – *Urethral stricture* – *Surgical over-correction of stress incontinence* – *Cystocele* – *Fecal impaction* • *Ineffective detrussor contractions* – *Pelvic irradiation* – *Autonomic dysfunction* • *Diabetic neuropathy* • *Spinal stenosis* • *Neurodegenerative diseases* • *DHIC*
Functional incontinence		• *Conditions causing immobility* • *Environmental barriers (eg, restraints or bedrails)* • *Excessive sedation* • *Psychological disorder* – *Refusal to go to toilet* – *Indifference to wetting self* • *Diuretics* • *Metabolic disorders causing polyuria* – *Hyperglycemia* – *Hypercalcemia*
Mixed incontinence	*23–33%*	

[a]The range in which the reported prevalence falls in most surveys of incontinent middle-aged and older adults.

[b]Prevalence is not available when not indicated.

GETTING STARTED

Many patients are embarrassed by UI and may not report it unless asked. The history is the most cost-effective diagnostic tool for detecting UI, although its sensitivity and specificity vary according to the way questions are asked and by the age-specific prevalence of incontinence subtypes.[5] A 7-day voiding diary can provide information about the frequency and circumstances of incontinent episodes, which can be especially helpful when ascertaining the dominant type in a patient reporting mixed symptoms (Figure 41–3). The voiding diary also can be used to track the effectiveness of interventions.

VOIDING DIARY

Name _____

Day _____

Date____/____/____
Mo   Day   Year

Instructions:

For each time period,

1. In the first column, mark how many times that you urinated in the toilet.
2. In the second column, check the box if you had an accident during that time period, then check whether it was a leak (small amount) or a large amount (soaking clothing or pad).
3. In the third column, write down the reason for the accident or the situation in which it occurred.
    For example,
    If you leaked after coughing, write down, "coughed."
    If you had an accident after having a strong urge to urinate, write "urge."
4. In the fourth column, write down about how much time passed in minutes between feeling a strong need to urinate and the time you had the accident. If it was instantaneous, write,"0".

Column #	1	2	3	4
Time Period	Times urinated in toilet	Check if accident happened	Reason or situation	Time between urge and accident
6-8 am		Accident ☐ Leak ☐ Large ☐		
8-10 am		Accident ☐ Leak ☐ Large ☐		
10-12 N		Accident ☐ Leak ☐ Large ☐		
12-2 pm		Accident ☐ Leak ☐ Large ☐		
2-4 pm		Accident ☐ Leak ☐ Large ☐		
4-6 pm		Accident ☐ Leak ☐ Large ☐		
6-8 pm		Accident ☐ Leak ☐ Large ☐		
8-10 pm		Accident ☐ Leak ☐ Large ☐		
10-12 MN		Accident ☐ Leak ☐ Large ☐		
Overnight		Accident ☐ Leak ☐ Large ☐		

Figure 41–3. Sample voiding diary.

> ### Establishing the presence of UI[6]
>
> *Tell me about any troubles you're having with your bladder.*
>
> *Tell me about any trouble you're having holding your urine (water).*
>
> *In the last 6 months, have you lost your urine when you didn't want to? (How often?)*
>
> *In the last 6 months, have you had to wear a pad or a protective undergarment to catch your urine?*
>
> ### Remember
>
> - *Use simple, easily understood terminology. The first open-ended request encourages the patient to report other bladder symptoms that may be related to the UI.*
> - *Specific questions can be used as part of a pre-visit screening questionnaire.*
> - *An odor of urine helps establish the presence of UI, but may also be a clue to self-neglect and unmet care needs.*

INTERVIEW FRAMEWORK

Incontinence is a symptom, not a diagnosis. The goal of the interview is to classify the UI in order to focus the physical examination, laboratory testing, and management. The following steps should be performed in nearly all patients presenting with UI:

- Document the frequency, severity, duration, and diurnal pattern of the UI. Severity can be measured indirectly by having the patient estimate the number of pads, incontinent briefs, or other protective devices used per day.
- Note *changes* in the frequency, severity, and diurnal pattern of UI for patients with a history of incontinence.
- Obtain a list of all prescription and nonprescription drugs and food supplements, as many common medications can affect bladder function.
- Note previous treatments for UI, their effectiveness, and side effects.
- Ask about previous pelvic surgery or radiation therapy; known vaginal prolapse, cystocele, or rectocele; obstetric history (especially vaginal deliveries); history of prostate surgery or disease; history of pelvic trauma; and new onset of diseases (eg, congestive heart failure).
- Identify other lower urinary tract and perineal symptoms (eg, frequency, nocturia, dysuria, hesitancy, dribbling, straining, hematuria, suprapubic or perineal pain).
- Inquire about the quantity and timing of fluid intake, especially of caffeine-containing beverages.
- Ascertain how the patient is currently managing the incontinence (eg, use of incontinence products, making sure that a bathroom is always nearby, stopping aerobic exercise).
- For older patients with new or worsening UI, assess the patient's functional and mental status (eg, mobility, recent falls, confusion).
- Ask about alterations in bowel habits or sexual function.
- Determine which urinary tract symptoms are the most bothersome and assess how the UI is affecting the patient's social functioning. Since UI is a major reason for institutionalization, also assess the reaction of the caregiver (if there is one).
- Learn the patient's expectations for outcomes of treatment.

IDENTIFYING ALARM SYMPTOMS

- In developmentally disabled and older adults, new or worsening UI may herald acute illness remote from the urinary tract (eg, pneumonia).
- In these patients, UI may be one of several recent changes in the patient's functional status, some of which may be serious (eg, falls, delirium).

Alarm symptoms	**Consider**
In older or developmentally disabled patient: new or worsening UI with or without other acute changes in the patient's functional or cognitive status	*Urinary tract or other infection* *Acute metabolic disturbance* *Stroke, myocardial infarction, or other acute medical condition*
Continuous leakage (every few minutes) with inability to urinate or sensation of full bladder	*Severe urinary retention with overflow (post-void residual mandatory to confirm retention)*
UI with dysuria	*Bacterial cystitis, urethritis from a sexually transmitted disease, atrophic urethritis from estrogen deficiency, nonbacterial cystitis*
UI with gross hematuria	*Hemorrhagic cystitis, bladder or urethral cancer*
UI with polyuria	*Metabolic disturbance (eg, hyperglycemia, hypercalcemia)*
UI with fecal matter or large air bubbles excreted during urination	*Vesicorectal (or vesicosigmoid) fistula as result of pelvic carcinoma or previous pelvic irradiation*
Consistent loss of urine in upright posture or with any action that produces a minimal increase in intra-abdominal pressure, despite bladder not feeling full	*Incompetent urethral sphincter or severe pelvic floor collapse*

FOCUSED QUESTIONS

These questions help you identify the type(s) of UI and contributing factors.

Questions	**Think about**
Quality	
In the past month, have you leaked urine	
• *While you were on your way to the toilet?*	*Urge incontinence*
• *Because you had to wait to use the toilet?*	*Urge incontinence*
• *When you delayed going to the toilet immediately after first feeling the need to urinate?*	*Urge incontinence*
Do you experience a warning (an urge to urinate)? Is the warning at least 1 minute before you leak urine?	
• *Yes to both questions*	*Urge incontinence*
• *No to both questions: urine just comes out*	*Detrussor disinhibition* *Overflow incontinence*
• *Yes to first and No to second question: experience a warning, but the urine comes out within a few seconds*	*Detrussor disinhibition* *Urge incontinence with short latency*
Do you ever leak urine while seated or lying without realizing it until later?	*Detrussor disinhibition* *Overflow incontinence*

(continued)

Quality	*Think About*
Have you wet yourself in the past month when you	
• Coughed, laughed, or sneezed?	Stress incontinence
• Lifted a heavy object?	Stress incontinence
• Stood up from a chair?	Stress incontinence
• Engaged in exercise (especially jumping or jogging)?	Stress incontinence
Are you unable to feel your bladder getting full before you experience a leakage of urine?	Autonomic neuropathy, causing urinary retention with overflow
	Detrussor disinhibition
When you leak urine, how large is the amount?	
• Moderate to large	Urge incontinence or detrussor disinhibition
• Small	Stress or overflow incontinence

Time course	*Think about*
Did the difficulty controlling your urine start or significantly worsen fairly suddenly, over hours to days?	
• Describe any symptoms that accompanied or immediately preceded the start or worsening of your urine leakage.	
– Symptoms of urge incontinence; see above	Acute urinary tract infection or urethritis producing urge incontinence
– Sudden onset of weakness or paralysis, suggestive of a stroke	Detrussor disinhibition
– Difficulty starting stream, dribbling (men), sensation of incomplete emptying of bladder	Urinary retention with overflow
• Describe any recent procedures that immediately preceded the start or significant worsening of your urine leakage.	
– Vaginal delivery	Stress incontinence
– Transurethral prostatectomy, other transurethral instrumentation	Stress incontinence
– Bladder catheter	Acute urinary tract infection producing urge incontinence
Did the difficulty controlling your urine come on gradually, over weeks to months?	Any incontinence subtype

Associated symptoms	*Think about*
Is it painful to urinate?	Urinary tract infection
	Atrophic urethritis (in women, associated with vaginal dryness, painful intercourse, sensitive labia)

Do you need to go frequently (urinary frequency)?	*Urinary tract infection*
	Atrophic urethritis
	Diuretics or conditions causing polyuria (eg, diabetes, hypercalcemia)
On average, how long is the interval between leakages?	
• *At least 1 hour*	*Urge or detrusor disinhibition*
• *Minutes or nearly continuous*	*Overflow incontinence*
• *Variable (depends on bladder volume plus maneuvers that increase intra-abdominal pressure)*	*Stress incontinence*
Do you experience constipation (eg, last bowel movement 3 or more days ago)?	*Fecal impaction, which may cause urge incontinence or urinary retention with overflow*
In the past month, have you wet the bed at night, or needed to use a pad or protective cover beneath you because of leaking while asleep?	*Detrussor disinhibition*
	Urge incontinence with short latency
	Functional incontinence (major difficulty getting to the toilet)
Do you need to strain or push to begin your stream? Is there a significant delay between trying to urinate and the urine starting to flow?	*Obstructive uropathy, which may cause a hyperactive bladder or urinary retention with overflow*
(Men) Is your stream weak or do you dribble?	*Obstructive uropathy, which may cause a hyperactive bladder or urinary retention with overflow*
When you urinate, do you feel that you are unable to completely empty your bladder?	*Urinary retention with overflow*
	DHIC in frail, older person
(Women) How many children have you had by vaginal delivery?	*Stress incontinence due to pelvic floor laxity (the greater the number, the higher the risk)*
After finishing urinating, do you need to return to the toilet in a few minutes because you feel the need to void again? If yes and you void again, what is the amount?	
• *None to a few drops*	*Urethritis or cystitis*
• *Small*	*Urinary retention with overflow*
• *Moderate to large*	*Large cystocele[a]*
	Diuretics, conditions causing polyuria (eg, diabetes)
(Directed to family member or caregiver) Has the patient been confused?	*Delirium or dementia causing detrussor disinhibition (In older persons, delirium and UI may signal an infection or metabolic disturbance; urinary retention may also cause delirium.)*
Have you been very depressed or lost interest in things? (To family member or caregiver) Has the patient seemed very depressed or lost interest in things?	*Detrussor disinhibition*
	Functional incontinence (patient indifferent to self-soiling)

(continued)

Associated symptoms	Think about
Do you require assistance to go to the toilet?	Functional incontinence
Do you have moderate or severe pain?	Overflow incontinence, due to inhibition of sphincter relaxation (from elevated serum catecholamines)

Modifying symptoms	Think about
Is the incontinence worse at night?	Excessive consumption of fluids or caffeinated beverages in the late afternoon or evening Taking diuretics in the evening
Is the incontinence worse during the day?	Excessive consumption of fluids or caffeinated beverages, use of diuretics or drugs that promote diuresis (eg, alcohol, theophylline)
Do you have a chronic cough that makes the incontinence worse?	Stress incontinence
Have you started a new medication or increased the dose?	
• A diuretic	Urge or functional incontinence
• α-Adrenergic blocker (terazosin, others)	Stress incontinence due to sphincter relaxation
• Anticholinergic drug (amitriptyline, diphenhydramine, oxybutynin, others)	Overflow incontinence due to impaired bladder contractility (usually in presence of preexisting bladder outlet obstruction or detrussor dysfunction)
• α-Adrenergic agonist (pseudoephedrine, others)	Overflow incontinence due to inadequate relaxation of sphincter (usually in presence of preexisting bladder outlet obstruction or detrussor dysfunction)
Have you been spending most of your time in bed?	Overflow incontinence from urinary retention due to prolonged bed rest

[a]A moderate amount of urine may be trapped inside a large cystocele during toileting but flows back into the main bladder cavity when the patient lies down, causing the patient to reexperience bladder fullness.

CAVEATS

- Because urinary incontinence is a symptom, a diagnostic approach aimed at solely identifying the type may preclude identification of serious underlying conditions or iatrogenic contributors.
- In elderly and disabled persons, UI may herald other functional impairments. Evaluation of UI should include an assessment of the patient's cognitive and physical functioning.
- Urge incontinence and detrussor disinhibition in elderly and disabled persons often persist as a chronic condition, which may have a negative impact on the patient's and caregiver's quality of life. Periodic reassessment of intervention strategies and patient and caregiver coping is an essential part of the ongoing management of UI.

PROGNOSIS

- Acute UI related to reversible causes generally has a good prognosis.
- Both urge and stress UI can improve with bladder retraining exercises, which may be as effective as medication.
- Newer surgical techniques and artificial sphincters have improved the prognosis for patients with severe UI due to pelvic floor dysfunction or sphincter incompetence.

REFERENCES

1. Hu T-W, Wagner TH, Bentkover JD, LeBlanc K, et al. Costs of urinary incontinence and overactive bladder in the United States: a comparative study. *Urology.* 2004;63:461–465.
2. Stewart WF, Van Rooyen JB, Cundiff GW, et al. Prevalence and burden of overactive bladder in the United States. *World J Urol.* 2003;20:327–336.
3. Miller YD, Brown WJ, Russell A, et al. Urinary incontinence across the lifespan. *Neurourol Urodyn.* 2003;22:550–557.
4. Parazzini F, Chiaffarino F, Lavezzari M, et al. Risk factors for stress, urge or mixed urinary incontinence in Italy. *BJOG.* 2003;110:927–933.
5. Kirschner-Hermanns R, Scherr PA, Branch LG, et al. Accuracy of survey questions for geriatric urinary incontinence. *J Urol.* 1998;159:1903–1908.
6. Fantyl JA, Newman DK, Colling J, et al. *Urinary Incontinence in Adults: Acute and Chronic Management. Clinical Practice Guideline No. 2, 1996 Update.* Rockville, MD: Agency for Health Care Policy and Research; March 1996. AHCPR Publication No. 96-0682.

SUGGESTED READING

Culligan PJ, Heit M. Urinary incontinence in women: evaluation and management. *Am Fam Physician.* 2000;62:2433–2444, 2447, 2452.

Griffiths DJ, McCracken PN, Harrison GM, Gormley EA, Moore KN. Urge incontinence and impaired detrusor contractility in the elderly. *Neurourol Urodyn.* 2002;21:126–131.

Kim YH, Frenkl T. Male urinary incontinence. *Med Health R I.* 2002;85:156–159.

Klausner AP, Vapnek JM. Urinary incontinence in the geriatric population. *Mt Sinai J Med.* 2003;70:54–61.

Miles TP, Palmer RF, Espino DV, et al. New-onset incontinence and markers of frailty: data from the Hispanic Established Populations for Epidemiologic Studies of the Elderly. *J Gerontol A Biol Sci Med Sci.* 2001;56:M19–24.

Ouslander JG. Geriatric urinary incontinence. *Disease-a-Month.* 1992;38:69–147.

Romanzi LJ. Urinary incontinence in women and men. *J Gend Specif Med.* 2001;4:14–20.

Wahle GR. Urinary incontinence after radical prostatectomy. *Semin Urol Oncol.* 2000;18:66–70.

Diagnostic Approach: Urinary Incontinence

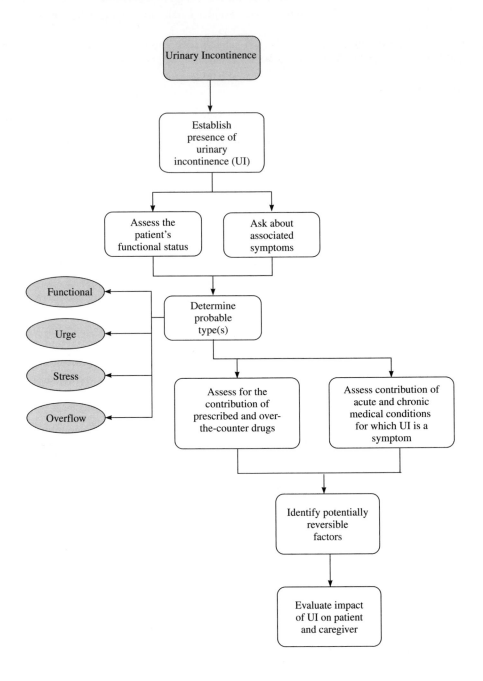

SECTION IX
Women's Health

Amenorrhea

Laura Pham, MD, & Tonya Fancher, MD, MPH

Amenorrhea is the absence of menses. This condition may be transient, intermittent, or permanent and usually results from congenital, neuroendocrine, or anatomic abnormalities. Amenorrhea is generally classified as either primary or secondary, which narrows the differential diagnosis and may simplify the diagnostic evaluation. However, the causes of primary and secondary amenorrhea may overlap.

KEY TERMS

Asherman syndrome	Intrauterine synechiae (adhesions) usually resulting from uterine instrumentation (eg, curettage or scraping of the uterine cavity to remove tissue).
Follicle-stimulating hormone (FSH) and luteinizing hormone (LH)	Pituitary hormones that stimulate the follicles of the ovary and assist in follicular maturation.
Gonadal dysgenesis (Turner syndrome)	The failure of the gonads to develop in the presence of an abnormal karyotype. Gonadal failure in the presence of a normal karyotype is termed gonadal agenesis.
Gonadotropin-releasing hormone (GnRH)	A hormone, secreted by the hypothalamus, which stimulates FSH and LH release.
Hypothalamic or functional amenorrhea	Disorder of GnRH release resulting in loss of the LH surge and anovulation.
Hypothalamic-pituitary-ovarian axis	The hormonal regulatory system that controls the menstrual/reproductive cycle.
Müllerian agenesis	The absence of the fallopian tubes, uterus, and internal portion of the vagina. Patients have normal female genotype, normal secondary sex characteristics (phenotype), and amenorrhea.
Polycystic ovary syndrome (PCOS)	Syndrome characterized by hirsutism (excessive body and facial hair), obesity, menstrual abnormalities, infertility, and enlarged ovaries.
Post-pill amenorrhea	Failure to resume ovulation 6 months after discontinuing hormonal contraception.

(continued)

KEY TERMS

Premature ovarian failure

Depletion of oocytes and surrounding follicles before age 40. Causes include chemotherapy, radiation, and autoimmune disease.

Primary amenorrhea

The absence of menses by age 16.

Secondary amenorrhea

The absence of menses for more than 3 menstrual cycles or 6 months in a woman who was previously menstruating.

ETIOLOGY

Differential Diagnosis: Primary Amenorrhea[1-4]	**Prevalence**[a]
Pregnancy	*Most common*
Anatomic and genetic abnormalities	
• *Gonadal dysgenesis (Turner syndrome)*	*45%*
• *Müllerian agenesis*	*15%*
• *Obstructed outflow tract (transverse vaginal septum, imperforate hymen)*	*5%*
Disorders of hypothalamic-pituitary-ovarian axis	
• *Physiologic delay of puberty*	*20%*
• *Hypothalamic dysfunction (see Secondary Amenorrhea below)*	
• *Pituitary dysfunction*	
• *Ovarian dysfunction*	
• *Other (hypothyroidism, androgen insensitivity, Kallman syndrome)*	

[a]Prevalence is unknown when not indicated.

Differential Diagnosis: Secondary Amenorrhea[1-4]	**Prevalence**[a]
Pregnancy	*Most common*
Anatomic abnormalities	
– *Asherman syndrome*	*7%*
Hypothalamic-pituitary-ovarian axis abnormalities	
• *Hypothalamic dysfunction*	
– *Abnormalities of height, weight, and nutrition (anorexia nervosa, bulimia)*	*15–54%*
– *Exercise*	*10%*
– *Psychosocial stress*	*10–21%*
– *Infiltrative diseases (sarcoidosis) or tumors (craniopharyngioma)*	*< 0.1%*

• *Pituitary dysfunction*	
– *Prolactin-secreting tumor*	*17%*
– *Empty sella syndrome*	*1%*
– *Sheehan syndrome*	*1%*
– *Adrenocorticotropic hormone–secreting tumor*	*< 1%*
– *Growth hormone–secreting tumor*	*< 1%*
• *Ovarian dysfunction*	
– *Premature ovarian failure*	*10%*
– *PCOS*	*30%*
– *Ovarian tumors*	*1%*
• *Other*	
– *Thyroid disease*	*1%*
– *Nonclassical adrenal hyperplasia*	*< 1%*
– *Drug-induced*	*1.5%*
– *Post-pill amenorrhea*	
– *Idiopathic*	*25%*

aPrevalence is unknown when not indicated.

GETTING STARTED

- Let the patient tell the story in her own words before asking more directed and focused questions.
- While interviewing the patient, try to get an overall impression of the patient's health status. Many specific medical conditions as well as poor overall health can cause amenorrhea.
- If the patient is not alone during your interview, set aside time to speak with her privately. Patients may feel uncomfortable discussing certain issues in front of a friend or family member.
- Although a thorough history is essential to the evaluation of amenorrhea, keep in mind that often laboratory tests and imaging will be required to make a diagnosis.

Questions	**Remember**
Tell me about your periods.	• *Listen to the patient's description*
At what age did your periods begin?	• *Don't rush the interview by interrupting or focusing the history too soon*
When did your last period begin?	
Do you have regular periods?	
What is your usual cycle length?	
Could you be pregnant?	

INTERVIEW FRAMEWORK

- In evaluating amenorrhea, first rule out pregnancy as a cause.
- Assess for alarm symptoms that will require urgent evaluation.

- Determine whether the patient has primary or secondary amenorrhea.
- Primary amenorrhea is usually caused by genetic or congenital disorders that may not become manifest until puberty. It is therefore important to ask about other developmental problems. Remember, development will be normal in patients with outflow tract defects.
- Secondary amenorrhea generally results from neuroendocrine or anatomic disorders. Begin with a detailed menstrual history that covers menarche to the present. Then use more focused questions to tease out patterns or clues to the etiology of the amenorrhea.

IDENTIFYING ALARM SYMPTOMS

Some causes of amenorrhea require prompt diagnosis and treatment.

Alarm signs and symptoms	Consider
Recent unprotected intercourse	*Pregnancy*
Headaches, galactorrhea, loss of peripheral vision	*Intracranial tumor*
Body weight 15% below ideal and impaired body image	*Anorexia*

FOCUSED QUESTIONS

Questions	Think about
Have you had unprotected intercourse?	*Pregnancy*
Have you had morning nausea?	*Pregnancy*
Have you noticed that most of your friends developed breasts and pubic hair before you?	*Hypogonadism* *Turner syndrome*
Are most of your friends (of similar age) taller than you?	*Hypogonadism* *Turner syndrome*
Have you recently lost or gained weight?	*Hypothalamic dysfunction* *Thyroid disease* *PCOS* *Occult malignancy*
Have you ever been told that you exercise too much?	*Hypothalamic dysfunction*
Have you recently lost weight?	*Hypothalamic dysfunction*
Have you been under greater than usual psychosocial stress?	*Hypothalamic dysfunction*
Do you have an impaired sense of smell?	*Kallman syndrome*
Have you ever been diagnosed with renal failure, thyroid disease, sarcoidosis, lymphoma, histiocytosis X, or juvenile rheumatoid arthritis?	*Many systemic illnesses may cause amenorrhea*
Do you have nipple discharge, impaired peripheral vision, or headaches?	*Pituitary tumor*

What medications are you taking?	*Medications such as oral contraceptives, dopamine antagonists (haloperidol, risperidone, metoclopramide, domperidone), or antihypertensive drugs which raise serum prolactin levels (methyldopa, reserpine), GnRH antagonists (danazol), and high-dose progestins may cause amenorrhea*
Have you taken oral contraceptives in the past year?	*Post-pill amenorrhea*
Have you ever had a uterine surgical procedure, infection, or abortion?	*Asherman syndrome*
Have you been pregnant recently?	*Postpartum amenorrhea*
If you were recently gave birth, were there any complications?	*Sheehan syndrome*
Have you ever been exposed to high doses of radiation (eg, for treatment of cancer)?	*Premature ovarian failure*
Have you ever received cancer chemotherapy?	*Premature ovarian failure*
Have you recently experienced hot flashes, night sweats, mood changes, or vaginal dryness?	*Premature ovarian failure*
Do you have excessive facial hair and acne?	*PCOS*
Do you have heat or cold intolerance, change in energy level, weight loss or gain, diarrhea or constipation, heart palpitations, change in skin or hair texture?	*Thyroid disease*
Have you had headaches, mood, or personality changes?	*Hypothalamic dysfunction due to infiltrative lesions*
Have you experienced fatigue, anorexia, weight loss, or fever?	*Lymphoma* *Sarcoidosis*
Do you have a chronic cough or difficulty breathing?	*Sarcoidosis*
Have you had weakness, weight loss, arthritis, or a change in skin color?	*Hemochromatosis*
Do you have a depressed mood, change in appetite, alteration of sleep patterns, or a lack of interest in things you normally enjoy?	*Depression*
Do you have recurring intrusive thoughts that cause you to engage in repetitive behaviors?	*Obsessive-compulsive disorder (medications)*
Do you see or hear things that others do not?	*Schizophrenia (medications)*

PROGNOSIS

Patients with amenorrhea often seek medical attention because they are concerned about the impact it will have on their future fertility. Recovery of normal menstrual cycles and reproductive ability varies greatly depending on the etiology of amenorrhea.

Reversible causes[5,6]

- *Imperforate hymen*
- *Asherman syndrome*
- *Polycystic ovarian syndrome*
- *Hyperprolactinemia*
- *Post-pill amenorrhea*
- *Drug-induced*
- *Exercise-, stress-, or weight-loss induced*
- *Systemic illness*

Irreversible causes[4,5]

- *Empty sella syndrome*
- *Cushing's syndrome*
- *Kallman syndrome*
- *Gonadal dysgenesis*
- *Müllerian defects*

Women with Turner syndrome and other genetic abnormalities are usually infertile. The few women who are able to successfully conceive experience high rates of miscarriage, stillbirth, and birth defects.[5]

Anatomic defects such as imperforate hymen and Asherman syndrome are often amenable to surgical correction.[6]

Amenorrhea associated with hormonal disturbances from PCOS and pituitary tumors may be corrected with normalization of hormone levels, using medical therapy alone or in conjunction with surgical procedures.[5]

Hypothalamic amenorrhea and amenorrhea due to systemic illness often resolve with treatment of the underlying condition.

REFERENCES

1. Barbieri RL. Amenorrhea. WebMD Scientific American Medicine. April 2002.

2. Reindollar RH, Novak M, Tho SPT, McDonough PG. Adult-onset amenorrhea: a study of 262 patients. *Am J Obstet Gynecol.* 1986;155:531–543.

3. Perkins RB, Hall JE, Martin KA. Aetiology, previous menstrual function and patterns of neuro-endocrine disturbance as prognostic indicators in hypothalamic amenorrhoea. *Hum Reprod.* 2001;16:2198–2205.

4. Hamilton-Fairly D, Taylor A. ABC of Subfertility: Anovulation. *BMJ.* 2003;327:546–549.

5. Abir R, Fisch B, Nahum R, Orvieto R, Nitke S, Ben Rafael Z. Turner's syndrome and fertility: current status and possible putative prospects. *Hum Reprod Update.* 2001;7:603–610.

6. Schenker JG. Etiology of and therapeutic approach to synechia uteri. *Eur J Obstet & Gynecol Reprod Biol.* 1996;65:109–113.

SUGGESTED READING

Falsetti L, Gambera A, Barbetti L, Specchia C. Long-term follow-up of functional hypothalamic amenorrhea and prognostic factors. *J Clin Endocrinol Metab.* 2002;87:500–505.

Timmreck LS, Reindollar RH. Contemporary issues in primary amenorrhea. *Obstet & Gynecol Clin North Am.* 2003;30:287–302.

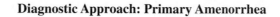

Diagnostic Approach: Primary Amenorrhea

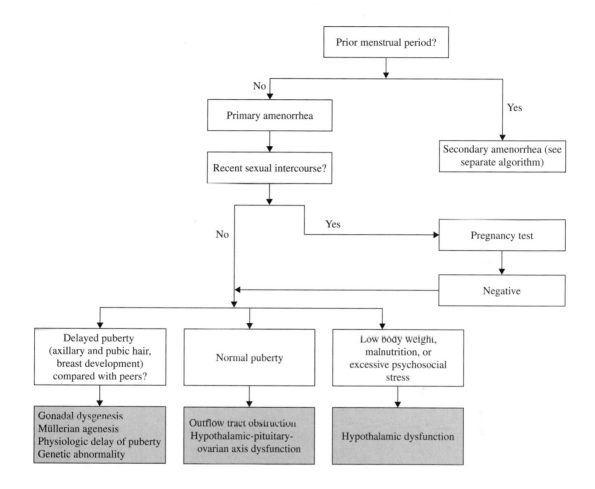

Diagnostic Approach: Secondary Amenorrhea

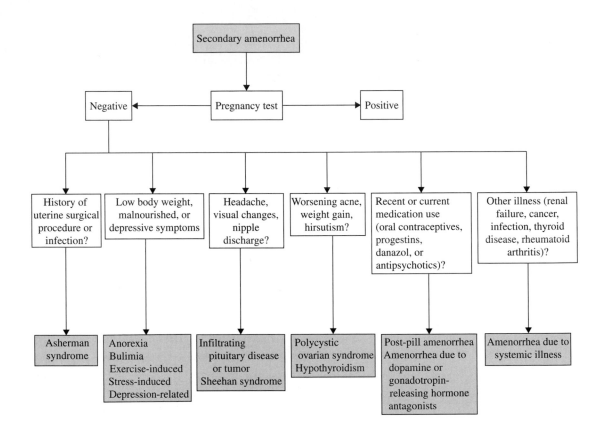

Breast Complaints

Helen K. Chew, MD

The 3 most common breast complaints are breast lumps, breast pain, and nipple discharge.[1,2] While most of these complaints prove to be due to a benign cause, the greatest fear among patients is the diagnosis of breast cancer. A delay in the diagnosis of breast cancer remains the leading cause of medical malpractice suits. Therefore, it is important to elicit features of the history that suggest a malignant process. The purposes of the physician evaluation are to rule out breast cancer and to address the underlying cause of the breast complaint.

KEY TERMS

Breast cancer	*Cancerous growth beginning in the ductal/lobular unit of the breast. If the cancer is confined to the ductal/lobular unit, it is referred to as ductal carcinoma in situ. If the cancer disrupts the basement membrane, it is referred to as invasive or infiltrating carcinoma.*
Duct ectasia	*The benign distention of subareolar ducts associated with breast discharge.*
Fibroadenoma	*A benign solid tumor with glandular and fibrous tissue, which is well defined and mobile.*
Fibrocystic changes	*An increased number of cysts or fibrous tissue in an otherwise normal breast. When these changes are accompanied by symptoms such as pain, nipple discharge, or lump(s), the condition is referred to as fibrocystic disease.*
Mastalgia	*Breast pain.*
Papilloma	*The growth of papillary cells from the wall of a duct or cyst into the lumen. This lesion is usually benign.*
Proliferative breast disease	*Premalignant changes in the breast including ductal hyperplasia, atypical ductal hyperplasia, and atypical lobular hyperplasia.*

ETIOLOGY

Most breast complaints prove to be due to a benign condition. However, the cause varies based on the particular symptom, the patient's age, and menopausal status. For example, fibroadenoma is more common in younger, premenopausal women. In contrast, the incidence of breast cancer increases with age.

Differential Diagnosis	Comments	Prevalence[a]
Fibrocystic disease	The most common cause of breast lumpiness and pain	Accounts for 20% of breast complaints in primary care clinics[1]
Fibroadenoma		The cause in 7–13% of breast lumps in a specialty clinic
Mastitis/breast abscess		Occurs in up to 13% of lactating post-partum women[3]
Stretching of Cooper's ligaments	Cyclical breast pain in women with large, pendulous breasts	
Papilloma	The most common cause of a bloody nipple discharge	50% of patients have nipple discharge without a palpable mass[4]
Breast cancer	The risk of developing breast cancer increases with age. For women up to age 39 years, the risk is 1 in 228; for women 40–59 years, the risk is 1 in 24; for women 60–79 years, the risk is 1 in 14.[5]	Found in < 10% of biopsies for lumps, pain, or discharge in primary care clinics[1]

[a]Prevalence is unknown when not indicated.

GETTING STARTED

- Review medication list prior to evaluation and confirm with patient.
- Determine whether patient is menopausal.

Questions	Remember
Tell me about your breast problem.	• Allow patient to use her (or his) own words.
How long have you had this breast problem?	• Determine the patient's anxiety level regarding breast cancer.
Is this problem in 1 or both breasts?	
Is there any relationship of this problem to your periods (if patient is premenopausal)?	
Is there any relationship of this problem to new medicines, including oral contraceptives or hormone replacement therapy?	
Are you worried about breast cancer?	

INTERVIEW FRAMEWORK

For any breast problem, a thorough history should focus on:

- The patient's breast cancer risk factors.
- Medications.
- Other medical problems.
- Relationship to the menstrual cycle.

Breast cancer risk factors include[6]:

- Increasing age.
- Early age at menarche (< 11).
- Older age at menopause (> 55).
- Nulliparity or age at first live birth > 35 years.
- Family history of breast cancer, particularly in first-degree relatives.
- Prior breast biopsies, especially showing atypia.
- Prior breast cancer.
- Prior neck or chest radiation.

Despite these established risk factors, 70% of patients in whom breast cancer has been diagnosed have no identifiable risk factor except for age.[7] Five to 10% of patients will have a family history suggestive of hereditary breast cancer.

Inquire about recent medications, even if already discontinued. Ask specifically about oral contraceptive pills (OCPs), transdermal estrogen formulations, and hormone replacement therapy (HRT) as the patient may overlook these. Exogenous estrogens may contribute to breast symptoms, including breast tenderness or breast lumps.

Ask about other medical problems, particularly hypothyroidism, pituitary problems, and the possibility of pregnancy or recent lactation. Also inquire about accompanying symptoms such as headaches or visual changes, which may be associated with less common causes such as hypothyroidism or pituitary adenomas.

Many breast complaints are cyclical and worse prior to menstruation. Ask about menstrual irregularities and infertility.

If a patient is over 35 years of age, determine whether she had breast imaging such as a mammogram.

IDENTIFYING ALARM SYMPTOMS

In the absence of a breast mass or radiographic abnormalities, the majority of breast complaints prove to be due to a benign cause. If the patient describes breast pain or discharge, ask directly about whether they feel a mass or if there are accompanying changes in the skin overlying the breast.

The prevalence of breast cancer in patients with breast complaints has not been well established. However, breast cancer was the diagnosis in less than 10% of women undergoing breast biopsy in primary care clinics.[1]

Serious Diagnoses

- Breast cancer

Alarm symptoms	Serious causes	Benign causes
Breast mass	*Breast cancer*	*Fibrocystic disease* *Fibroadenoma*
Skin ulceration, thickening	*Inflammatory breast cancer* *Breast abscess*	*Mastitis*

(continued)

Alarm symptoms	Serious causes	Benign causes
Axillary mass	Breast cancer	Benign adenopathy
Bloody nipple discharge	Breast cancer	Papilloma Physiologic conditions
Strong family history of breast and/or ovarian cancer	Hereditary breast cancer	Sporadic cancer history
Systemic symptoms, including new respiratory symptoms, bone pain, headaches	Metastatic breast cancer	Unrelated symptoms (eg, respiratory infection, arthritis, migraines, etc)

FOCUSED QUESTIONS

Questions

Breast lump or skin changes	Think about
How quickly did this change come on? Did it begin gradually or all of a sudden?	Chronic lumpiness may be due to fibrocystic breasts. A long-standing breast mass in a young woman may be a fibroadenoma.
Is this lump movable?	Cancer is more of a concern when masses are immobile or are fixed to surrounding structures.
Is this the only lump or are there many?	Cancer is more of a concern when nodules are discrete and solitary. Diffuse lumpiness is usually benign.
Is this lumpiness in 1 breast or both?	Bilateral breast cancer is extremely rare and accounts for 1% of all presenting breast cancers. Bilateral breast lumpiness is usually due to fibrocystic changes.
Are you taking hormones for any reason?	Hormonal changes in the breast are common and associated with OCPs and HRT.
Does this lump change with your periods?	Cyclical lumps are usually due to hormonal surges prior to menstruation.

Breast pain, sensitivity, or soreness	Think about
Can you feel a mass or lump in the area of pain?	Breast cancer or fibroadenoma
Does the pain change with your periods?	Cyclical breast sensitivity is usually due to hormonal surges prior to menstruation. Chronic pain may be due to large, pendulous breasts and the stretching of Cooper's ligaments.
Did the pain begin suddenly?	Mastitis, cellulitis, or other infection. Thrombosis of the lateral thoracic vein (Mondor disease) is extremely rare.
Have you hurt yourself in the chest, been in an automobile accident, or had recent surgery?	Trauma
Have you had a fever or is the skin warm?	Mastitis, cellulitis, or other infection

Does caffeine make it worse?	Fibrocystic breasts may be more sensitive to caffeine.
Is the pain severe, interfering with life?	Reassure if other work-up negative and consider treatment for mastalgia.[8]
Breast discharge[9]	**Think about**
Can you feel a mass or lump in the breast?	Breast cancer
Is this in 1 breast or both?	Bilateral discharge is almost always due to physiologic or endocrine etiologies.
If in 1 breast, is the discharge from 1 part of the nipple (1 duct) or from all parts of the nipple?	Discharge from 1 duct is more likely due to a problem with a specific duct such as papilloma or less commonly in situ cancer. Discharge from multiple ducts is more likely due to a physiologic cause such as medications or lactation.
Does the discharge come out by itself or do you have to express it?	Cancer is more of a concern when discharge is spontaneous.
Describe the color of your discharge.	Cancer or papilloma is more of a concern when discharge is bloody serosanguinons. Green, black, brown, or other colored discharge is usually due to a benign problem such as duct ectasia or normal physiologic discharge.
Does this discharge change with your period?	Physiologic discharge may be due to hormonal surges prior to menstruation.
Is there a recent change in bra?	Constrictive clothing may stimulate breast discharge.
Do you have headaches or changes in your vision?	Pituitary adenoma may cause galactorrhea.
Time course	**Comment**
Is the lump/pain/discharge associated with your period?	Most causes of benign breast disease are cyclical in nature.
Did you notice this symptom after starting a new medication?	Hormonal therapy may increase lumpiness or tenderness and cause discharge. Dopamine antagonists (eg, phenothiazines, haloperidol) and other medications may be associated with discharge.
Have you recently stopped/started nursing?	It is not unusual to have discharge last up to several months after prior lactation.
Associated and modifying symptoms	**Think about**
Do you have headaches, nausea and vomiting, or vision changes?	Pituitary pathology
Have you had fevers?	Infection may lead to skin changes
Have you had prior breast surgery?	Scar tissue, recent trauma

DIAGNOSTIC APPROACH

- Determine whether there is an underlying mass. Most complaints of pain or discharge without a palpable mass or radiographic abnormality are due to benign conditions and the patient can be reassured.[10]

- What is the patient's risk of breast malignancy? Is this an older postmenopausal woman with a new lump or skin changes (more likely to have cancer) or a young woman with cyclical lumpiness (more likely to be fibrocystic disease)?
- If the patient is over 35 years and hasn't had a mammogram, imaging should be considered to evaluate a new breast complaint.
- See Figure, Diagnostic Approach: Breast Complaints.

CAVEATS

- Although breast cancer risk assessment may be helpful in stratifying patients, keep in mind that most patients in whom breast cancer develops do not have these risk factors.
- If a patient complains of a discrete mass, this needs to be worked up completely (eg, breast biopsy) even with a "normal" or unremarkable mammogram.
- Breast pain or discharge in the absence of a mass or radiographic abnormality is unlikely due to cancer.
- Increase your suspicion of breast cancer in patients who are postmenopausal or have had prior breast cancer or a prior breast biopsy showing atypia.

PROGNOSIS

- Fibrocystic disease does not increase the risk of developing breast cancer.
- Cyclical breast pain is more likely to respond to medical treatment than noncyclical mastalgia.[8]
- The prognosis for breast cancer varies with stage. Five-year survival is 97% for patients with localized disease, 79% for patients with regional involvement, and only 23% for those who have distant (metastatic) disease. Fortunately, only 10% of patients have distant disease at presentation, according to the American Cancer Society and SEER database at www.cancer.org.

REFERENCES

1. Barton MB, Elmore JG, Fletcher SW. Breast symptoms among women enrolled in a health maintenance organization: frequency, evaluation, and outcome. *Ann Intern Med.* 1999;130:651–657.
2. Williams RS, Brook D, Monypenny IJ, Gower-Thomas K. The relevance of reported symptoms in a breast screening programme. *Clin Radiol.* 2002;57:725–729.
3. Foxman B, D'Arcy H, Gillespie B, Bobo JK, Schwartz K. Lactation mastitis: occurrence and medical management among 946 breastfeeding women in the United States. *Am J Epidemiol.* 2002;155:103–114.
4. Florio MG, Manganaro T, Pollicino A, Scarfo P, Micali B. Surgical approach to nipple discharge: a ten-year experience. *J Surg Oncol.* 1999;71:235–238.
5. Jemal A, Murray T, Samuels A, Ghafoor A, Ward E, Thurn MJ. Cancer Statistics, 2003. *CA Cancer J Clin.* 2003;53:5–26.
6. Gail MH, Brinton LA, Byar DP, et al. Projecting individualized probabilities of developing breast cancer for white females who are being examined annually [see comments]. *J Natl Cancer Inst.* 1989;81:1879–1886.
7. Madigan MP, Ziegler RG, Benichou J, Byrne C, Hoover RN. Proportion of breast cancer cases in the United States explained by well-established risk factors. *J Natl Cancer Inst.* 1995;87:1681–1685.
8. Gateley CA, Miers M, Mansel RE, Hughes LE. Drug treatments for mastalgia: 17 years experience in the Cardiff Mastalgia Clinic. *J R Soc Med.* 1992;85:12–15.
9. King TA, Carter KM, Bolton JS, Fuhrman GM. A simple approach to nipple discharge. *Am Surg.* 2000;66:960–965; discussion 965–966.
10. Morrow M. The evaluation of common breast problems. *Am Fam Physician.* 2000;61:2371–2378, 2385.

SUGGESTED READING

Armstrong K, Eisen A, Weber B. Assessing the risk of breast cancer. *N Engl J Med.* 2000;342:564–571.

Diagnosis and management of benign breast disease. In: Harris JR et al, editors. *Diseases of the Breast.* Lippincott Williams & Wilkins; 2000.

Diagnostic Approach: Breast Complaints

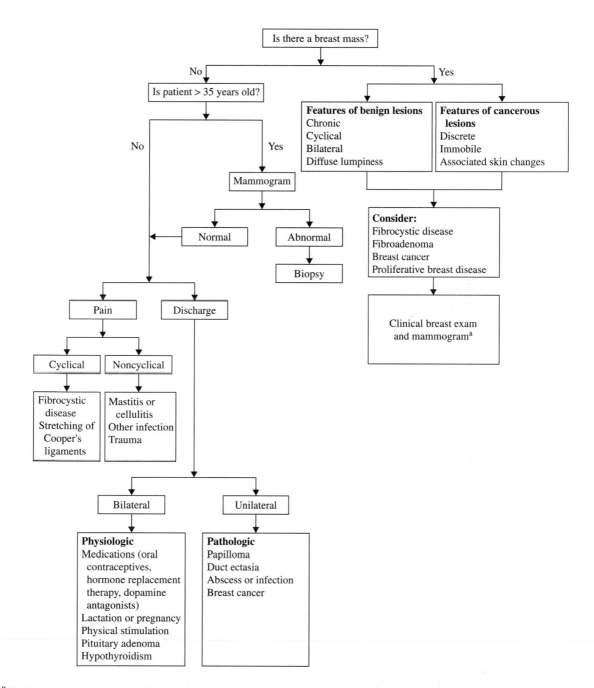

[a]Physical exam and radiographic features are imperative in the diagnostic evaluation. A persistent mass must be thoroughly evaluated even if radiography is unremarkable.

Pelvic Pain

Francesca C. Dwamena, MD

Pelvic pain is a common problem plaguing 39% of women in primary care[1] and 15% of community women in the United States.[2] In a study of 284,162 women aged 12 to 70 years, the annual prevalence of chronic pelvic pain (CPP) was similar to that of migraine, asthma, and back pain.[3] CPP accounts for up to10% of outpatient gynecologic referrals and is the primary reason for 10–35% of laparoscopies and 10–12% of hysterectomies performed in the United States at an estimated cost of more than $2 billion annually.[4,5]

KEY TERMS

Acute pelvic pain (APP)	_Pain symptoms below the umbilicus that have been present for less than 3 months._
Chronic pelvic pain (CPP)	_Nonmenstrual pain below the umbilicus of at least 3 months' duration._
Cyclic pelvic pain	_Pain below the umbilicus that is exacerbated before and during menses._
Dysmenorrhea	_Recurrent crampy, lower abdominal pain during menses._
Negative likelihood ratio (LR–)	_The increase in the odds of a particular diagnosis if a factor is absent._
Positive likelihood ratio (LR+)	_The increase in odds of a particular diagnosis if a factor is present._

ETIOLOGY

The most serious causes of pelvic pain present acutely (< 3 months) and can be classified as pregnancy-related causes, gynecologic disorders, and nonreproductive disorders.[6] The relative frequencies of these disorders in patients with APP have not been elucidated and clinical diagnosis has been notoriously difficult. For example, no abnormality was found in 23% of patients with a clinical diagnosis of pelvic inflammatory disease (PID) on laparoscopic examination; 12% were found to have a different diagnosis, including ectopic pregnancy, endometriosis, acute appendicitis, and complications of ovarian cysts.[7] Similarly, laparoscopy confirmed PID in only 46% of cases clinically diagnosed as PID,[8] and only 37.8% of cases with a clinical diagnosis of adnexal torsion were confirmed by surgery in another series.[9]

Diagnosis of CPP is even more challenging. Although laparoscopic studies have suggested pelvic adhesions and endometriosis as the most important findings,[10] other controlled studies suggest that these may be incidental rather than causal.[11] Moreover, no visible gynecologic pathology is evident on laparoscopy in up to 36% of patients with CPP.[4] In such patients, CPP may be functional (eg, myofascial pain or irritable bowel syndrome) or psychogenic (eg, depression, anxiety, somatization).[11]

Differential Diagnosis of APP

Pregnancy related

Ectopic pregnancy

Abortion

Intrauterine pregnancy with corpus luteum bleeding

Gynecologic

Acute PID

Endometriosis

Ovarian cyst (hemorrhage or rupture)

Adnexal torsion

Uterine leiomyoma (degeneration or torsion)

Tumor

Nongynecologic, gastrointestinal

Acute appendicitis

Inflammatory bowel disease

Mesenteric adenitis
Irritable bowel syndrome

Diverticulitis

Nongynecologic, urinary tract

Urinary tract infection

Renal calculus

Medically unexplained

Differential Diagnosis of CPP

Prevalence[a]

Cyclic or recurrent pelvic pain

Primary dysmenorrhea

Mittelschmerz

Endometriosis

Adnexal torsion

Müllerian duct anomalies

Noncyclic CPP (laparoscopic findings)[b]

	Prevalence[a]
Endometriosis	37%
Pelvic adhesions	26%
Cystic ovaries	1%
Normal laparoscopy	36%

[a]Prevalence is unknown when not indicated.
[b]CPP may also be functional or psychogenic.

GETTING STARTED

- Let the patient tell the pelvic pain story in her own words before asking more directed and focused questions.
- Be sure to elicit patient's personal and emotional story to establish the relationship and to assess whether there is primary or comorbid psychological disease.
- Understand the patient's agenda. Patients often seek medical care due to concern about a serious cause.

Open-ended questions

Tell me about your pelvic pain
Is this pain the same pelvic pain you've had before or is it different in some way?

When did the pelvic pain first start?
Give me an example of your most recent pelvic pain; tell me what you experienced from beginning to end.

Why did you choose to see me for the pelvic pain today?

Remember

- *Listen to the story.*
- *Don't try to rush the interview by interrupting and focusing the history too soon.*
- *Reassure the patient when possible.*

- *This question determines whether pain is acute, chronic, or both. Chronic pelvic pain is usually benign.*

- *Determine the patient's primary agenda for the visit and most concerning feature.*

INTERVIEW FRAMEWORK

- The first goal is to determine whether the pelvic pain is acute or chronic, cyclic or noncyclic.
- Inquire about pain characteristics using the cardinal symptom features:
  - Onset
  - Duration
  - Frequency
  - Pain character
  - Location of pain
  - Associated features
  - Precipitating and alleviating factors
  - Change in frequency or character over time.

IDENTIFYING ALARM SYMPTOMS

Serious Diagnoses

Serious diagnoses in patients with pelvic pain are rare. The relative frequencies of the conditions shown below in all patients with pelvic pain are unknown but are likely to be lower than reported.

After the open-ended portion of the history, determine whether pelvic pain is acute (< 3 months) or chronic (> 3 months). If not clear, then specifically ask about the presence of the alarm symptoms to assess for the possibility of a serious cause for pelvic pain.

Diagnosis	Population	Frequency
Acute PID	Age 15–39	1–1.3%[12]
	Age 20–24	2%[12] (incidence)
Ectopic pregnancy	All reported pregnancies in the United States (in 1992)	2%[a] (prevalence)
Adnexal torsion	Gynecologic surgical emergencies	2.7%[9] (prevalence)
Acute appendicitis	Patients suspected of acute appendicitis	0.84%[13] (incidence)

[a]http://www.cdc.gov/mmwr/preview/mmwrhtml/00035709.htm

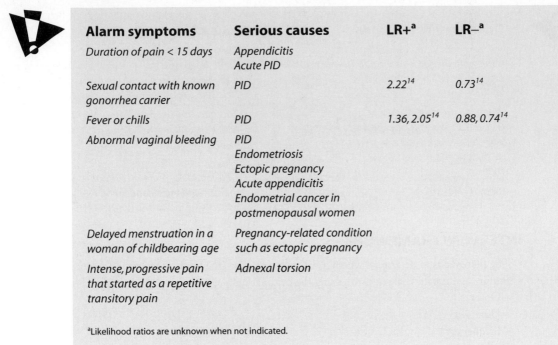

Alarm symptoms	Serious causes	LR+[a]	LR–[a]
Duration of pain < 15 days	Appendicitis Acute PID		
Sexual contact with known gonorrhea carrier	PID	2.22[14]	0.73[14]
Fever or chills	PID	1.36, 2.05[14]	0.88, 0.74[14]
Abnormal vaginal bleeding	PID Endometriosis Ectopic pregnancy Acute appendicitis Endometrial cancer in postmenopausal women		
Delayed menstruation in a woman of childbearing age	Pregnancy-related condition such as ectopic pregnancy		
Intense, progressive pain that started as a repetitive transitory pain	Adnexal torsion		

[a]Likelihood ratios are unknown when not indicated.

FOCUSED QUESTIONS

After hearing the patient's story in her own words and considering possible alarm symptoms, ask the following questions, if not already answered, to begin to narrow the differential diagnosis.

Questions	Think about
How old are you?	Young age (15–25 years) is a risk factor for PID
Menstrual history	
• How old were you when you first started your periods? • How long do your periods last? • What is the length of your cycle? • How heavy are your periods? How many times do you have to change your pads or tampons?	Excessive bleeding suggests uterine fibroids or adenomyosis
Obstetric history	
• Have you ever been pregnant? • Have you had any problem becoming pregnant?	A history of infertility and dysmenorrhea suggests endometriosis
Have you been sexually involved with a partner in the past 6 months? If yes, ask the following questions:	Sexual abstinence rules out pregnancy-related disorder, although a pregnancy test is suggested in all patients

• With women, men, or both?	A male sexual partner with symptoms of urethritis increases the risk for PID
• Have you had more than 5 sexual partners in your lifetime?	Multiple sexual partners increase the risk of PID
• When did you last have sex with a partner?	A woman who has been sexually abstinent in the months preceding the onset of pain is unlikely to have a pregnancy-related etiology
• What is your method of contraception?	Use of an intrauterine contraceptive device (IUD) is a risk factor for PID and ectopic pregnancy. Conversely, risk for PID is reduced by 50% in patients taking oral contraceptives (OCP) or using a barrier method; and reliable use of combined OCP decreases risk for ectopic pregnancy and complications of functional ovarian cysts. Pregnancy in a woman who has undergone tubal ligation has a 30-fold risk of being ectopic.[6]
• Do you have pain with intercourse?	Deep dyspareunia suggests endometriosis.[6]
Has anyone ever hit you or forced you to have sex? How old were you?	Childhood sexual abuse before the age of 15 is associated with the later development of CPP

Quality

What does the pain feel like?

Think about

• Constant and burning?	Neuropathic pain such as pudendal neuralgia (pain in area supplied by the pudendal nerve such as external genitalia, urethra, anus, and perineum)

Where is the pain located?

• It started in the epigastrum or periumbilical area and migrated to right lower quadrant	Appendicitis
• Pain is unilateral	Adnexal torsion
• Pain is bilateral	PID Ruptured or hemorrhagic ovarian cyst
• Colicky flank pain that radiates to the anterior abdomen	Urinary stone disease

On a scale of 1 to 10, with 10 being the worst pain you ever had in your life, how severe is your pain?

Time course

Tell me about how the pain started and progressed.

Think about

Symptoms associated with infection usually develop progressively over a few days.
Pain occurs suddenly with rupture or torsion, and the patient can usually tell precisely at what time symptoms began.[15]

(continued)

Associated symptoms	Think about
Have you noticed any urgency or increased frequency of urination?	Patients with interstitial cystitis report urgency and increased frequency as the most distressing symptoms.
Have you noticed any blood in your stool?	Bloody diarrhea suggests inflammatory bowel disease.
Modifying factors	**Think about**
Have you found that anything in particular worsens or improves your pelvic pain?	
• Rest makes it better	Musculoskeletal or adnexal torsion

DIAGNOSTIC APPROACH

The first step is to determine whether pelvic pain is acute or chronic and to distinguish old from new pain. The history should include a thorough review of the gynecologic, gastrointestinal, urologic, and psychological systems.

PROGNOSIS

The prognosis of CPP is excellent. In a retrospective cohort study of 86 females with pelvic pain and negative ultrasound, 77% of patients reported improvement or resolution of symptoms after a mean follow-up period of 15 months.[5] In that study, those with APP were more likely to report improvement than those with CPP (86% vs 50%); and only 4 of 11 patients who had subsequent laparoscopies were found to have significant abnormality (eg, endometriosis, adenomyosis, pelvic adhesions). Similarly, Baker et al[16] reported improved pain scores after 6 months in 58 of 60 patients with CPP and negative laparoscopy. However, Richter et al[17] found high incidence of anxiety, depression, physical worries, and marital problems in both laparoscopy-positive and laparoscopy-negative women with CPP even after long-term follow-up, despite modest improvement of pain. This emphasizes the importance of a multidisciplinary approach to these patients.

REFERENCES

1. Jamieson DJ, Steege JF. The prevalence of dysmenorrhea, dyspareunia, pelvic pain, and irritable bowel syndrome in primary care practices. *Obstet Gynecol.* 1996;87:55–58.

2. Mathias SD, Kuppermann M, Liberman RF, et al. Chronic pelvic pain: prevalence, health-related quality of life, and economic correlates. *Obstet Gynecol.* 1996;87:321–327.

3. Zondervan KT, Yudkin PL, Vessey MP, et al. Prevalence and incidence of chronic pelvic pain in primary care: evidence from a national general practice database. *Br J Obstet Gynaecol.* 1999;106:1149–1155.

4. Reiter RC. A profile of women with chronic pelvic pain. *Clin Obstet Gynecol.* 1990;33:130–136.

5. Harris RD, Holtzman SR, Poppe AM. Clinical outcome in female patients with pelvic pain and normal pelvic US findings. *Radiology.* 2000;216:440–443.

6. Quan M. Diagnosis of acute pelvic pain. *J Fam Pract.* 1992;35:422–432.

7. Jacobson L, Westrom L. Objectivized diagnosis of acute pelvic inflammatory disease. Diagnostic and prognostic value of routine laparoscopy. *Am J Obstet Gynecol.* 1969;105:1088–1098.

8. Chaparro MV, Ghosh S, Nashed A, Poliak A. Laparoscopy for the confirmation and prognostic evaluation of pelvic inflammatory disease. *Int J Gynaecol Obstet.* 1978;15:307–309.

9. Hibbard LT. Adnexal torsion. *Am J Obstet Gynecol.* 1985;152:456–461.

10. Kresch AJ, Seifer DB, Sachs LB, Barrese I. Laparoscopy in 100 women with chronic pelvic pain. *Obstet Gynecol.* 1984; 64:672–674.

11. Walker E, Katon W, Harrop-Griffiths J, et al. Relationship of chronic pelvic pain to psychiatric diagnoses and childhood sexual abuse. *Am J Psychiatry.* 1988;145:75–80.

12. Westrom L. Incidence, prevalence, and trends of acute pelvic inflammatory disease and its consequences in industrialized countries. *Am J Obstet Gynecol.* 1980;138(7 Pt 2):880–892.

13. Korner H, Soreide JA, Pedersen EJ, et al. Stability in incidence of acute appendicitis. A population-based longitudinal study. *Dig Surg.* 2001;18:61–66.

14. Kahn JG, Walker C, Washington AE, et al. Diagnosing pelvic inflammatory disease. A comprehensive analysis and considerations for developing a new model. *JAMA.* 1991;266:2594–2604.

15. Goldstein DP. Acute and chronic pelvic pain. *Pediatr Clin North Am.* 1989;36:573–580.

16. Baker PN, Symonds EM. The resolution of chronic pelvic pain after normal laparoscopy findings. *Am J Obstet Gynecol.* 1992;166:835–836.

17. Richter HE, Holley RL, Chandraiah S, Varner RE. Laparoscopic and psychologic evaluation of women with chronic pelvic pain. *Int J Psychiatry Med.* 1998;28:243–253.

SUGGESTED READING

Hewitt GD, Brown RT. Acute and chronic pelvic pain in female adolescents. *Med Clin North Am.* 2000;84:1009–1025.

Lifford KL, Barbieri RL. Diagnosis and management of chronic pelvic pain. *Urol Clin North Am.* 2002;29:637–647.

Milburn A, Reiter RC, Rhomberg AT. Multidisciplinary approach to chronic pelvic pain. *Obstet Gynecol Clin North Am.* 1993; 20:643–661.

Quan M. Diagnosis of acute pelvic pain. *J Fam Pract.* 1992;35:422–432.

Diagnostic Approach: Pelvic Pain

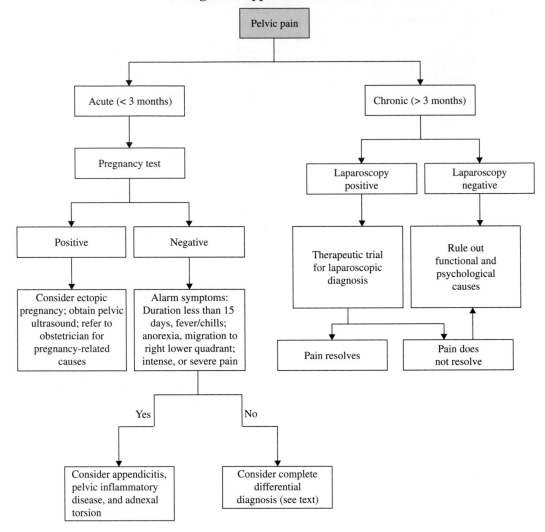

Vaginitis

Carol Bates, MD, & Michele Coviello, MD

Vulvovaginal symptoms are among the most common reasons that patients consult a primary care physician. It is difficult to assess the actual prevalence of vulvovaginitis because many patients treat their own symptoms with over-the-counter medications and never seek medical advice.

While not usually life-threatening, recurrent or chronic vulvovaginal complaints often involve significant discomfort, sexual dysfunction, and emotional distress. Most patients will ultimately prove to have a benign cause of vaginitis, but vaginal symptoms may indicate more serious upper genital tract disease requiring urgent evaluation and treatment. Clinicians should not rely upon history alone and should confirm the suspected diagnosis with pelvic examination and microscopy.

KEY TERMS

Cervicitis	Irritation or infection that primarily involves the cervix and can cause vaginal discharge. Usually the vulva is spared.
Dyspareunia	Discomfort during intercourse. The discomfort may be superficial (pain on initial penetration or with attempted penetration) or deep (related to deep penetration only).
Dysuria	Pain or burning with urination.
Pelvic inflammatory disease (PID)	Infection involving the uterus, fallopian tubes and ovaries, which can lead to peritonitis.
Pruritus	Itching.
Sexually transmitted disease (STD)	Infection anywhere in the genital tract transmitted via interpersonal genital contact. Includes infection with chlamydia, gonorrhea, syphilis, herpes simplex, trichomonas.
Toxic shock syndrome (TSS)	Life-threatening syndrome of fever, hypotension, multiorgan failure, and rash caused by enterotoxins produced by Staphylococcus aureus or group A streptococcus. Associated with the use of highly absorbent tampons or foreign bodies left in the vagina for prolonged periods.
Upper and lower genital tract	The upper genital tract includes the ovaries, fallopian tubes, and uterus. The lower genital tract includes the vagina, vulva, and other external structures. The cervix is in the lower tract but is the portal to the upper tract and so may be involved in upper tract processes.

(continued)

KEY TERMS

Vaginal discharge

Vaginal fluid composed of cervical mucus, exfoliated epithelial cells, bacteria, and vaginal secretions. Normally, it is odorless and white or clear in appearance. The appearance and amount of vaginal discharge varies with estrogen and progesterone levels, irritation, and infection.

Vaginitis

Inflammation of the vagina characterized by vaginal soreness and/or itching, usually but not always accompanied by vaginal discharge. A summative term used to describe a variety of vaginal complaints.

Vulvitis

Symptoms of irritation felt externally in the vulva. The irritation is not always accompanied by an increase or change in vaginal discharge.

Vulvovaginitis

Irritation felt externally in the vulva and internally in the vagina.

ETIOLOGY

Approximately 90% of all vulvovaginitis is infectious and is due to candidiasis, trichomoniasis, or bacterial vaginosis.[1–3] The remaining 10% of vulvovaginitis results from noninfectious causes such as irritants, low estrogen states, and dermatologic disorders.

Differential Diagnosis	Prevalence[a]
Infections	
• Candidiasis	20–24% in urban STD clinic[3,4]
• Bacterial vaginosis	20–33% in urban STD clinic[3,5]
• Trichomoniasis	10–15% in urban STD clinic[3,6]
• Cervicitis	20–25% in urban STD clinic[3]
Atrophic vaginitis	8–47% of postmenopausal women[7]
Dermatologic disorders	
Irritant vaginitis (ie, latex, chemical vaginitis from douche)	
Physiologic discharge	

[a]Prevalence is unknown when not indicated.

GETTING STARTED

It is important to realize that small amounts of vaginal discharge are normal. Between 1 mL and 4 mL of fluid is produced daily. Normal vaginal discharge may be colorless, white, or pale yellow. Vaginal discharge increases normally at ovulation when the thick and viscid cervical mucous plug is expelled.

Vaginal complaints can be very difficult for women to discuss. Be patient and try to let the woman tell her story in her own words.

Many women do not examine their vulvas or vaginas and so cannot pinpoint the location of their symptoms. Gently encourage the patient to be specific about symptoms.

Taking a detailed sexual history is paramount. Remember to obtain the history in an open and non-judgmental manner. Patients may be concerned about sexually transmitted diseases and about their partners' fidelity.

Questions	Remember
Tell me what the discharge looks and feels like.	*Elucidate the color, consistency, odor, and amount of the discharge.*
Is there discomfort or itching? If so, where?	
Are you currently involved in a sexual relationship?	

INTERVIEW FRAMEWORK

- Assess for alarm symptoms.
- Ascertain sexual history including number of sexual partners and specific sexual practices (see Focused Questions below).
- Inquire about contraceptive use.
- Ask about prior episodes of vaginitis and their treatment.
- Determine history of prior STDs.
- Take a menstrual history.
- Explore use of any vaginal topical or douching products.
- Review medication history.
- Inquire about history of systemic illness, particularly dermatologic and gastrointestinal problems.
- Inquire about exact anatomic location of discomfort.

IDENTIFYING ALARM SYMPTOMS

Serious Diagnoses

While vulvovaginitis causes discomfort and irritation, it does not cause acute systemic illness. Serious symptoms (eg, fever, abdominal pain, dizziness, or fainting) warrant consideration of upper genital tract disease or TSS. If fever and abdominal pain predominate, consider PID.

Diagnosis	Prevalence
PID	55% of adolescents in 1 series with laparoscopically confirmed PID reported vaginal discharge[8]
TSS	Relative risk of 2.1 of TSS in women with antecedent vaginitis[9]
Erythema multiforme major	Rare
Urinary tract infection	Common
Malignancy (vulvar, vaginal, cervical)	Rare. Relative risk of 6.1 of vaginal cancer in women with prior vaginitis[10]
Foreign body (ie, retained tampon)	Common
Rectovaginal fistula	Rare

Alarm symptoms	Serious causes	Benign causes
Lower abdominal pain	PID Urinary tract infection	Irritable bowel syndrome (unrelated to vaginitis)
Bleeding	Trauma Malignancy Foreign body	Menses
Fever	PID TSS Urinary tract infection Erythema multiforme major	Coincident viral syndrome
Dizziness or near syncope	TSS	Vasovagal syncope
Rash	TSS Erythema multiforme major	Unrelated dermatoses
Muscle pain	TSS	Overuse injury
Confusion, lethargy	TSS	
Nausea and vomiting	TSS Pregnancy PID	Gastroenteritis
Urinary frequency, hematuria	Urinary tract infection Renal stone	
Fetid or feculent discharge	Rectovaginal fistula	
Vaginal sores and discharge	Herpes infection Dermatoses (pemphigus, pemphigoid, erythema multiforme major, Behçet syndrome)	Local trauma from scratching

FOCUSED QUESTIONS

Questions	Think about
Do you engage in sexual activities with men, women, or both? With how many partners are you currently sexually active? How many sexual partners have you had in the past year?	Helps assess the risk for sexually transmitted infection.
Do you engage in oral sex?	Candidal vulvovaginitis
Do you have vulvar itching or soreness?	Candidal vulvovaginitis Trichomoniasis
Are you postmenopausal?	Atrophic vaginitis
If postmenopausal, are you using estrogen products (orally or topically)?	Candida vaginitis

Quality

Do you notice an odor to the discharge?

What color is the discharge?

Is the vaginal discharge clumped?

Time course

When did the discharge occur in relation to menstrual cycle?

Have you recently been treated with antibiotics?

Does discharge occur after sexual intercourse?

Does discharge occur after condom use?

Associated symptoms

Do you notice itching?

Is the itching internal or external?

Do you notice odor?

Do you notice burning with urination?

Do you have pain with intercourse? If so, does the pain occur with initial penetration or with deeper thrusting?

Are blisters present in the vagina or on the vulva that accompany discharge?

Modifying symptoms

Have you tried over-the-counter yeast preparations? If so, do they help?

Think about

Bacterial vaginosis
Trichomoniasis

White suggests candidiasis; gray suggests bacterial vaginosis; yellow or green suggests trichomoniasis

Candidal vulvovaginitis

Think about

Premenstrual suggests candidiasis
Postmenstrual suggests trichomoniasis

Candidal vulvovaginitis

Bacterial vaginosis
Trichomoniasis
Candidal vulvovaginitis

Latex allergy or other irritant (nonoxynol 9, propylene glycol)

Think about

Candidal vulvovaginitis
Lichen sclerosis
Lichen planus
Lichen simplex chronicus
Psoriasis

Internal and external itching suggests candidal infection
Isolated external itching suggests dermatologic cause

Bacterial vaginosis
Trichomoniasis
Foreign body

Internal burning suggests urinary tract infection
External suggests vulvar irritation

If superficial dyspareunia, consider vulvovaginal condition
If deep dyspareunia, consider upper genital tract problem (endometriosis, fibroids, etc)

Pemphigus
Cicatricial pemphigoid
Behçet syndrome
Herpes infection
Erythema multiforme major

Think about

If consistently relieved with topical treatment, consider candidiasis

DIAGNOSTIC APPROACH

The first step is to rule out serious upper genital tract disease. The presence of fever, abdominal pain, deep dyspareunia, or weight loss suggests a serious diagnosis.

CAVEATS

- Differentiate between lower and upper tract symptoms.
- Not all vaginal discharge is pathologic or due to infection.
- Not all infectious vulvovaginitis is sexually transmitted; candida and bacterial vaginosis are generally not sexually transmitted.
- The diagnosis of any STD should prompt investigation for other sexually transmitted infections and patient education about measures to prevent new infections.
- Vulvar edema only occurs in candidiasis, trichomoniasis, or dermatologic disorders
- Deep dyspareunia most often occurs with conditions other than vaginitis, implying pain with movement of deeper structures such as the uterus, ovaries, fallopian tubes, or bladder.
- Distinguish external dysuria (pain experienced in the vulva as urine passes over the skin) from internal dysuria (pain felt deeper in the pelvis in the area of the bladder or urethra). External dysuria most often results from a vulvovaginal problem.
- Be aware that mixed genital infections occur frequently.
- In the postmenopausal or postpartum woman, strongly consider atrophic vaginitis as the etiology of discharge. However, infectious causes remain common after menopause.
- Refine all diagnostic impressions based on history with a careful genital examination, wet preparation, and potassium hydroxide (KOH) microscopy of vaginal secretions.

PROGNOSIS

Infectious causes of vulvovaginitis are easily treated. Recurrent infections with *Candida* and bacterial vaginosis are very common. Atrophic vaginitis may be a chronic problem but generally responds well to topical estrogen therapy. Dermatologic disorders of the vulva (eg, lichen sclerosis) may be more difficult to manage and require prolonged courses of treatment. Recognition of upper tract infections is important because these infections may cause significant morbidity and require urgent systemic antibiotic therapy.

REFERENCES

1. Schaaf M, Perez-Stable E, Borchardt K. The limited value of symptoms and signs in the diagnosis of vaginal infections. *Arch Intern Med.* 1990;150:1929–1933.
2. Kent H. Epidemiology of vaginitis. *Am J Obstet Gynecol.* 1991;165:1168–1176.
3. Fleury F. Adult vaginitis. *Clin Obstet Gynecol.* 1981;24:407–438.
4. Eckert L, Hawes S, Stevens C, et al. Vulvovaginal candidiasis: clinical manifestations, risk factors, management algorithm. *Obstet Gynecol.* 1998;92:757–765.
5. Moi H. Prevalence of bacterial vaginosis and its association with genital infections, inflammation, and contraceptive methods in women attending sexually transmitted disease and primary health clinics. *Int J STD AIDS.* 1990;1:86–94.
6. Wolner-Hanssen P, Krieger J, Kiviat N, et al. clinical manifestations of vaginal trichomoniasis. *JAMA.* 1989;261:571–576.
7. Spinillo A, Bernuzzi AM, Cevini C, et al. The relationship of bacterial vaginosis, Candida and Trichomonas infection to symptomatic vaginitis in postmenopausal women attending a vaginitis clinic. *Maturitas.* 1997;27:253–260.
8. Freij B. Acute pelvic inflammatory disease. *Semin Adolesc Med.* 1986;2:143–153.
9. Lanes S, Poole C, Dreyer NA, Lanza LL. Toxic shock syndrome, contraceptive methods and vaginitis. *Am J Obstet Gynecol.* 1986;154:989–991.
10. Brinton L, Nasca PC, Mallin K, et al. Case-control study of in situ and invasive carcinoma of the vagina. *Gynecol Oncol.* 1990;38:49–59.

SUGGESTED READING

Egan M, Lipsky M. Diagnosis of vaginitis. *Am Fam Physician.* 2000;62:1095–1104.

Sobel J. Vaginits. *N Engl J Med.* 1997;337:1896–1903.

Sexually Transmitted Diseases Treatment Guidelines 2002. Centers for Disease Control and Prevention. *MMWR Recomm Rep.* 2002:51(RR6):1–78.

The V Book. Stewart E. 2002.

Genital Skin Disorders. Fisher B, Margesson L. 1998.

Diagnostic Approach: Vaginitis

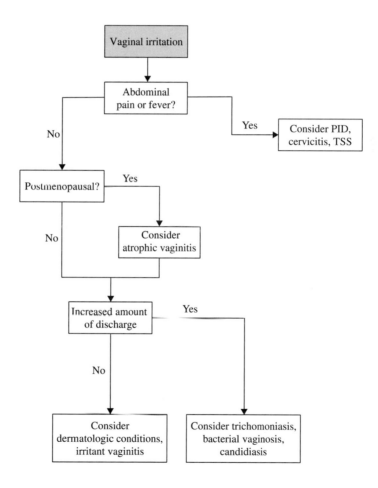

PID, pelvic inflammatory disease; TSS, toxic shock syndrome.

Abnormal Vaginal Bleeding

46

Amy N. Ship, MD

Abnormal vaginal bleeding is one of the most common clinical problems in women's health. Statistics regarding the frequency of various causes of abnormal vaginal bleeding are not available. Abnormal vaginal bleeding may be categorized as independent of or related to hormonal cycles. Normal menstrual bleeding lasts an average of 4 days (ranging from 2 to 7 days), and involves loss of about 30–60 mL of blood. Vaginal bleeding related to the menstrual cycle is considered abnormal if it varies from normal menstrual bleeding in volume, frequency, or timing. Otherwise, abnormal vaginal bleeding may result from hormonal abnormalities or structural abnormalities anywhere along the genital tract. The likely source depends on the age and reproductive status of the woman.

KEY TERMS

Dysfunctional uterine bleeding (DUB)	*Abnormal uterine bleeding that is hormonal in nature and not due to structural or systemic disease.*
Menometrorrhagia	*Irregular or excessive bleeding during menstruation and between periods.*
Menorrhagia	*Bleeding of excessive flow and duration that occurs at regular intervals.*
Metrorrhagia	*Bleeding that occurs at irregular intervals.*
Oligomenorrhea	*Bleeding that occurs at intervals > 35 days.*
Ovulation bleeding	*A single episode of spotting between regular menstrual periods.*
Polymenorrhea	*Bleeding that occurs at intervals < 21 days.*
Positive likelihood ratio (LR+)	*The increase in the odds of a particular diagnosis if a given factor is present.*

ETIOLOGY

The etiology of abnormal vaginal bleeding depends on the age and reproductive status of the patient. Although the vast majority of abnormal bleeding is dysfunctional uterine bleeding, it remains a diagnosis of exclusion. Pregnancy, abnormalities of the reproductive tract, systemic diseases, and medications (eg, oral contraceptive pills [OCPs]) may all cause abnormal vaginal bleeding; clinicians must consider these diagnoses before assigning a diagnosis of DUB.

Differential Diagnosis	Prevalence[a]
Complications related to pregnancy	
Normal intrauterine pregnancy	
Ectopic pregnancy	
Gestational trophoblastic disease	
Spontaneous abortion (threatened, incomplete, or missed)	
Placenta previa	
Retained products of conception after therapeutic abortion	
Abnormalities of the reproductive tract	*67% of women referred for hysteroscopy[1]*
Benign lesions (cervical, endometrial, adenomyosis)	
Malignant lesions (cervical, endometrial)	*5% of postmenopausal women[2]*
Infection (cervicitis, endometritis)	
Trauma (laceration, abrasion, foreign body)	
Systemic disease	
Endocrinopathy (hypothyroidism, hyperprolactinemia, Cushing disease, polycystic ovarian syndrome, adrenal dysfunction/tumor)	
Coagulopathy • *von Willebrand disease*	*19% of adolescent patients[3]; 11% of patients aged 18–45 years[4]*
• *Thrombocytopenia*	
• *Leukemia*	
Renal disease	
Hepatic disease	
Iatrogenic factors/medications	
Anticoagulation therapy	
Intrauterine device	
Hormone therapy (oral, topical, or injection contraceptives; estrogen replacement therapy; selective estrogen receptor modulators)	
Psychotropic agents	
DUB	

[a]Among women with abnormal menstrual bleeding in the specific population described; prevalence is unknown when not indicated.

GETTING STARTED

- Establish how long the abnormal bleeding has been present and how excessive it is.
- Remember that although worrisome to patients, abnormal vaginal bleeding does not indicate serious disease in the vast majority of patients.
- Consider pregnancy in any woman of reproductive age.

INTERVIEW FRAMEWORK

- After determining the patient's age, focus questions based on bleeding issues common in the appropriate age group.
- Assess whether bleeding has normal intervals and volume or is erratic and excessive.
- If the patient is premenopausal, establish her normal menstrual pattern. If she is postmenopausal, obtain a brief menstrual history, including when cycles stopped and previous intervals.
- Establish that the source of bleeding is vaginal rather than from the gastrointestinal or urinary tract.
- Inquire about bleeding characteristics including the following:
  - Onset
  - Precipitating factors
  - Nature of bleeding (temporal pattern, duration, postcoital, quantity)
  - Associated symptoms
  - Patient's medical history
  - Medication use and history
  - Personal or family history of bleeding disorder.

IDENTIFYING ALARM SYMPTOMS

While abnormal vaginal bleeding may be caused by worrisome diseases, only 2 life-threatening conditions must be considered: ectopic pregnancy and intrauterine hemorrhage from various causes. Women with life-threatening vaginal hemorrhage will usually seek medical attention at urgent care settings and appear ill due to marked, dramatic blood loss with tachycardia, hypotension, lightheadedness, dizziness or syncope. Ectopic pregnancy can present with classic symptoms of severe abdominal pain and bleeding in the setting of a known pregnancy, or more subtly with only mild abdominal discomfort and light bleeding.

Serious Diagnoses

- Ectopic pregnancy
- Gynecologic cancer
- Severe bleeding diathesis
- Vaginal hemorrhage

Alarm features	Serious causes	LR+	Benign causes
Dizziness, lightheadedness, syncope, palpitations, tachycardia	*Hemorrhage*		*Anxiety* *Arrhythmia*
Abdominal pain and known pregnancy	*Ectopic pregnancy*	*1.4–6.1*[5]	*Normal pregnancy* *Fibroid* *Benign gastrointestinal source*
Weight loss	*Endometrial cancer*		*Lifestyle change* *Thyroid abnormality*
Bloating, increasing abdominal girth	*Ovarian cancer*		*Hormonal change* *Thyroid abnormality* *Inactivity*

FOCUSED QUESTIONS

Questions	Think about
Are your menstrual cycles regular?	Provides a baseline against which bleeding can be assessed
What is the usual interval between periods?	DUB if interval doesn't fall between 25 and 31 days
What was the first day of your last period?	Establishing baseline for irregular bleeding
Is your period late?	Pregnancy
Do you have bleeding occurring	
• Irregularly between menstrual cycles?	OCPs Breakthrough bleeding Uterine lesions Cervicitis
• After sexual intercourse?	Irritation Cervical mass or lesion
• Midway between periods? Associated with dull aching pain?	Midcycle bleeding (mittelschmerz) associated with ovulation
• A few days before the onset of your normal cycle?	Premenstrual spotting, a variant of metrorrhagia
Does the bleeding occur irregularly? Is it unpredictable as to amount and duration?	DUB Perimenopause (if patient is 45–55 years old) Stress Illness Polycystic ovarian syndrome Breakthrough bleeding
Duration of menses	***Think about***
What is the duration of flow?	
• 2–7 days?	Normal
• More than 7 days?	Menorrhagia Uterine lesions
• Prolonged and with irregular inter-menstrual bleeding?	Menometrorrhagia Chronic anovulation
Amount of blood loss	***Think about***
What is the amount of menstrual blood loss?	
• Increased? Excessive?	Hypermenorrhea Abnormality of reproductive tract Bleeding diathesis
• Spotty? Light? With regular predictable menstruation?	Hypomenorrhea Obstruction of outflow tract Scarring
How many tampons or pads do you use daily?	A poor estimate of blood loss; normal use varies widely
Are you passing any clots?	Heavy bleeding

Accompanying symptoms	*Think about*
Do you have	
• The following symptoms a few days before the onset of menstrual flow: breast fullness or tenderness, abdominal bloating, low back pain, weight gain, or mood changes?	Premenstrual symptoms suggestive of ovulatory bleeding
• Abdominal cramping with or just prior to your menstruations?	Dysmenorrhea; more common during ovulatory cycles
• Dull aching pain at midcycle?	Ovulatory bleeding (mittelschmerz)
• Chronic pain in the lower abdomen increased during menstruation?	Fibroids Infection Pelvic inflammatory disease (PID) Endometriosis
• Fever?	PID
• Vaginal discharge or itching?	Vaginal infection
• Milky nipple discharge?	Pregnancy Hyperprolactinemia
• Easy bruising or bleeding from other sites?	Bleeding diathesis or clotting disorder
• Hot flashes or night sweats?	Vasomotor instability associated with menopause in patient of appropriate age
• Heat or cold intolerance?	Thyroid disorder

Additional issues	*Think about*
What medications are you taking?	Medication-associated bleeding (ie, warfarin, enoxaparin, OCPs, hormone preparations)
Do you use OCPs? Recently started? Missed pill?	Inadequate dosing or a missed pill may cause "breakthrough bleeding"
Are you having sexual intercourse?	Pregnancy PID Trauma
Have you had any recent change in weight, chronic illness, or stress?	DUB
Have you recently stopped taking hormonal therapy?	In postmenopausal woman, estrogen withdrawal bleeding
Are you pregnant?	Implantation bleeding Ectopic pregnancy Abortion (threatened or incomplete)
Have you had a previous ectopic pregnancy or PID?	Ectopic pregnancy
Have you had a recent pregnancy? A recent abortion?	Retention of gestational products
Have you been forced to have sexual relations or have you had sex that was rough or painful?	Trauma
Are you having abnormal bleeding from any other site? Have you bruised easily recently?	Bleeding diathesis

DIAGNOSTIC APPROACH

Once alarm symptoms have been excluded, the first step is to determine whether the patient is premenopausal or postmenopausal. In any woman of reproductive age, bleeding must be considered a possible complication of pregnancy until proven otherwise. If premenopausal and not likely to be pregnant, determine whether a specific source for the bleeding is suggested by the history (trauma, infection, medication use, systemic disease) or whether DUB is likely. In the postmenopausal population, evaluate for use of hormone replacement therapy before considering an anatomic source.

CAVEATS

- Establish the patient's age and menopausal status in order to move correctly through the diagnostic algorithm.
- Consider pregnancy in any woman of reproductive age. Unless the woman is not sexually active with men, pregnancy must be excluded.
- Make sure to establish the patient's sexual history, including recent sexual intercourse, potential for sexual trauma, history of sexually transmitted diseases, and prior pregnancy history.
- Irregular bleeding is acceptable during the first 6 months of hormone replacement therapy; if bleeding persists after 6 months it should be investigated further.
- Consider the less likely causes of abnormal vaginal bleeding (eg, hepatic and renal disease) in women with risk factors or other suggestive symptoms.
- Consider coagulopathy in adolescent women with heavy abnormal vaginal bleeding.
- Consider pelvic lesions in women without other sources of bleeding whose history suggests ovulatory bleeding (cyclic symptoms including breast tenderness, moodiness, abdominal bloating).
- Remember that DUB is a diagnosis of exclusion, which is most often due to anovulation. It is more common at the extremes of reproductive age (postmenarchal and perimenopausal periods).

PROGNOSIS

In the absence of vaginal hemorrhage or ruptured ectopic pregnancy, abnormal vaginal bleeding has a favorable prognosis in the vast majority of cases. Although postmenopausal vaginal bleeding may suggest a gynecologic cancer, vaginal atrophy is 6 times more likely, and cancers identified are often at an early treatable stage.

REFERENCES

1. Motashaw ND, Dave S. Diagnostic and therapeutic hysteroscopy in the management of abnormal uterine bleeding. *J Reprod Med.* 1990;35:616–620.
2. MacMahon B. Overview of studies on endometrial cancer and other types of cancer in humans: perspectives of an epidemiologist. *Semin Oncol.* 1997;24(suppl 1)S1–122.
3. Claessens EA, Cowell CA. Acute adolescent menorrhagia. *Am J Obstet Gynecol.* 1981;139:277–280.
4. Dilley A, Drews C, Miller C et al. von Willebrand disease and other inherited bleeding disorders in women with diagnosed menorrhagia. *Obstet Gynecol.* 2001;97:630–636.
5. Buckley RG, King KJ, Disney JD, et al. History and physical examination to estimate the risk of ectopic pregnancy: validation of a clinical prediction model. *Ann Emerg Med.* 1999;34:664–667.

SUGGESTED READING

Goodman AK. Terminology and differential diagnosis of genital tract bleeding in women. UpToDate online, 2003. Available at http://www.uptodateonline.com

Kilbourn CL, Richards, CS. Abnormal uterine bleeding; diagnostic considerations, management options. *Postgrad Med.* 2001; 109:137–138, 141–144, 147–150.

Oriel KA, Schrager,SA. Abnormal uterine bleeding. *Am Fam Physician.* 1999;60:1371–1382.

Diagnostic Approach: Abnormal Vaginal Bleeding

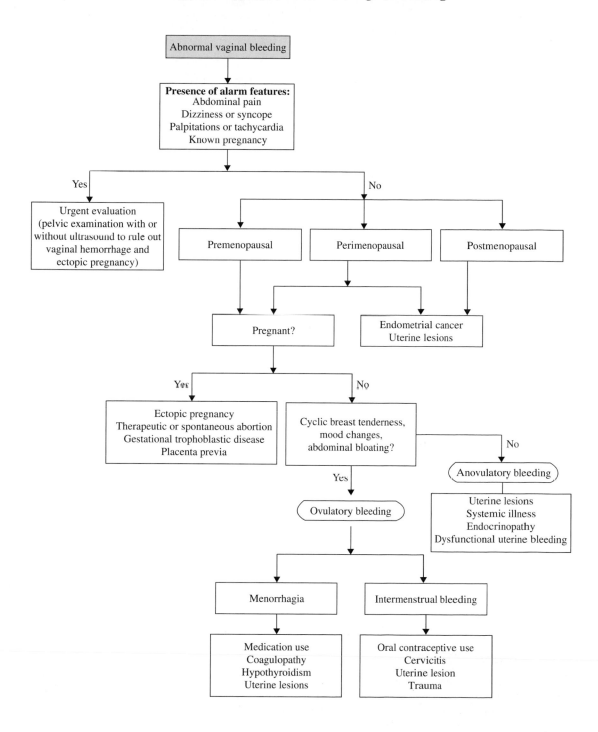

SECTION X
Musculoskeletal System

Neck Pain

47

John D. Goodson, MD

Neck pain can be categorized by location and onset. Most neck pain originates in the back (posterior) portion of the neck in the muscular, neurologic, or bony structures. Patients may also describe pain as most intense in the neck or shoulders, or upper extremities along the distribution of a cervical nerve root.[1]

Pain arising from muscular, vascular, and glandular structures, as well as the trachea and esophagus, may localize to the front (anterior portion) of the neck. Finally, pain may be referred from other parts of the body.

KEY TERMS

Anterior neck pain	Pain in the front of the neck. May originate from cervical lymph nodes, sternoclavicular muscles, trachea, pharynx, carotid arteries, thyroid, or esophagus. Referred pain from the heart, lungs, or pericardium generally occurs in the anterior neck.
Carotidynia	Pain in the anterior neck overlying the carotid artery.
Cervical radiculopathy	Pain or numbness in the distribution of 1 or more of the cervical nerve roots (see Figure 47–1 and in "Motor function for select cervical spine myotomes"). Patients may report little or no neck pain per se. Focal weakness may also occur. Impingement can result from disk herniation or from nerve root entrapment due to degenerative arthritis of the facet joints.
Complex regional pain syndrome	A combination of pain, swelling, and dysautonomic symptoms such as flushing or warmth in an anatomic region such as an extremity or part of an extremity (Chapter 49).
Dermatome	The cutaneous sensory distribution of an individual spinal nerve bundle or root.
Neck stiffness	A generalized decrease in neck mobility. This usually results from facet joint arthritis or neck injury with associated neck muscle or trapezius muscle spasm. Other causes include polymyalgia rheumatica (PMR), localized infection, and meningitis.
Occipital neuralgia	Pain located at the base of the skull at the juncture of the occiput and the first cervical vertebral body (atlas). Pain may radiate to the back of the head in the distribution of the second cervical nerve root. Pain is commonly referred to the vertex of the head and forehead.

(continued)

KEY TERMS

Posterior neck pain   *Pain located in 1 or both paraspinous muscles or the trapezius muscle. Causes include cervical disk herniation, nerve root impingement, hypertrophy or thickening of the facet joints, and congenital spinal stenosis.*

Thoracic outlet syndrome   *Mechanical compromise of the neurovascular bundle to an upper extremity by bone or soft tissue structures (eg, neck or shoulder muscles).*

Whiplash   *A rapid acceleration/deceleration injury to the soft tissue or bony structures of the neck.*

ETIOLOGY

Many acute and chronic illnesses cause neck pain. Posterior neck pain is common and is the only type that has been well studied from an epidemiologic standpoint. For example, in a United Kingdom survey of 5752 adults in 3 general practices, the prevalence of posterior neck pain was 18%, of which roughly 5% was intense, disabling, and chronic.[2]

Differential Diagnosis	**Prevalence**[a]
Posterior neck pain	18% in a primary care setting[2]
Cervical radiculopathy with or without pain	0.5% in patients with traumatic neck pain in an emergency department[3]
Anterior neck pain	
Neck stiffness	
Occipital neuralgia	

[a]Prevalence is unknown when not indicated.

GETTING STARTED

- Determine whether a life-threatening or disabling condition is present. If the neck is mechanically stable and no immediate risk of cord injury or airway compromise exists, stratify the pain based on location (eg, anterior or posterior neck pain).
- Patients often localize anterior neck pain to a specific part of the neck. If the patient cannot localize the pain, consider the possibility of referred pain from the lungs, upper chest, heart, or mediastinum.

Questions	**Remember**
Describe your neck pain to me.	• *Allow the patient to describe the nature and location of the pain.*
How did the pain start? What were you doing when you first noticed your neck pain?	• *Ask about positions or repetitive motions that provoke the pain.*
How severe is the pain on a scale from 1 to 10, where 10 is severe pain?	• *Observe the patient's neck movement to determine the extent of limitation and severity.*

INTERVIEW FRAMEWORK

- Encourage the patient to identify the location by pointing to the site of the neck pain (Figure 47–1).
- Ask about:
  - Onset of the pain, including the time and date of onset and the circumstances
  - History of recent and past neck trauma
  - Duration of pain
  - Frequency of pain
  - Any radiation of the pain
  - Positions or postures that both worsen and improve the symptoms.
- Review the patient record to determine whether the patient has a history of neck complaints or problems.

IDENTIFYING ALARM SYMPTOMS

Symptoms of airway obstruction or spinal cord impingement require immediate diagnosis and treatment. Consider spinal cord impingement in patients with the following features: acute injury such as whiplash, acute worsening of chronic neck pain, weakness in an extremity, or change in bowel or bladder function.

In a large multicenter study of patients seeking medical attention at an emergency department with blunt neck injury, the following combination of features had a 99.9% negative predictive value for cervical spine injury[3,4]:

- Absence of midline cervical tenderness
- Absence of focal neurologic deficit

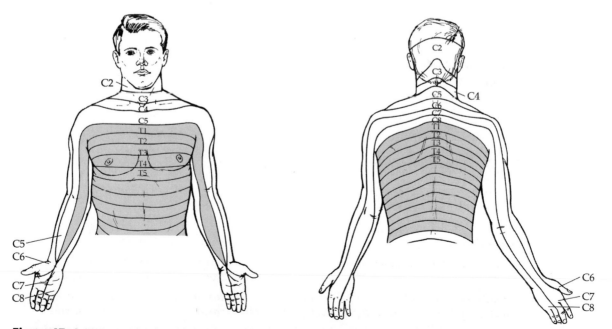

Figure 47–1. Dermatome distribution for cervical and high thoracic spine. (Reprinted from Nakano KK. Neck pain. In: McCullough K, Burton C, editors. *Textbook of Rheumatology*, 3rd ed. Philadelphia: WB Saunders Company; 1989:475)

- Normal alertness
- No evidence of intoxication
- No other clinically apparent pain that might distract the patient from the pain of the neck injury per se.

In certain patient populations, such as the elderly and those with connective tissue diseases (eg, rheumatoid arthritis, ankylosing spondylitis) or cervical spinal stenosis, even minor trauma can cause bony and soft tissue shifts putting the cervical spinal cord at risk for injury.

In patients with acute injury or recent deterioration of chronic neck pain, assess for peripheral nerve damage and loss of sensory or motor function in the distribution of 1 or more cervical nerve roots. The sensory distribution and the motor effects of damage to different cervical nerve roots are shown in Figure 47–1 and in "Motor function for select cervical spine myotomes".

Serious Diagnoses	Prevalence[a]
Airway obstruction	
Cervical spinal cord injury	
Peripheral motor or sensory nerve injury	< 0.5%[3]
Cervical spine fracture	2.4–2.6%[3,4]

[a]Among patients presenting to an emergency department with neck pain; prevalence is unknown when not indicated.

Alarm symptoms	Serious causes	Benign causes
Dyspnea	Airway obstruction Aspiration of a foreign body	Anxiety Gastroesophageal reflux disease (GERD)
Sensation of having something stuck in throat	Airway obstruction Aspiration of a foreign body	Anxiety GERD
Inability to talk	Airway obstruction Aspiration of a foreign body	Anxiety GERD
Weakness in arms or legs Tingling in hands or feet Tingling up and down spine when neck is flexed or extended (Lhermitte sign)	Myelopathy due to: • Central cervical disk herniation • Vertebral osteomyelitis • Epidural abscess • Cervical spinal stenosis • Multiple sclerosis	
Weakness in shoulders, arms, or hands	Impingement or entrapment of 1 or more cervical nerve roots	Carpal tunnel syndrome Cubital fossa syndrome
Loss of sensation in arms or hands (see Figure 47–1)	Impingement or entrapment of 1 or more cervical nerve roots	Carpal tunnel syndrome Cubital fossa syndrome
Dropping things	Impingement or entrapment of 1 or more cervical nerve roots	Carpal tunnel syndrome Cubital fossa syndrome
Intense pain (following an injury)	Cervical spine fracture	Paraspinous muscle spasm

Motor Function for Select Cervical Spine Myotomes

	Motor	**Reflex**
C5	Arm elevation (deltoid) Elbow flexion (biceps)	Biceps
C6	Wrist extension (extensor carpi)	Forearm
C7	Elbow extension (triceps) Finger extension	Triceps

FOCUSED QUESTIONS

Direct questions toward the most likely anatomic location of the neck symptoms.

Questions	**Think about**
Is the pain located in the back of the neck or in the muscles between your neck and shoulder (trapezius)?	Mild whiplash Chronic overuse PMR
Does the pain spread from your neck (or trapezius) to the shoulder or arm?	Cervical radicular pain Complex regional pain syndrome Thoracic outlet syndrome
Is the pain exclusively located in the shoulder or arm?	Cervical radicular pain Complex regional pain syndrome Thoracic outlet syndrome
Is the pain located on the side or the front of the neck?	Painful lymphadenopathy Spasm or pain in the sternoclavicular muscle Temporomandibular joint pain Carotidynia Carotid artery dissection Acute or chronic pharyngitis Acute or chronic tracheitis Acute or chronic esophagitis Foreign body in airway Inflammation of thyroid cartilage Polychondritis Painful thyroiditis Herpes zoster Pericarditis Aortic dissection Angina
Associated symptoms	**Think about**
Do you have numbness or tingling in the arms, shoulders, or hands?	Cervical radiculopathy Complex regional pain syndrome Thoracic outlet syndrome

(continued)

Associated symptoms	**Think about**
Can you reproduce the pain by touching or pressing on parts of your neck:	
• Front of the neck (anterior cervical lymph nodes)?	Lymphadenitis
• The area of your jaw in front of the ears (parotid gland)?	Parotitis Temporomandibular joint disorder
• The neck artery pulsation?	Carotidynia Carotid dissection
• The low front of the neck (the thyroid cartilage and thyroid gland)?	Relapsing polychondritis Rheumatoid arthritis Painful thyroiditis
Is the pain associated with chewing?	Parotitis Temporomandibular joint disorder Temporal arteritis
Have you had fever?	Acute pharyngitis Epiglottis Meningitis Osteomyelitis Discitis
Do you have a painful rash?	Herpes zoster
Have you noticed any neck lumps?	Malignancy, usually lymphoma or squamous cell carcinoma
Is the pain at the base of the occiput?	Occipital neuralgia Migraine
Is there fever, cognitive change, or photophobia?	Meningitis

Quality	**Think about**
Is the pain intense, 6 or greater (on a scale of 1 to 10)?	Acute whiplash Acute exacerbation of a chronic neck arthritis Acute exacerbation of a chronic neck overuse syndrome
Is the pain mild, 3 or less (on a scale of 1 to 10)?	Chronic neck arthritis Chronic overuse syndrome
Is the neck stiff?	Chronic neck arthritis Chronic overuse syndrome
Where does the pain radiate?	See Figure 47–1 for the sensory distribution of the cervical nerve roots.

Time course	**Think about**
Did the pain occur after an acute injury?	Acute whiplash Acute exacerbation of chronic neck arthritis

Did the pain occur after a minor injury or event such as falling asleep in an unusual posture?	Chronic neck arthritis Chronic overuse syndrome
Has the pain been intermittent for weeks or months?	Chronic neck arthritis Chronic overuse syndrome
Modifying symptoms	**Think about**
Does the pain worsen with neck movement?	Chronic neck arthritis Chronic overuse syndrome PMR
Does the pain worsen with activity or exertion?	Angina
Are there radicular symptoms that occur with neck movement, such as numbness or pain over 1 of the cervical nerve root dermatomes?	Whiplash Chronic neck arthritis Chronic overuse syndrome
Does the pain occur with swallowing?	Pharyngitis Esophagitis Relapsing polychondritis Rheumatoid arthritis

DIAGNOSTIC APPROACH

The first step is to localize the pain to the front or back of the neck or to the base of the skull. Ask if the pain is dominant on one side. Next, inquire about trauma and the relationship of symptoms to a specific event or to specific repetitive activities. Ask about motions or positions that worsen the pain. Encourage the patient to point and describe what is happening to the pain as you watch to determine what mechanical activities worsen the pain. Inquire about the radiation of pain and any symptoms of localized weakness.

Associated symptoms such as fever or dysphagia may be important elements of the history. Ask about any relevant work or leisure activities that might cause chronic irritation of bony or soft tissue structures in the neck.

CAVEATS

- Nearly all adults have wear and tear changes of the neck structures resulting from the normal aging process and the twisting, turning, and bending of modern life.
- Hyperreflexia in all 4 extremities suggests cervical spinal cord compression and myelopathy.
- Chronic neck problems frequently result from overuse. Examples include chronic neck hyperextension, such as when individuals work above their heads repeatedly or hyperextend their necks in order to bring reading glasses into focus. People who hold phones, especially small cellular phones, between the shrugged shoulder and the angle of the jaw, are also at risk for mechanical nerve root impingement.
- When evaluating a whiplash-type injury, recognize that significant injury to the bony and soft tissue structures may not be readily apparent. Muscle spasm in the neck is protective.

- Neck manipulation by chiropractors and physical therapists can create rather significant additional morbidity, including carotid artery dissection and exacerbation of underlying arthritis.[5]
- Neck pain may be the presenting feature of shoulder joint impingement syndromes.[6]
- PMR is a subtle inflammatory condition that causes pain and stiffness in the neck and shoulders. It may also be associated with a more worrisome inflammatory condition involving the arteries, giant cell arteritis (GCA). GCA is a medical emergency that can lead to stroke or blindness.
- Torticollis is a tonic contraction of the neck muscles that causes the head to turn uncontrollably. It is a sign of an underlying neuromuscular disorder, such as dystonia or cervical nerve root damage.
- Upper extremity complex regional pain syndrome, formally known as reflex sympathetic dystrophy, is an inflammatory condition that can affect the arm, usually after mechanical trauma. Symptoms include severe pain with swelling, erythema, and skin temperature changes.

PROGNOSIS

Most patients with both acute and chronic neck pain from soft tissue and or bony abnormalities improve with time as long as the neck is protected from further injury or damage. The most common impediment to recovery is the continued irritation of the neck by repeated misuse, especially flexion, extension, or lateral bending. The prognosis of an unrecognized and untreated cervical spine fracture is poor.

Even patients with significant nerve root compression with resultant motor and sensory loss will improve over time; however, such patients need to be closely monitored.

REFERENCES

1. Anderson BC, Sheon RP. Evaluation of the patient with neck pain. UpToDate (serial online 11.2) 2003 April (21 screens). Available from: http://uptodateonline.com/appilcation/topic/print.asp?file

2. Webb R, Brammah T, Lunt M, et al. Prevalence and predictors of intense, chronic, and disabling neck and back pain in the UK general population. *Spine*. 2003;28:1195–1202.

3. Stiell IG, Clement CM, McKnight RD, et al. The Canadian C-spine rule versus the NEXUS low-risk criteria in patients with trauma. *N Engl J Med*. 2003;349:2510–2518.

4. Hoffman JR, Mower WR, Wolfson AB, et al. Validity of a set of clinical criteria to rule out injury to the cervical spine in patients with blunt trauma. *N Engl J Med*. 2003;343:94–99.

5. Smith WS, Johnston SC, Skalabrin EJ, et al. Spinal manipulative therapy is an independent risk factor for vertebral artery dissection. *Neurology*. 2003;60:1424–1428.

6. Devereaux MW. Neck and lower back pain. *Med Clin North Am*. 2003;87:643–662.

SUGGESTED READING

Barnsley L. Neck pain. In: Klippel JH, Dieppe PA, editors. *Rheumatology*, 2nd ed. London: Mosby International; 1998:4.1–4.12.

Glazer PA, Taft K. The cervical spine. In: Gates SJ, Mooar PA, editors. Musculoskeletal primary care. Philadelphia: Lippincott, Williams & Wilkins; 1999:48–74.

Hoppenfeld S. *Physical examination of the spine and extremities*. New York: Appleton-Century-Crofts. A publishing division of Prentice-Hall, Inc.; 1976.

Nakano KK. Neck pain. In: McCullough K, Burton C, editors. *Textbook of Rheumatology*, 3rd ed. Philadelphia: WB Saunders Company; 1989:471–490.

Diagnostic Approach: Neck Pain

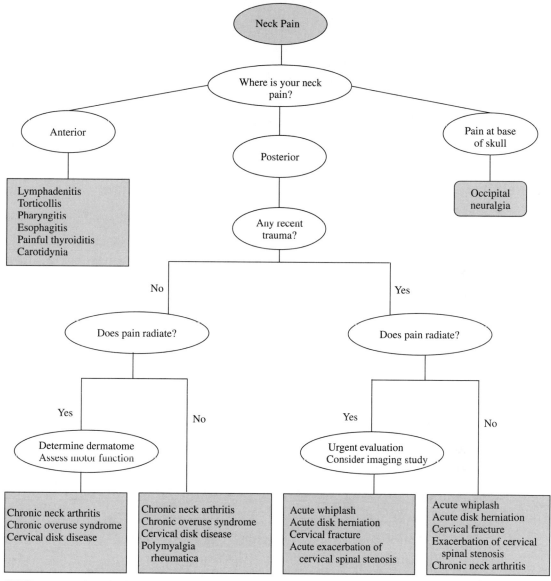

GERD, gastroesophageal reflux disease.

Shoulder Pain

48

John Wolfe Blotzer, MD

Musculoskeletal disease represents one of the most common reasons for a patient to seek primary care attention. Incidence and prevalence figures vary depending on the population studied and the site of care.[1] In Great Britain, shoulder pain is the third most common musculoskeletal complaint and represents 5% of musculoskeletal general practice visits.[2,3] Reaching a peak in the fourth to sixth decades of life, the incidence of shoulder pain is somewhere between 6.6 and 25 per thousand in Great Britain and the Netherlands.[4–7] In a community survey of patients over the age of 70, the prevalence of shoulder pain was 21% with fewer than 40% seeking medical attention.[6]

Because patients often think of the shoulder as a region of the body, the clinician must be careful not to equate *shoulder pain* with *shoulder joint pain* or, more narrowly, *glenohumeral joint pain*. Many nonmusculoskeletal disorders refer pain to the shoulder. Furthermore, shoulder range of motion involves 4 articulations: glenohumeral, acromioclavicular, sternoclavicular, and scapulothoracic as well as the associated ligaments, tendons, bursae, and muscles responsible for motion.

Evidence-based literature on history in the diagnosis of specific shoulder disorders is virtually nonexistent. Nevertheless, most shoulder pain can be diagnosed by history and physical examination.

Structural causes of primary shoulder pain	Possible source
Bones	Scapula
	Humerus
	Clavicle
Joints	Glenohumeral
	Acromioclavicular
	Sternoclavicular
Ligaments	Acromioclavicular
	Coracoclavicular
	Glenohumeral
Muscles	Trapezius
	Deltoid
	Levator scapulae
	Rhomboids
	Rotator cuff
	Triceps
	Serratus anterior
	Pectoralis
	Teres major
	Latissimus dorsae

(continued)

Structural causes of primary shoulder pain	Possible source
Tendons	Biceps
	Supraspinatus
	Infraspinatus
	Subscapularis
	Teres minor
Bursae	Subacromial
	Subcoracoid
Nerves	Subscapular
	Long thoracic
	Dorsal scapular

KEY TERMS

Bicipital tendinitis	*Overuse syndrome of the bicipital tendon usually producing anterior shoulder pain and occurring in association with impingement or glenohumeral instability.*
Calcific tendinitis	*Calcification of a rotator cuff tendon, usually the supraspinatus, proposed to be part of the degenerative process of rotator cuff tendinitis. It may be acute or chronic.*
Frozen shoulder (capsulitis/ adhesive capsulitis)	*Painful restriction of range of motion of the glenohumeral joint in all planes of motion both actively and passively.*
Impingement syndrome (rotator cuff tendinitis)	*Encroachment of the rotator cuff by the acromion, coracoacromial ligament, coracoid process, or acromioclavicular joint resulting in shoulder pain from edema, tendinitis, fibrosis, tears, rupture, and osteophytosis. It can be divided into 3 pathologic stages:* • *Stage 1 is characterized by edema and hemorrhage* • *Stage 2 is characterized by fibrosis and partial tear* • *Stage 3 represents a full thickness tear. It is the most common cause of chronic intrinsic shoulder pain.* *Symptoms do not correlate with pathologic stage.*
Moving parts pain	*Pain exacerbated by movement and relieved by rest and attributable to the bones, joints, muscles, bursae, tendons, and ligaments that comprise the shoulder joint; primary shoulder pain or intrinsic shoulder joint pain—opposite of referred pain.*
Referred shoulder pain	*Pain from a process in a nonshoulder area or organ perceived as shoulder discomfort; typically its intensity and relief is unrelated to movement of the shoulder. Carpal tunnel syndrome and cervical spondylosis, diseases of the chest (eg, lung, heart and mediastinum) may refer pain to the shoulder. Irritation of the diaphragm from thoracic or abdominal structures may refer pain to the shoulder. Secondary shoulder pain or extrinsic shoulder pain—opposite of moving parts pain.*

Rotator cuff	*Musculotendinous structure blending into the glenohumeral joint capsule that provides range of motion and strength. It is composed of the insertions of the supraspinatus, infraspinatus, teres minor, and subscapularis tendons.*
Subacromial bursitis	*Occurs as part of the impingement process and coexists with rotator cuff tendinitis.*

ETIOLOGY[1–9]

Although most shoulder pain arises from articular and periarticular structures, the shoulder is also a common location for referred pain. The differential diagnosis and determination of referred pain versus primary pain is critical because many of the disorders producing referred pain are life-threatening. The range of problems that can refer pain to the shoulder make the evaluation of shoulder pain challenging. Cervical spine disease is the most common cause of pain referred to the shoulder.

The most common cause of shoulder pain is the impingement syndrome and related disorders and rotator cuff tears. These disorders are periarticular and may be associated with each other or part of the overall process of impingement. Much less commonly, the shoulder can be affected by inflammatory arthritis. Occasionally, systemic disorders, such as rheumatoid arthritis, can present first in the glenohumeral joint although subsequent involvement in other joints will usually lead to the correct diagnosis. Gout and pseudogout, while possible in the glenohumeral or sternoclavicular joints, seldom occur there without preexisting degenerative disease. Septic arthritis uncommonly occurs in the shoulder but should always be considered. Polymyalgia rheumatica may present mainly with shoulder pain and occasionally be difficult to distinguish from early frozen shoulder or capsulitis. Shoulder symptoms are rarely the first manifestation of primary or metastatic tumors.

Differential Diagnosis: Referred Pain

Cervical spine disease	*Abdominal and pelvic disorders*	*Neurologic disorders*
Chest disorders	*Ectopic pregnancy*	*Spinal cord lesions*
Myocardial infarction	*Splenic infarction*	*Brachial plexopathy*
Angina pectoris	*Splenic rupture*	*Entrapment neuropathy*
Pericarditis	*Hepatic hematoma or abscess*	*Herpes zoster*
Aortic dissection	*Subphrenic abscess*	
Pulmonary embolism	*Cholecystitis*	
Pneumothorax	*Ruptured abdominal viscus*	
Pneumonia	*Aneurysm*	
Pleuritis	*Intra-abdominal hemorrhage*	
Pancoast tumor	*Vascular insufficiency including arteritis*	
Mesothelioma	*Venous thrombosis*	
Mediastinal neoplasm	*Peptic ulcer*	
Esophageal disease	*Pancreatitis*	
	Abdominal neoplasms	
	Splenic and hepatic flexure syndromes	

Differential Diagnosis: Primary Pain	Prevalence[a]
Impingement syndrome/rotator cuff tendinitis (includes full and partial tears)	*48–72%*
Calcific tendinitis	*6%*
Rotator cuff tears	
Bicipital tendinitis	
Glenohumeral instability	
Acromioclavicular syndromes	
Frozen shoulder/capsulitis	*16–22%*
Glenoid labral tear	
Inflammatory arthritides including rheumatoid, crystal-associated, reactive, etc	
Infection of joint or soft tissues	
Osteoarthritis	
Polymyalgia rheumatica	
Osteonecrosis	

[a]In primary care setting[5,10]; prevalence is unknown when not indicated.

GETTING STARTED

- Most shoulder pain is due to trauma and rotator cuff impingement, a process that begins with edema and hemorrhage, and ultimately leads to fibrosis and tears. Important historical issues include an inciting event, the patient's occupation and avocations, and any changes in activity as a consequence of the shoulder pain.
- Include basic questions about onset, severity on a scale of 1 to 10, quality, course, radiation, and ameliorating and exacerbating factors.
- Young patients tend to have impingement, tendinitis, trauma and instability; while older patients are more likely to have rotator cuff tears and more significant disability.

Open-ended questions	Tips for effective interviewing
Where is your pain?	*Ask the patient to point to the area where it hurts:*
What were you doing when you first noted the pain?	• *Lateral deltoid pain suggests impingement and rotator cuff tendinitis*
Can you describe the pain?	• *Anterior shoulder pain suggests acromioclavicular joint, glenohumeral joint, or anterior tendon disease (eg, biceps tendinitis)*
	• *Demonstrate shoulder range of motion for the patient to determine which motion accentuates the pain*
What activities make the pain worse, and what activities make it better?	• *Shoulder pain aggravated by reaching overhead suggests impingement syndrome or rotator cuff tendinitis*

INTERVIEW FRAMEWORK

- Determine the character of the pain, specifically whether it is exacerbated by movement (primary shoulder pain) versus referred pain.
- Ascertain whether there is a history of trauma or an occupation that stresses the glenohumeral joint.
- Ask about other joint complaints or history of other joint disease.
- Determine whether there are alarm symptoms.
- Determine how the patient's ability to function is affected.

IDENTIFYING ALARM SYMPTOMS

Serious Diagnoses

- Local infection: septic glenohumeral arthritis, osteomyelitis or soft tissue abscess
- Cervical radiculopathy (referred pain)
- Referred pain of any type (refer to Etiology section)
- Glenohumeral joint arthritis
- Shoulder dislocation
- Complete rotator cuff tear
- Fracture

Alarm symptoms	Consider
Visible swelling	All causes of arthritis (including infection)
	Malignant tumors
	Amyloidosis
Fever and chills	Infection (septic arthritis, soft tissue abscess)
Constant and progressive pain	Referred pain
	Infection
	Tumor
Axillary pain	Referred pain from the mediastinum
Night pain	Infection
	Fracture
	Major tear
	Neoplasm
Numbness or tingling	Radiculopathy
	Neuropathy
	Myelopathy
Inability to abduct or maintain abduction	Rotator cuff rupture
Shoulder pain aggravated by neck motion	Cervical radiculopathy (see Chapter 47)
Shoulder pain unrelated to arm movement	Referred pain
Symptoms of vascular impairment (eg, claudication)	Thoracic outlet syndrome
	Vascular occlusion
Weight loss	Neoplasm or infection
Dyspnea	Heart disease (cardiac ischemia)
	Pulmonary disease

FOCUSED QUESTIONS

Focused questions are used to determine whether the pain is referred or not, whether there is trauma or an occupation or recreation that stresses the glenohumeral joint and its muscles, ligaments and tendons, and whether there is arthritis or infection. If the pain is clearly referred, extensive questioning will be required to determine the nature of an underlying neck, thoracic, or abdominal problem referring the pain.

If answered in the affirmative	Think about
Is your pain affected by moving your arm?	Impingement or tear of the rotator cuff Arthritis Polymyalgia rheumatica If the patient notes no exacerbation with movement, then pain is most likely referred pain.
Did you injure your shoulder recently or fall?	Tendon tears Contusion Fracture
Was the onset sudden?	Trauma Tendon tears Infection Acute arthritis Serious acute referred pain (eg, ruptured viscus, acute cardiac disease, ectopic pregnancy)
Is your shoulder pain worsened by all shoulder movements or only certain ones?	Arthritis and capsulitis (eg, frozen shoulder) are affected by all movements Tendinitis and impingement are worsened by movements of a particular tendon responsible for the movement
Is your pain aggravated by reaching over your head?	Impingement syndrome (found in 75% of patients)
Do you notice any swelling of your shoulder?	Arthritis or hemorrhage into the joint
Do you notice any associated symptoms such as fever, night sweats, or weight loss?	Referred pain from the chest or abdomen A systemic disorder Local infection or neoplasm
Do you have stiffness relieved by activity and worsened by rest? (gelling)	Polymyalgia rheumatica or systemic arthritis (eg, rheumatoid arthritis)
Do you have stiffness in the morning lasting greater than 60 minutes that improves with activity? (morning stiffness)	Polymyalgia rheumatica or systemic arthritis (eg, rheumatoid arthritis)
Is your shoulder constantly stiff?	Frozen shoulder
Have you taken high doses of glucocorticoids?	Osteonecrosis
Is your shoulder weak?	Large rotator cuff tear
Do your arms feel weak? Do you notice numbness, tingling, a sensation of burning, or a pins and needles sensation?	Cervical radiculopathy or neuropathy

What kind of work do you do? What kind of recreations do you pursue?	*Impingement syndrome, tendinitis, and tendon and muscle tears are associated with activities that involve lifting the arms frequently. Examples include welding, pitching, painting, conducting a symphony orchestra, and tennis.*
Is your shoulder unstable? Does it slip or "pop out?"	*Subluxation or dislocation*
Does your shoulder catch or lock?	*Labral tear* *Loose body*
Do you have any other health problems?	*Frozen shoulder is common in diabetics. Gout and pseudogout may manifest in the shoulder, but this typically occurs later in their course.*

It is also important to assess the patient's function. The following 12 questions will help determine severity and demonstrate concern for the repercussions of the patient's problem[11]:

1. Is your arm comfortable with your arm at rest by your side?
2. Does your shoulder allow you to sleep comfortably?
3. Can you reach the small of your back to tuck in your shirt/blouse with your hand?
4. Can you place your hand behind your head with the elbow straight out to the side?
5. Can you place a coin on a shelf at the level of your shoulder without bending your elbow?
6. Can you lift 1 lb. (a full pint container) to the level of the top of your head without bending your elbow?
7. Can you lift an 8 lb (a full gallon) container to the level of the top of your head without bending your elbow?
8. Can you carry 20 lb at your side with the affected extremity?
9. Do you think you can throw a softball underhand 10 yards with the affected extremity?
10. Do you think you can throw a softball overhand 20 yards with the affected extremity?
11. Can you wash the back of your opposite shoulder with the affected extremity?
12. Would your shoulder allow you to work fulltime at your usual job?

More simply you might ask if the patient can comb their hair, brush their teeth, fasten a bra, put on a sweater, or get their arm into a blouse or shirt, or pull a wallet out of a back pocket.

DIAGNOSTIC APPROACH

Most shoulder pain is due to impingement of the rotator cuff, which is suggested by the patient's age and clinical history. Older patients are more likely to have rotator cuff disease, rotator cuff tears, and secondary osteoarthritis. The physical examination is critical to the diagnosis of shoulder disorders and is superior to the history for most glenohumeral joint and periarticular problems. The most critical part of the history is determining whether the pain is referred or not.

CAVEATS

- Early rheumatoid arthritis and polymyalgia rheumatica can be difficult to distinguish from impingement in older patients.
- Referred pain to the shoulder is uncommon and most often due to cervical radiculopathy; however, it may represent serious thoracic, cardiac, or abdominal disease.

- The hallmark of rotator cuff tears is weakness; however, the history is often inadequate for distinguishing weakness secondary to pain from true weakness. Physical examination and strength testing after local anesthetic injection into the joint may be required.

PROGNOSIS

The prognosis of shoulder pain depends on the nature of the specific problem. Periarticular disorders, such as impingement, may be self-limited and respond to rest, analgesics, and range of motion and strengthening exercises. Impingement syndrome can be chronic and recurrent and associated with morbidity from the development of full thickness tears and secondary osteoarthritis. By middle age, asymptomatic rotator cuff tears are common. Large tears can often lead to loss of abduction and decreased strength and function.

REFERENCES

1. Walker-Bone KE, Palmer KT, Reading I, Cooper C. Soft-tissue rheumatic disorders of the neck and upper limbs: prevalence and risk factors. *Semin Arthritis Rheum.* 2003;33:185–203.

2. Croft P. Soft tissue rheumatism. In: Silman AJ, Hochberg MC, editors. *Epidemiology of the rheumatic diseases.* Oxford University Press; 1993:375–421.

3. Unwin M, Symmons D, Allison T, et al. Estimating the burden of musculoskeletal disorders in the community: the comparative prevalence of symptoms at different anatomical sites, and the relation to social deprivation. *Ann Rheum Dis.* 1998; 57:649–655.

4. Peters D, Davies P, Pietroni P. Musculoskeletal clinic in general practice: a study of one year's referrals. *Br J Gen Pract.* 1994; 44:25–29.

5. van der Windt D A W M, Koes BW, Jong de BA, Bouter LM. Shoulder disorders in general practice: incidence, patient characteristics, and management. *Ann Rheum Dis.* 1995;54:959–964.

6. Chard MD, Hazleman R, Hazleman BL, et al. Shoulder disorders in the elderly: a community survey. *Arthritis Rheum.* 1991; 34:766–769.

7. Liesdek C, van der Windt D A W M, Koes BW, Bouter LM. Soft-tissue disorders of the shoulder. A study of inter-observer agreement between general practitioners and physiotherapists and an overview of physiotherapeutic treatment. *Physiotherapy.* 1997;83:12–17.

8. Winter de AF, Jans MP, Scholten R J P M, et al. Diagnostic classification of shoulder disorders: interobserver agreement and determinants of disagreement. *Ann Rheum Dis.* 1999;58:272–277.

9. Blanchard TK, Bearcroft PW, Constant CR, Griffin DR, Dixon AK. Diagnostic and therapeutic impact of MRI and arthrography in the investigation of full thickness rotator cuff tears. *Eur Radiol.* 1999;9:638–642.

10. Stevenson JH, Trojian T. Evaluation of shoulder pain. *J Fam Pract.* 2002;51:605–610.

11. Matsen FA III, Lippitt SB, Sidles JA, Harryman DT II. *Practical Evaluation and Management of the Shoulder.* Saunders, 1994:6–15.

SUGGESTED READING

Anderson BC. *Office Orthopedics for Primary Care: Diagnosis and Treatment,* 2nd ed, WB Saunders; 1999.

Dalton S. The shoulder. In: Hochberg MC, Silman AJ, Smolen JS, Weinblatt ME, Weisman MH, editors. *Rheumatology,* 3rd ed. Mosby; 2003:615–630.

Rockwood CA Jr, Matsen FA III, Wirth MA, Harryman DT II, eds. *The Shoulder,* 2nd ed. WB Saunders; 1998.

Sheon RP, Moskowitz RW, Goldberg VM. *Soft Tissue Rheumatic Pain: Recognition, Management and Prevention,* 3rd ed. Lippincott Williams & Wilkins; 1996.

Wirth MA, Orfaly RM, Rockwood CA Jr, Shoulder. In: Greene WB (editor). Essentials of Musculoskeletal Care, 2nd ed. American Academy of Orthopedic Surgeons, 2001, 104-160.

Diagnostic Approach: Shoulder Pain

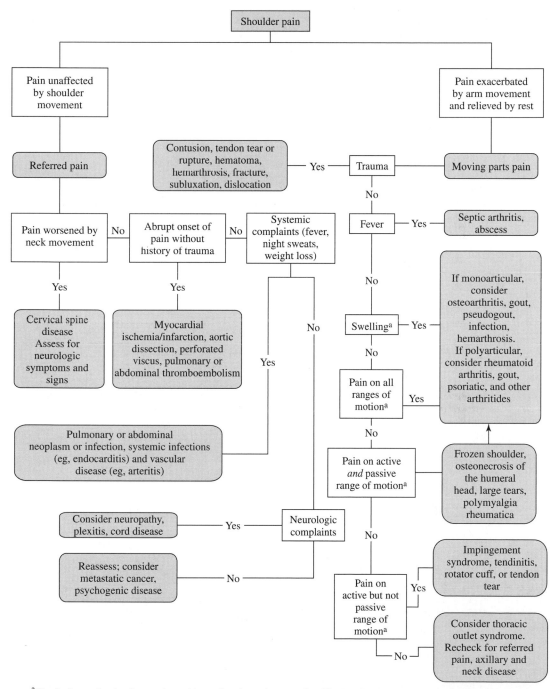

^aPhysical examination is superior to history but the patient may be able to answer.

Arm and Hand Pain

49

Robert D. Ficalora, MD

Pain in the upper extremities may result from diseases of the blood vessels or peripheral nerves, local infection, or be referred from embryologically linked structures in the chest. However, musculoskeletal sources are the most common cause. Deep pain, arising from vessels, fascia, joints, tendons, periosteum, and supporting structures, is often poorly localized and dull and may be accompanied by the perception of joint stiffness and deep tenderness. Pain that arises from adjacent or supporting structures may be attributed to the joints in the absence of any true joint pathology. Pain due to disorders of the more proximal joints (elbow and wrist) is usually related to local inflammation from overuse syndromes or work-related activities (1% of work-related injuries affect the forearm and 55% of work-related injuries affect the wrist). Pain in the joints of the hand is often a consequence of degenerative or inflammatory disease.

Painful intermittent vasospasm in the hands (Raynaud's phenomenon) is commonly attributed to digital artery vascular instability in young female patients but occurs in all age groups. It occurs less commonly in men. A variety of medications have been implicated as exacerbating this phenomenon. Obstruction of vessels by atherosclerosis occurs rarely in the upper extremity, usually in the setting of systemic vascular disease. Pain caused by diseases of the peripheral nerves or by entrapment neuropathies, such as carpal or ulnar tunnel entrapment, is accompanied by motor (weakness), reflex, and other sensory changes (burning or tingling).

Rarely, neuropathic pain in the upper extremity may result from reflex sympathetic dystrophy/chronic regional pain syndrome (RSD/CRPS), a poorly understood condition that can result from local trauma, stroke, or spinal cord injury. Irritation of the cervical nerve roots (herniated nucleus pulposus, osteoarthritis) can cause pain in the upper extremities. Pain in the upper extremity caused by compression of the nerves and blood vessels as they exit the thorax (thoracic outlet syndrome) is frequently associated with evidence of vascular compression. Referred pain, originating from structures of the chest, such as thoracic outlet syndrome, ischemic heart disease, or gastroesophageal reflux disease (GERD), may radiate to the inner surfaces of the arm.

KEY TERMS

Bursitis	*Pain and inflammation of the structure containing the fluid that lubricates a joint or tendon sheath.*
Degenerative joint disease	*Painful, noninflammatory changes in a joint that result from "wear and tear" of chronic use and abuse.*
Entrapment neuropathy	*Pain and loss of function resulting from a nerve passing through a physiologic space that is narrowed secondary to acute or chronic trauma or inflammation.*
Epicondylitis	*Pain and inflammation of the area where bone and tendon connect.*

(continued)

KEY TERMS

Neuropathic pain	*Pain in a region as a result of nerve inflammation, trauma, or neurologic disease.*
Overuse syndrome	*Pain and inflammation resulting from intense or repetitive use of regional anatomic structures in the course of occupational or recreational activities.*
Referred pain	*Pain originating in 1 structure that is perceived in the area of another, usually because of physiologic or embryologic links between the 2 structures.*
Tendinitis	*Pain and inflammation of a tendon or tendon sheath.*
Vasospasm	*Spontaneous contraction or closure of a blood vessel.*

ETIOLOGY

Differential Diagnosis: Forearm and Elbow Pain

Diagnosis	*Explanation*	*Prevalence*
Lateral epicondylitis (tennis elbow)	*A strain of the wrist extensor attachments at the humerus, usually in tennis players with poor technique.*	*1–3% in the general population* *40–50% of tennis players, especially those over age 30[1]*
Medial epicondylitis (golfer's elbow)	*Any strain of the common flexor tendon can cause this injury.* *Involvement of the nearby ulnar nerve may result in tingling.*	*2.5% of workers[2]*
Olecranon bursitis	*Inflammatory fluid accumulating in the bursa often following local trauma; may be spontaneous in patients with gout, pseudogout or rheumatoid arthritis. When resulting from infection within the bursa, this is called septic olecranon bursitis.*	*0.718% of the mentally retarded* *Up to 1% of rheumatoid patients[3]*
Ulnar tunnel syndrome or Guyon tunnel syndrome	*The ulnar (Guyon) tunnel is a space at the elbow between the bones of the joint through which the ulnar nerve travels surrounded by a ligament. If this ligament hardens, the nerve is compressed into the ulnar groove or "entrapped," causing pain and tingling in the arm between the elbow and fingers.*	*1.7–2.5% of industrial workers* *25% of patients with carpal tunnel syndrome also have ulnar tunnel syndrome[4]*
Referred pain from chest structures	*Ischemic or irritative pain from the organs adjacent to the diaphragm (heart, stomach), and structures in and near the diaphragmatic hiatus (hiatus hernia, esophagus) refer pain to the lateral forearm and elbow.*	*0.6% of general population* *20% of angina patients have pain referred to their left arm[5]*

Cubital tunnel syndrome	Ulnar nerve is compressed as it crosses the elbow, resulting in pain that is like "hitting your funny bone." Persons who perform repetitive bending of the elbow by pulling levers, reaching, or lifting are at risk.	9% of musicians[6]
RSD/CRPS	A chronic progressive neurologic condition that affects a region, such as an arm or a leg. Can also occur after a minor injury, such as a sprain. In some cases, there is no precipitating event. Pain begins in 1 area or limb and then spreads. RSD/CRPS is characterized by burning pain, excessive sweating, swelling, and sensitivity to touch.	2–5% of peripheral nerve injury patients 12–21% of patients with hemiplegia (paralysis on 1 side of the body) 1–2% of bone fracture patients[2]

Differential Diagnosis: Wrist Pain

Diagnosis	*Explanation*	*Prevalence*
Carpal tunnel syndrome	Compression of the median nerve inside of the carpal tunnel of the wrist with pain and loss of function of the first 2 or 3 digits of the hand. May be related to overuse, pregnancy, or hypothyroidism.	2.7% of the general population[6]
de Quervain tenosynovitis	The abductor pollicis longus and extensor pollicis longus run in a tunnel along the side of the wrist above the thumb. Repeatedly grasping, pinching, squeezing, or wringing may lead to a tenosynovitis. This causes swelling, which further hampers the smooth gliding action of the tendons within the tunnel. Soreness on the thumb side of the forearm is the initial symptom. Pain spreads up the forearm or down into the wrist and thumb. The tendons may actually squeak as they move through the constricted tunnel.	0.46% of working adults[7]
Intersection syndrome (tenosynovitis at the wrist)	Tendinitis in the first and second dorsal compartments of the wrist. The tendons cross at a 60-degree angle proximal to the wrist joint on the dorsal aspect. It has also been described as a stenosing tenosynovitis of the tendon sheath where it crosses the bellies of the abductor pollicis longus and extensor pollicis brevis muscles.	12% of Alpine skiers[8]

Differential Diagnosis: Hand Pain

Diagnosis	Explanation	Prevalence
Trigger finger	Irritation from the tendon sliding through the pulley causes the tendon to swell and create a nodule. Pain at the bottom of the digit and a clicking sensation occur when the digit is bent and straightened. Can be a complication of diabetes.	2.6% in nondiabetic patients over 30 years of age 16–42% in diabetics[9]
Hand osteoarthritis	Hand pain, aching, or stiffness and 3 or 4 of the following features: • Enlargement of 2 or more of 10 joints • Enlargement of 2 or more distal interphalangeal joints • Fewer than 3 swollen metacarpophalangeal joints • Deformity of at least 1 of 10 joints.	Symptomatic in persons over 70 years: women, 26.2%; men, 13.4% Radiographic evidence in persons over 70 years 36%[10]
Rheumatoid arthritis	The cause is unknown. Hand involvement can be particularly debilitating. Synovial tissue and joint destruction occur early in the disease often before classic deformities develop.	2% in persons older than 60 years[11]
Raynaud disorder	Vasospasm of the digital vessels causes the characteristic 3-color changes of the digits—blanching (white), cyanosis (blue), numbness and rubor (red)—after cold exposure and rewarming.	15% of the general population[12]
Thoracic outlet syndrome	Compression of the nerves and vessels to the arm at the shoulder associated with repetitive motion of the arms held overhead or extended forward. Pain, weakness, numbness and tingling, swelling, fatigue or coldness of the arm and hand can mimic a herniated cervical disk, ulnar tunnel, or carpal tunnel syndromes.	0.1% of the general population[13]

GETTING STARTED

- Upper extremity complaints are usually localized and commonly related to an injury, inciting event, or recreational or occupational overuse.
- Basic questions about the onset, location, quality, and aggravating or ameliorating factors are most useful.
- An occupational and leisure time history is essential.

Questions	**Remember**
Where is the pain?	• *Most patients will not be able to adequately describe the location of the pain, so pointing is helpful.*
When did it start?	• *Physical demonstrations of typical activities may be valuable adjuncts to the history.*
Can you describe it for me? Is it dull? Sharp? Burning? Does it ever change?	• *Trying to be helpful, patients often group unrelated symptoms. Make sure that you understand each individual symptom or sign completely before moving on.*
Is there swelling?	
Is there a rash or discoloration?	
What makes it better or worse?	
Show me how you use your arms at work. Tell me about your leisure time activities.	

INTERVIEW FRAMEWORK

- Assess for alarm symptoms.
- Identify activities that put the patient at risk.
- Systematically identify complaints that relate to differential diagnoses of the joints, soft tissues, nerves and neuropathic disorders, and cervical and thoracic structures that refer pain to the upper extremity.

IDENTIFYING ALARM SYMPTOMS

Serious Diagnoses

- Septic olecranon bursitis
- Ischemic heart disease
- Cervical nerve root or spinal cord disorders

Alarm symptoms	**Serious causes**	**Benign causes**
Arm complaints (especially on the left side) associated with dyspnea, chest pain, dizziness, or palpitations	*Ischemic heart disease or other cardio-pulmonary conditions*	*Fatigue* *Anxiety* *GERD*
Persistent sensory abnormalities, such as numbness, burning or tingling, especially with associated neck complaints	*Acute cervical nerve root or spinal cord disorders*	*Muscle strain* *Anxiety* *GERD* *Entrapment neuropathy*
Painful redness, swelling, weeping or draining lesions with fever, fatigue, or malaise (especially related to trauma)	*Septic olecranon bursitis or other soft tissue infections*	*Crystalline arthropathies (eg, gout or pseudogout)*

FOCUSED QUESTIONS

After listening to the patient's complaint, put the description in a context of related risks and activities. Patients may have an idea of the cause of their symptoms from the media, friends, or the Internet, but they often won't be able to put all the pieces together.

Since most upper extremity disorders are not primary physiologic derangements but rather the effects of overuse or injury, narrowing down the differential diagnosis begins with defining the patient's activities.

Questions	**Think about**
What is your occupation?	
• *Work on an assembly line or keyboard operation*	*Thoracic outlet syndrome from repetitive shoulder movements*
• *Sewing, operating computers*	*Carpal tunnel syndrome due to repetitive wrist motion*
• *Chain saw or pneumatic drill operators*	*Raynaud's syndrome from chronic exposure to vibration*
• *Hammer, saw, or screwdriver use*	*DeQuervain tendinitis* *Trigger finger*
Tell me about your leisure time activities.	
• *Do you play golf or tennis?*	*Medial epicondylitis* *Lateral epicondylitis*
• *Are you a home improvement enthusiast who uses hammers and screwdrivers only on the weekends?*	*Medial epicondylitis* *DeQuervain tendinitis* *Trigger finger*
• *Do you drink? If so, how much?*	*Olecranon bursitis (drinker's elbow) from repeated trauma secondary to leaning on a curb or bar*
• *Are you a professional musician?*	*Cubital tunnel syndrome (especially saxophone playing)*
• *Are you a skier?*	*Intersection syndrome*
• *Do you lead a sedentary lifestyle? Do you smoke?*	*Coronary artery disease*
Quality	***Think about***
Is the pain	
• *Steady?*	*Rheumatoid arthritis* *Osteoarthritis* *Infection*
• *Aching?*	*Overuse syndrome or referred pain*
• *Shooting? sharp?*	*Entrapment neuropathy*
• *Burning?*	*Neuropathic pain*
• *Severe?*	*Arthritis (at rest)* *Osteomyelitis (with motion)* *Gout* *Infection* *Trauma*
• *Throbbing?*	*Inflammatory or vascular disorder*

Location	Think about
Where do you have pain?	
• In or around what joint?	Pain resulting from an articular disorder is perceived as coming directly from the joint not from the bones around the joints
• Elbows?	Septic arthritis Crystalline arthropathies (eg, pseudogout, gout) Trauma Neuropathic pain from entrapment neuropathy Medial epicondylitis Lateral epicondylitis
• Wrists?	Entrapment neuropathy (median nerve or tendinitis)
• Metacarpophalangeal joints?	Rheumatoid arthritis Occasionally in gout
• Proximal interphalangeal joints?	Rheumatoid arthritis (nontender Bouchard nodes in osteoarthritis)
• Distal interphalangeal joints?	Osteoarthritis (Heberden nodes; often painless) Psoriatic arthritis
• Carpometacarpal joint of thumb?	Osteoarthritis
• In an area adjacent to a joint?	Periarticular structures (tendinitis, bursitis, bone)
• In the first 3 fingers?	Carpal tunnel syndrome: compression of the median nerve at the wrist
• At the ulnar aspect of the hand?	Ulnar nerve lesion (commonly at the elbow) or of the brachial plexus
• In the fingers or at the finger tips? (on exposure to cold)	Raynaud's phenomenon or disease
• Along the limb spanning joint and muscle areas?	Lesion of nerve or blood vessels Nerve root compression Thoracic outlet syndrome Peripheral nerve lesion Referred pain Ischemic heart disease

Time course	Think about
Is the pain related to an activity?	Overuse syndromes may come on after hours, days, or weeks of a repetitive activity or after resumption of an activity after some time away from it
Does the pain wax and wane?	Overuse syndromes are often better on weekends, worse on Fridays Carpal tunnel syndrome may be most painful at night Epicondylitis can be most symptomatic the day after the activity

(continued)

Time course	Think about
Was the onset of pain	
• *Sudden? (minutes to hours)*	*Acute infectious process* *Trauma* *Crystalline arthropathies* *Vascular processes* *Referred pain* *Inflammatory processes (eg, rheumatoid arthritis)*
• *Gradual?*	*Arthritis* *Tendinitis* *Bursitis* *Rheumatoid arthritis* *Neuropathic pain*

Associated symptoms	Think about
Is there swelling	
• *In the area of the pain?* • *Around or near it?*	*In rheumatoid and crystalline arthritis, the joints are painful and swollen.* *In RSD/CRPS, the entire region may be swollen.* *In carpal tunnel syndrome, the wrist swelling may be hard to appreciate but more distal swelling is often obvious.*
Is the skin red?	*Tendinitis may have erythema (redness) over the affected tendon* *Infected structures often have surrounding erythema*
Does the skin change colors?	*Vasomotor processes (Raynaud's), although the classic 3-color changes not always be present*

Modifying factors	Think about
Is joint pain	
• *Present only with movements?*	*Suggests effusion, such as in osteoarthritis*
• *Present at rest?*	*Inflammation (eg, rheumatoid arthritis)*
• *Increased by motion? Activity?*	*Abnormalities of the tendons or bursae* *Typical of overuse syndromes*
Is your arm pain induced or made worse	
• *By sneezing? Coughing? Hyperextension of the neck? Shaving under the chin?*	*Cervical radiculopathy or cervical nerve root involvement*
• *Upon rotating the head? Or upon laterally flexing the neck?*	*Cervical spine lesion*
• *When elevating the arm above the head? With exertion?*	*Referred pain: ischemic heart disease* *Thoracic outlet syndrome*
• *After a meal?*	*GERD*
• *By light touch?*	*Neuropathic pain (eg, entrapment neuropathy)*

Does the pain occur	
• *When grasping an object for a prolonged time?*	*Carpal tunnel syndrome* *Intersection syndrome*
• *At night?*	*Carpal tunnel syndrome*
• *After activity is over?*	*Epicondylitis* *Tendinitis*
• *With exposure to cold?*	*Raynaud's phenomenon*
How do you use your arm?	***Think about***
Are you unable to remove a ring? Wear a watch? Slip the hand into an old glove?	*Diffuse swelling of the hand may indicate an inflammatory disorder (eg, rheumatoid arthritis, Raynaud's disease, neurovascular compression syndrome)*
Are you unable to drive a car? To dress? Eat?	*Related to pain, rather than restricted motion at the elbow (the shoulder is able to compensate for most limitation of elbow motion)*
Are you unable to lift with the hands? Shave? Sew? Open jars?	*Disability related to disorders of the wrist or hand*
Is the pain	
• *Greatest in the morning?*	*Rheumatoid arthritis, also referred to as "morning gel"*
• *Worse with prolonged use of the joint?*	*Osteoarthritis*
Do you have	
• *Fever? Chills?*	*Septic arthritis or bursitis*
• *Numbness, tingling, burning in the arm?*	*Neuropathic pain such as entrapment neuropathy, thoracic outlet syndrome* *Peripheral neuropathy*
• *Chest pain on exertion?*	*Ischemic heart disease with referred pain to the arm*

DIAGNOSTIC APPROACH

- Characterize the pain: type, onset, associated complaints.
- Localize the pain: joints, tendons, soft tissues, hints that the pain is referred or neuropathic.
- Examine the functional anatomy of the pain: specific movements that cause, exacerbate, or relieve the pain.
- Identify potential causes: occupation, activity, habits, and lifestyle.

CAVEATS

Significant morbidity from upper extremity musculoskeletal disorders is rare. However, life- or limb-threatening disease can result from joint or soft tissue infection, and cardiopulmonary diseases may present as upper limb discomfort. These entities should always be considered.

Neuropathic pain is the great mimicker. While investigation of the painful structure is necessary, do not ignore inflamed nerves, nerve roots, or pain referred from other structures.

Descriptions are useful, but in an easily accessible area like the upper extremity there is no substitute for pointing to the area in question, and performing the movement that causes the pain or demonstrating the inducing work-related activity.

PROGNOSIS

Most primary causes of upper extremity pain resolve spontaneously or with cessation of the inciting activity. Physical therapy helps many patients. More aggressive treatment is reserved for patients in whom conservative treatment fails. Learning ergonomically safe ways to accomplish a task, such as perfecting a tennis swing, limits recurrences. Permanent disability is unusual.

REFERENCES

1. Cooke AJ, Roussopoulos K, Pallis JM, Haake S. Correlation between racquet design and arm injuries. 4th International Conference of the Engineering of Sport. September 2002.

2. National Institute for Occupational Safety and Health Report (NIOSH). 1997.

3. A Critical Review of Epidemiologic Evidence for Work-Related Musculoskeletal Disorders of the Neck, Upper Extremity, and Low Back. Cincinnati, Public Health Service, Centers for Disease Control and Prevention National Institute for Occupational Safety and Health. 1997.

4. Gibbons RJ, Chatterjee K, Daley J, et al. ACC/AHA/ACP-ASIM Guidelines for the management of patients with chronic stable angina: a report of The American College of Cardiology/American Heart Association Task Force on Practice Guidelines (Committee on Management of Patients With Chronic Stable Angina). *J Am Coll Cardiol.* 1999;33:2092–2197.

5. Brandfonbrener AG. Musicians with focal dystonia. *Med Probl Perform Art.* 1991;6:132–136.

6. Atroshi I, Gummesson C, Johnsson R, et al. Prevalence of carpal tunnel syndrome in a general population. *JAMA.* 1999; 282:153–158.

7. Tanaka S, Petersen M, Cameron L. Prevalence and risk factors of tendinitis and related disorders of the distal upper extremity along U.S. workers: comparison to carpal tunnel syndrome. *Am J Ind Med.* 2001;39:328–335.

8. Servi JT. Wrist pain from overuse: detecting and relieving intersection syndrome. *Phys Sportsmed.* 1997;25.

9. Gorsche R, Wiley JP, Renger R, et al. Prevalence and incidence of stenosing flexor tenosynovitis (trigger finger) in a meatpacking plant. *J Occup Environ Med.* 1998;40:556–560.

10. Altman R, Alarcon G, Appelrouth D, et al. The American College of Rheumatology criteria for the classification and reporting of osteoarthritis of the hand. *Arthritis Rheum.* 1990;33:1601–1610.

11. Rasch EK, Hirsch R, Paulose-Ram R, Hochberg MC. Prevalence of rheumatoid arthritis in persons 60 years of age and older in the United States: effect of different methods of case classification. *Arthritis Rheum.* 2003;48:917–926.

12. Zhang Y, Niu J, Kelly-Hayes M, et al. Prevalence of symptomatic hand osteoarthritis and its impact on functional status among the elderly: The Framingham Study. *Am J Epidemiol.* 2002;156:1021–1027.

13. Edwards DP, Mulkern E, Raja AN, Barker P. Trans-axillary first ribs excision for thoracic outlet syndrome. *J R Coll Surg Edinb.* 1999;44:362–365.

SUGGESTED READING

Greene WB (editor). *Essentials of Musculoskeletal Care,* 2nd ed. American Academy of Orthopaedic Surgeons, American Academy of Pediatrics; 2001.

McCue FC III. *The Injured Athlete,* 2nd ed. JB Lippincott Co; 1992.

Low Back Pain

Garth Davis, MD

Low back pain (LBP) is among the most common complaints encountered in the outpatient setting. While LBP may herald the recurrence of cancer and other serious diagnoses, in unselected ambulatory patients with LBP, less than 1% will have serious underlying disease.[1]

The overwhelming majority of patients with LBP will experience a benign self-limited course. Neurologic impairment is the most serious complication of back pain. Fortunately, patients with back pain usually seek medical attention long before signs and symptoms of nerve root or spinal cord compression develop.

KEY TERMS

Cauda equina syndrome	*Acute compressive radiculopathy of the sacral nerve roots that comprise the cauda equina. Symptoms include severe back pain, urinary and fecal incontinence, saddle anesthesia, and leg weakness. Most commonly results from a large midline disk herniation but can complicate any process that leads to spinal canal narrowing at the level of the cauda equina.*
Pseudoclaudication	*Pain typically located in the low back, buttocks, and proximal thighs associated with spinal stenosis. Pain is brought on by exercise and improves with rest, sitting, or leaning forward.*
Sciatica	*Syndrome characterized by pain radiating down the leg, past the knee, in the distribution of the sciatic nerve. Most commonly due to compression of the L4, L5, or S1 nerve roots.*
Spinal stenosis	*Narrowing of the spinal canal leading to compression of the spinal cord or cauda equina. Most commonly seen in older patients with severe degenerative changes of the spine.*

ETIOLOGY

Despite the popular acceptance of terminology such as **herniated disk** and **slipped disk,** the etiology of back pain is less clear in clinical practice. Less than 2% of patients with LBP manifest true radicular symptoms or sciatica from nerve root compression or irritation.[2] Intervertebral disk herniation is common, demonstrated on magnetic resonance imaging (MRI) of the spine in upwards of 30% of asymptomatic adults.[3,4] Only 36% of asymptomatic patients evaluated with MRI had normal disks at all levels.[5] In addition, patients with LBP and disk herniation recover in a similar fashion to patients without demonstrable herniation.[6] Weak correlation between symptoms, results of imaging studies, and pathologic findings leave the vast majority of patients with the somewhat murky diagnosis of "musculoskeletal" or "nonspecific" LBP.[2] Compression fractures are diagnosed in less than 5% of unselected patients with LBP. Malignancy, infection, and inflammatory disorders of the spine account for less than 1% of patients.[7]

Differential Diagnosis[8]	Prevalence[a]
Mechanical LBP	**~ 99%**
Nonspecific or musculoskeletal	80%
Degenerative	10%
Disk herniation	4%
Osteoporotic compression fracture	4%
Spinal stenosis	3%
Spondylolisthesis	2%
Traumatic vertebral fracture	< 1%
Congenital disease	< 1%
Nonmechanical LBP	**~ 1%**
Neoplasia	0.7%
Inflammatory arthritis (eg, ankylosing spondylitis)	0.3%
Infection (eg, Osteomyelitis)	0.01%
Paget's disease of bone	< 0.01%

Referred pain from visceral disease

• Aortic aneurysm

• Renal disease
– Nephrolithiasis
– Pyelonephritis
– Perinephric abscess

• Gastrointestinal disease
– Pancreatitis
– Cholecystitis
– Perforating peptic ulcer

• Urogenital
– Endometriosis
– Chronic pelvic inflammatory disease
– Prostatitis

[a]Prevalence is unknown when not indicated.

GETTING STARTED

As with any complaint of pain, have the patient elaborate on the duration, character, severity, alleviating and exacerbating factors, and associated symptoms.

Questions	Remember
Can you describe how it started?	*Start with open-ended questions. Let the patient describe the symptoms rather than choosing from a list.*

When is the pain most severe?	Helps differentiate mechanical (pain worsened with use) from inflammatory (symptoms worsened with rest) etiologies.
How are you limited by your back pain?	Provides insight into the degree of disability experienced by the patient.

INTERVIEW FRAMEWORK

Since it is often difficult to determine a specific cause for LBP, it will be more useful to focus the evaluation on answering the following 3 questions:

1. Is a systemic disease causing the symptoms?
2. Is there evidence of a serious neurologic deficit?
3. Is this really a back problem or is it referred pain from a visceral structure?

IDENTIFYING ALARM SYMPTOMS

Alarm symptoms are more commonly associated with serious underlying disease than with benign disorders. Present, they increase the pretest probability of serious disease; unfortunately, their absence doesn't necessarily rule out serious disease.

Serious Diagnoses

Neurologic complications can result from any process that leads to compression of the spinal cord or nerve roots. Intervertebral disk herniation and degenerative disease of the spine can cause significant neurologic impairment requiring surgical intervention. However, the majority of neurologic emergencies associated with LBP are limited to the conditions listed below.

Serious nonmechanical causes of LBP are rare, comprising less than 1% of ambulatory patients. Thorough questioning to elicit alarm symptoms can help reduce the risk of missing serious disease. Focused questioning can help identify patients at increased risk for serious diagnoses.

Serious Diagnosis	Prevalence[a]
Malignancy	0.7%[1]
Infection	0.01%[7]
Compression fracture	4%[9]
Cauda equina syndrome	0.0004%[9]

[a]In ambulatory patients with LBP.

Alarm symptoms	Serious causes	Positive likelihood ratio (LR+)[a]	Benign causes
Pain at rest	Malignancy Ankylosing spondylitis		Mechanical LBP

(continued)

Alarm symptoms	Serious causes	Positive likelihood ratio (LR+)[a]	Benign causes
Pain that has already prompted an evaluation	Malignancy	3.0[1]	Mechanical LBP
Duration of episode > 1 month	Malignancy	2.6[1]	Mechanical LBP
Unexplained weight loss	Malignancy	2.7[1]	
Fever	Osteomyelitis Paravertebral abscess	25[10,11]	Pyelonephritis Mechanical LBP Viral syndrome
Urinary retention with incontinence (overflow)	Cauda equina syndrome	18[9]	Medications
Fecal incontinence	Cauda equina syndrome		
Saddle anesthesia	Cauda equina syndrome		
Extremity weakness	Malignancy		
Trauma	Compression fracture		
Severe lower extremity pain	Spinal stenosis	2[12]	Sciatica Intermittent claudication
No pain when seated	Spinal stenosis	6.6[12]	
Wide based gate	Spinal stenosis	14[12]	Peripheral neuropathy
Improvement with exercise	Ankylosing spondylitis	1.3–7.5[13]	
Pain makes patient get out of bed at night	Ankylosing spondylitis	3.1[13]	
Morning stiffness of back	Ankylosing spondylitis	0.9–2.3[13]	

[a]Each LR applies to the adjacent serious cause.

FOCUSED QUESTIONS

Questions	Think about
Do you have a personal history of cancer?	Malignancy—in patients with a personal history of cancer, new back pain should be considered malignant until proven otherwise (LR+ 14.7)[1]
Over 50 years of age?	Malignancy (LR+ 2.7)[1]
Have you been treated with corticosteroids for more than 1 month?	Vertebral compression fracture[1]
Any recent trauma?	Vertebral compression fracture[9]
Age over 70?	Vertebral compression fracture[9]
Does the pain keep you awake?	Malignancy Spondyloarthropathy

Does the pain steadily increase with walking?	Spinal stenosis
Is the pain improved with sitting or bending forward?	Spinal stenosis
Have you recently used injection drugs?	Vertebral osteomyelitis Paraspinous abscess
Are you taking immunosuppressant medication?	Vertebral osteomyelitis Paraspinous abscess
Have you recently had an indwelling venous catheter?	Vertebral osteomyelitis Paraspinous abscess
Have you recently had a urinary (bladder) catheter?	Vertebral osteomyelitis Paraspinous abscess
Do you have significant morning stiffness?[a]	Spondyloarthropathy
Does the pain improve with exercise?[a]	Spondyloarthropathy
Did symptoms progress gradually over time?[a]	Spondyloarthropathy
Symptoms ongoing for at least 3 months?[a]	Spondyloarthropathy
Symptoms started before age 35?[a]	Spondyloarthropathy

Quality	**Think about**
Is the pain shock-like?	Disk herniation
Does the pain radiate down the leg past the knee?	Sciatica (irritation or compression of the L4–5, S1 roots usually from disk herniation)
Does the pain have a tearing or ripping quality?	Aortic dissection
Is it localized?	Fracture
Is the pain constant or does it fluctuate in severity?	Mechanical LBP is usually constant and worsened with movement; nonmechanical LBP is constant but worse with rest. Colicky pain may implicate a visceral etiology.

Time course	**Think about**
Was the onset abrupt?	Mechanical back pain Fracture (traumatic, osteoporotic, or pathologic)
Has the pain been evaluated in the last month for failure to improve? Has it gradually increased in severity over months?	Malignancy Spondyloarthropathy
Is there an association with menstrual cycle?	Endometriosis

Associated symptoms	**Think about**
Do you have	
• Nausea or vomiting?	Perforated peptic ulcer Pyelonephritis
• Abdominal pain?	Pyelonephritis Retrocecal appendicitis Diverticular abscess

(continued)

Associated symptoms	Think about
• Fever?	Osteomyelitis
	Paraspinous abscess
	Pyelonephritis
• Dysuria?	Pyelonephritis
	Nephrolithiasis
Modifying symptoms	**Think about**
Is the pain improved with sitting?	Spinal stenosis
Does pain increase with movement?	Compression fracture
	Disk herniation
	Mechanical LBP
Does pain increase with walking?	Spinal stenosis

[a]Any 4 affirmative answers have a positive LR of 6.3 for spondyloarthropathy.[13]

CAVEATS

- Mechanical LBP can occasionally be *severe.*
- Patients with metastatic disease of the spine may be symptomatic for months and often have already been evaluated for back pain.
- Even though the severity of back pain may seem unimpressive, its etiology can still be malignant. Remember the important historical clues and warning signs.
- "I was lifting a box of books when the pain started." Although this sounds like a reasonable mechanical explanation for LBP, it may also represent serious underlying pathology. While muscular strains often present in this fashion, so do pathologic fractures.

PROGNOSIS

For most patients, LBP is a self-limited disorder and rapid recovery is the norm. In patients with mechanical LBP, as many as 90% are better at 2 weeks; more conservative estimates would indicate recovery by 6 weeks for approximately 67% of patients. Unfortunately, as many as 40% of patients will have recurrent symptoms by 6 months. It is not uncommon for such patients to evolve to a more chronic disease state with waxing and waning symptoms. Patients with documented disk herniation usually recover with conservative management, and fewer than 10% undergo back surgery for intractable pain or neurologic dysfunction.[8]

Patients with spinal stenosis tend to progress over time. Pain and limitation are triggered by ever decreasing activity and patients can suffer severe disability from pseudoclaudication. Compression fractures may cause significant pain, sometimes for months after the original injury. Therapy was previously limited to immobilization and analgesics but newer therapies, such as interventional vertebroplasty, will hopefully reduce the burden of suffering. Spinal and paraspinal infections cause significant morbidity and mortality, the best outcomes occurring with prompt diagnosis and medical and surgical intervention. Metastatic disease of the spine bears the already grim prognosis of any advanced malignancy. However, development of lower extremity paralysis from a progressive spinal metastasis in a patient with already limited survival is devastating, tragic, and often preventable. Early identification of patients with metastatic disease of the spine allows for effective treatment to protect the patient from progressive spinal cord injury.

REFERENCES

1. Deyo RA, Diehl AK. Cancer as a cause of back pain: frequency, clinical presentation, and diagnostic strategies. *J Gen Intern Med.* 1988;3:230–238.

2. Frymoyer JW. Back pain and sciatica. *N Engl J Med.* 1988;318:291–300.

3. Wiesel SW, Tsourmas N, Feffer HL, et al. A study of computer-assisted tomography. I. The incidence of positive CAT scans in an asymptomatic group of patients. *Spine.* 1984;9:549–551.

4. Boden SD, Davis DO, Dina TS, et al. Abnormal magnetic-resonance scans of the lumbar spine in asymptomatic subjects. a prospective investigation. *J Bone Joint Surg Am.* 1990;72:403–408.

5. Jensen MC, Brant-Zawadzki MN, Obuchowski N, et al. Magnetic resonance imaging of the lumbar spine in people without back pain. *N Engl J Med.* 1994;331:69–73.

6. Bell GR, Rothman RH. The conservative treatment of sciatica. *Spine.* 1984;9:54–56.

7. Liang M, Komaroff AL. Roentgenograms in primary care patients with acute low back pain: a cost-effectiveness analysis. *Arch Intern Med.* 1982;142:1108–1112.

8. Deyo RA, Weinstein JN. Low back pain. *N Engl J Med.* 2001;344:363–370.

9. Deyo RA, Rainville J, Kent DL. What can the history and physical examination tell us about low back pain? *JAMA.* 1992;268:760–765.

10. Baker AS, Ojemann RG, Swartz MN, et al. Spinal epidural abscess. *N Engl J Med.* 1975;293:463–468.

11. Sapico FL, Montgomerie JZ. Pyogenic vertebral osteomyelitis: report of nine cases and review of the literature. *Rev Infect Dis.* 1979;1:754–776.

12. Katz JN, Dalgas M, Stucki G, et al. Degenerative lumbar spinal stenosis. Diagnostic value of the history and physical examination. *Arthritis Rheum.* 1995;38:1236–1241.

13. Calin A, Porta J, Fries JF, Schuman DJ. Clinical history as a screening test for ankylosing spondylitis. *JAMA.* 1977;237:2613–2614.

SUGGESTED READING

Rosomoff HL, Rosomoff RS. Low back pain. Evaluation and management in the primary care setting. *Med Clin North Am.* 1999;83:643–662.

Diagnostic Approach: Lower Back Pain

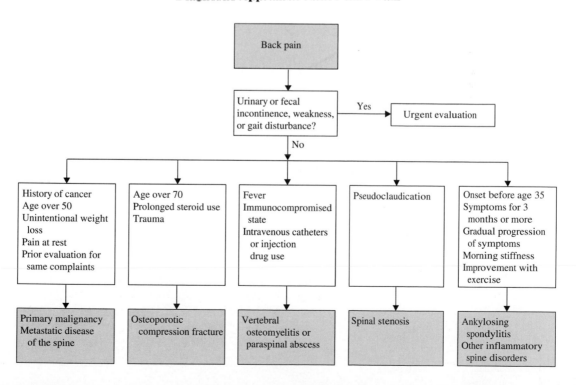

Buttock, Hip, and Thigh Pain

51

Robert D. Ficalora, MD

Pain in the proximal lower extremities may result from diseases of the blood vessels, peripheral nerves, local infection, or may be referred from local structures, such as hip pain referred to the ipsilateral knee. Disorders of use and abuse, particularly sports-related disorders predominate in this area.

Deep pain arising from vessels, fascia, joints, tendons, periosteum, and supporting structures is often poorly localized and dull and may be accompanied by the perception of joint stiffness and deep tenderness. The close proximity of structures and the complicated functional anatomy of the region make localization of the pain and identification of the affected structure even more difficult. Pain that arises from adjacent or supporting structures may be attributed to the joints in the absence of any true joint pathology.

Pain due to disorders of the tendons, muscles, and bursae of the buttock and thigh are common sites of inflammation due to athletic injuries. Pain in the hip is often a consequence of degenerative or inflammatory conditions. Pain caused by diseases of the peripheral nerves or by entrapment neuropathies, such as meralgia paresthetica, can be difficult to sort out by history. Neuropathic pain may result from reflex sympathetic dystrophy/chronic regional pain syndrome (RSD/CRPS), a poorly understood condition that can result from local trauma, stroke, or spinal cord injury. Irritation of the lumbar nerve roots (herniated nucleus pulposus, osteoarthritis) can cause pain in the lower extremities and may complicate the diagnosis of more local disorders such as trochanteric bursitis and peripheral sciatic nerve inflammation.

There are complex functional relationships that may obscure primary and secondary etiologies of pain. Gait abnormalities can result from disorders in this region and can also be etiologic in others: degenerative hip joint disease may result in a gait disorder that causes piriformis syndrome or trochanteric bursitis. Obstruction of vessels by atherosclerosis usually occurs in the setting of systemic vascular disease and rarely is an isolated phenomenon. Deep venous thrombosis (DVT) requires immediate identification and action.

KEY TERMS

Bursitis	Pain and inflammation of the structure that contains the fluid that lubricates a joint or tendon sheath.
Degenerative joint disease	Characteristic painful, noninflammatory changes in a joint that result from "wear and tear" of chronic use and abuse.
Entrapment neuropathy	Pain and loss of function resulting from a nerve passing through a physiologic space that is narrowed secondary to acute or chronic trauma or inflammation.
Neuropathic pain	Pain in a region as a result of nerve inflammation, trauma, or neurologic disease.

(continued)

KEY TERMS

Overuse syndrome	*Pain and inflammation resulting from intense or repetitive use of regional anatomic structures in the course of occupational or recreational activities.*
Radiculopathy	*Pain caused by irritation or compression of a nerve in or near the spinal column. It produces symptoms in the area of innervation.*
Referred pain	*Pain originating in 1 structure that is perceived in the area of another, usually because of physiologic or embryologic links between the 2 structures.*
Strain	*Micro-tears of muscle fibers; can be indistinguishable from muscle tear and the terms are often used interchangeably.*
Tendinitis	*Pain and inflammation of a tendon or tendon sheath.*

ETIOLOGY

Differential Diagnosis: Buttock Pain

Diagnosis	*Explanation*	*Prevalence*
Coccydynia	*Pain at the base of the spine that represents a collection of conditions that have different causes ranging from hypermobility of the sacral vertebra to neuropathic pain as a result of multiple traumatic events. Coccydynia can follow falls, childbirth, repetitive strain, or surgery.*	*Up to 20% of women after difficult deliveries[1]*
Sciatica	*Pain, weakness, numbness, and other discomfort along the path of the sciatic nerve; often accompanies low back pain. It indicates a problem at some point along the sciatic nerve, such as herniated disk, spinal stenosis, obturator foramen stenosis or hernia, and piriformis syndrome.*	*5.7% of workers with low back pain[2]*
Hamstring/ischial tuberosity syndrome	*Pain in the posterior thigh, particularly during and following activities like running. Hamstring injuries occur in sports that require bursts of speed or rapid acceleration, such as track, soccer, and football. Predisposing factors include improper warm-up, fatigue, previous injury, strength imbalance, and poor flexibility.*	*2–11% of all injuries in athletes annually[3,4]*
Piriformis syndrome	*Spasm of a small buttock muscle through which the sciatic nerve runs. Pain and leg symptoms are attributed to entrapment of the sciatic nerve. Occurs primarily in individuals with gait abnormalities, weakness of postural muscles, and pregnancy. May occur concurrently with trochanteric bursitis.*	*Up to 13% of patients with symptoms of sciatica[5]*

| RSD/CRPS | A chronic progressive neurologic condition that affects a region, such as an arm or a leg. Can also occur after a minor injury, such as a sprain. In some cases, there is no precipitating event. Pain begins in 1 area or limb and then spreads. RSD/CRPS is characterized by burning pain, excessive sweating, swelling, and sensitivity to touch. Marked osteopenia is noted in bones within the nerve distribution. | 2–5% of peripheral nerve injury patients
12–21% of patients with hemiplegia (paralysis on 1 side of the body)
1–2% of bone fracture patients[6] |

Differential Diagnosis: Thigh Pain

Diagnosis	*Explanation*	*Prevalence*
Lateral femoral cutaneous nerve (LFCN) syndrome or meralgia paresthetica	Damage to the LFCN from surgery on the iliac crest, hysterectomy, laparoscopic herniorrhaphy, aortic valve surgery, coronary artery bypass surgery; diabetic neuropathy; restrictive clothing; and tightly worn, wide weight-lifting belts.	Varies widely but has been reported in up to 20% of some surgical procedures[7]
Quadriceps muscle strain or tear	The quadriceps muscles consist of the vastus lateralis, vastus medialis, vastus intermedius, and the rectus femoris. Any of these muscles can strain (or tear), but the most common is the rectus femoris. Occurs in football/soccer players, skaters, runners and older athletes whose exercise program is primarily walking.	US Military Academy at West Point data is as follows: rugby, 4.7%; karate and judo, 2.3%; football, 1.6%; all other sports, < 1%.[8]
Hamstring strain	Hamstrings are long muscles that extend down the back of the thigh. Because hamstrings work to pull back the leg and bend the knee, they can be injured during running, kicking, or jumping. Patients may feel a "pop," usually at the back of the thigh, when the muscle tears.	Unknown[9]
Trochanteric bursitis	Inflammation of 1 or more of the 4 bursae usually present around the greater trochanter; 3 are constant—2 major and 1 minor. These bursae function as a gliding mechanism for the anterior portion of the gluteus maximus tendon as it passes over the greater trochanter to insert into the iliotibial band (ITB). Any inflammation or irritation of these bursae can result in symptoms of trochanteric bursitis. Seen typically with disorders of gait due to hip, knee, or low back problems; obesity; or pregnancy.	Unknown[10]

(continued)

Diagnosis	Explanation	Prevalence
Lumbar radiculopathy (L2, L3), lumbar facet syndrome	A sensory or motor nerve exiting the spinal column may be irritated or entrapped by arthritis of the foramina or the facet or compressed by a herniated disk, with pain referring to the lateral thigh.	2% of the population Of these, 10–25% develop symptoms that persist for more than 6 weeks[2]
Iliopsoas bursitis/tendinitis Iliopsoas syndrome "snapping hip syndrome"	Pain and snapping in medial groin or thigh. Acute injury and overuse are the 2 main causes. The acute injury involves an eccentric contraction of the iliopsoas muscle or direct trauma. Overuse injury occurs in activities involving repeated hip flexion or external rotation of the thigh. Seen in dancers, gymnasts, cheerleaders, and runners.	43.8% of ballet dancers with hip pain[11]
Hip adductor strain or "groin pull" also called "gracilis strain," which is a misnomer since all the hip adductor muscles can be involved	A bruise or strain of the muscles that run from the front of the hip bone to the inside of the thigh. These muscles stabilize the hip and leg during all sporting activities that involve running. Pain and stiffness in the groin region occur in the morning and at the beginning of athletic activity. May abate after warming up but often recurs after athletic activity.	62% of groin injuries; accounts for 5% of all soccer injuries and 2.5% of karate injuries[12]
ITB syndrome "runner's knee"	Lateral hip, thigh, or knee pain, snapping as ITB passes over the greater trochanter. The most common overuse syndrome of the knee. It is caused by repetitive friction of the ITB on the lateral femoral condyle during flexion-extension, resulting in an inflammatory reaction.	Unknown; occurs mainly in athletes, especially runners and cyclists[13]
DVT of the thigh	Characterized by unilateral warmth, erythema, swelling and tenderness of the calf and thigh, in which a large vein is occluded by thrombus.	5% of patients with lower limb orthopedic conditions without prophylaxis. Can be significantly increased in persons with hypercoagulable states[14]
Entrapment neuropathies involving the subcostal, and the lateral cutaneous branches of the iliohypogastric nerves	Causes pain in the proximal anterior thigh and occurs after abdominal surgical procedures (eg, appendectomy, herniorrhaphy).	Unknown[15]

Differential Diagnosis: Hip Pain

Diagnosis	Explanation	Prevalence
Aseptic necrosis of the femoral head	Vascular supply to the femoral head is precarious and easily compromised. A large portion of the total surface is covered with articular cartilage through which vessels do not penetrate. The blood supply enters through a restricted space, and there is limited collateral circulation. Risk factors include fracture, corticosteroid therapy, alcohol, gout, diabetes, sickle cell anemia, and Gaucher disease.	0.72% of general population Corticosteroids increase risk significantly[13]
Hip fracture	A fracture of the femur above a point 5 cm below the distal part of the lesser trochanter. An intracapsular fracture occurs proximal to the point at which the hip joint capsule attaches to the femur. Subtrochanteric fractures occur in the most distal part of the proximal femoral segment (below the lesser trochanter). Extracapsular fractures occur distal to the hip joint capsule.	0.11% of the general population Prevalence increases from about 3 per 100 women aged 65–74 to 12.6 per 100 women aged 85 or older[16]
Hip osteoarthritis	Osteoarthritis is a mechanically stimulated, chemically mediated process in which attempted repair results in abnormal bone structure. Risk factors include aging, obesity, occupation, and gender.	70% of the general population over 65 years[17]
Rheumatoid arthritis	The cause is unknown. Hip involvement, since it compromises mobility, can be particularly debilitating. Synovial tissue and joint destruction can occur early in the disease process, before classic deformities develop.	2% in persons older than 60[18]

GETTING STARTED

- Lower extremity complaints are usually localized and commonly related to an injury, inciting event, recreational or occupational overuse.
- Anatomic and functional relationships are complex and require careful investigation.
- Basic questions as to the onset, location, qualities, and aggravating or ameliorating factors are most useful.
- An occupational and leisure time (especially athletic) history is essential.

Questions

Where is the pain?

When did it start?

Can you describe it for me? Is it dull, sharp, or burning? Does it ever change?

Is there swelling?

Is there a rash or discoloration?

What activity makes it better or worse?

Can you bear weight?

Can you show me how you use your legs at work, or when you play?
Tell me about your leisure time activities.

Remember

- *Most patients will not be able to adequately describe the location of the pain, so pointing is helpful.*
- *Physical demonstrations of typical activities, or descriptions of sports-related movements may be valuable adjuncts to the history.*
- *Trying to be helpful, patients often group unrelated symptoms. Make sure that each individual symptom or sign is understood completely before moving on.*

INTERVIEW FRAMEWORK

- Assess for alarm symptoms.
- Identify activities that put the patient at risk.
- Systematically identify complaints that relate to differential diagnoses of the joints; soft tissues, including tendons, bursae, and muscle groups; nerves and neuropathic disorders; and lumbar structures that refer pain to the lower extremity.

IDENTIFYING ALARM SYMPTOMS

Serious Diagnoses

- Acute disk herniation
- Hip fracture
- Aseptic necrosis of the femoral head
- DVT
- Primary or metastatic tumor

Alarm symptoms	Serious causes	Benign causes
Loss of bowel or bladder control or persistent sensory abnormalities (eg, numbness, burning, or tingling), especially those associated with back complaints	*Lumbar nerve root or spinal cord disorders, especially acute lumbar disk herniation* *Epidural metastasis*	*Anxiety (may be a side effect of medications)*
Inability to bear weight	*Hip fracture or aseptic necrosis of the femoral head*	*Pain from tendinitis or bursitis or degenerative joint disease may be so intense that patients refuse to bear weight*
Painful redness and swelling of the thigh, particularly over the common femoral vein	*Thigh DVT has a high risk of pulmonary embolism and cardiopulmonary complications*	*Local trauma or skin infection*

FOCUSED QUESTIONS

After hearing a description of the complaint, put the description in a context of related risks and activities. Patients may have an idea of the causes of their disorder from the media, friends or the Internet, but they often won't be able to put all the pieces together. Since most disorders of the lower extremity are not primary physiological derangements, but rather the effects of overuse or injury (work related or athletic), narrowing the differential diagnosis begins with the defining the patient's activities.

Questions	Think about
Tell me about your work.	
Do you perform repetitive activities such as unloading trucks or work on an assembly line?	*Repetitive motion of the hip and lower back, as well as lifting, increases the risk of several forms of tendinitis or bursitis, lumbar radiculopathy, and disk herniation.*
Do you wear a lumbar support belt, weight-lifting belt, or other constrictive clothing?	*Meralgia paresthetica or lateral femoral cutaneous nerve syndrome (LFCN) is an entrapment neuropathy that can result from tight, restrictive clothing.*
Do you jump off trucks, platforms, or heavy equipment?	*Osteoarthritis results from chronic minor trauma to the hip.*
Tell me about your leisure time activities.	
Do you play football or soccer? Run track?	*Hamstring/ischial tuberosity syndrome from improper or inadequate stretching or warm up.*
Do you play football or soccer? Skate? Run? Practice judo or karate? Do you walk (in older patients)?	*Quadriceps muscle strain or tear* *Hip adductor strain*
Do participate in gymnastics or football?	*Hamstring tear, from kicking or jumping, after feeling a "pop" in the back of the thigh.*
Have you taken any long car rides or airplane trips?	*Inactivity without hourly stretching or movement of the legs is a major risk for DVT.*

Quality	*Think about*
Is the pain	
• *Steady?*	*Rheumatoid arthritis* *Osteoarthritis* *Infection*
• *Aching?*	*Overuse syndrome or referred pain*
• *Shooting? sharp?*	*Entrapment neuropathy*
• *Burning?*	*Neuropathic pain*
• *Severe?*	*Arthritis (at rest)* *Gout* *Infection* *Trauma* *Tumor*
• *Throbbing?*	*Inflammatory or vascular (DVT)*
• *Related to activity?*	*Tendinitis or bursitis*

(continued)

Location	**Think about**
Where do you have pain?	
• *In or around what joint?*	*Pain resulting from an articular disorder is perceived as coming directly from the joint, not from the bones between the joints. True hip pain is felt in the groin. Patients describe lateral thigh pain as "hip" pain which is usually a soft tissue problem*
• *Buttock?*	*Coccydynia, sciatica (with radiation down leg), piriformis syndrome*
• *Hip?*	*Osteoarthritis* *Hip fracture or aseptic necrosis* *Rheumatoid arthritis*
• *Anterior thigh?*	*Entrapment neuropathies* *Meralgia paresthetica (LFCN syndrome)* *Lumbar (L2/L3) radiculopathy* *Quadriceps muscle strain/tear* *Hip adductor strain*
• *Lateral thigh?*	*Trochanteric bursitis* *Entrapment neuropathies*
• *Medial thigh*	*DVT* *Iliopsoas bursitis or tendinitis*
• *Posterior thigh?*	*Hamstring strain* *Ischial tuberosity syndrome*
• *Along the limb spanning joint and muscle*	*Lesion of blood vessels such as DVT* *Nerve root compression*
Time course	**Think about**
Is the pain related to an activity?	*Overuse syndromes may come on after hours, days, or weeks of a repetitive activity, or after resumption of an activity after some time away from it*
Does the pain wax and wane?	*Work-related overuse syndromes are often better on weekends and worse on Fridays* *While sports-related overuse syndromes may have the reverse or a variable pattern* *Bursitis is most painful at night*
Was the onset of pain • *Sudden? (minutes to hours)*	*Acute infectious process* *Trauma* *Vascular processes* *Referred pain* *Inflammatory processes (eg, rheumatoid arthritis)*
• *Gradual?*	*Arthritis* *Tendinitis* *Bursitis* *Rheumatoid arthritis* *Neuropathic pain*

Associated symptoms	Think about
Is there swelling	
• In the area of the pain?	In rheumatoid arthritis, the joints are painful and swollen
• Around or near it?	In RSD, the entire region may be swollen. In the deep structures of the hip and buttocks, stiffness or immobility may be the only clue to deep tissue swelling.
Is the skin red?	Tendinitis may have erythema (redness) over the affected tendon. Infected structures often have surrounding erythema as does DVT

Modifying factors	Think about
Is the joint pain	
• Present only with movements?	Suggests effusion such as in osteoarthritis
• Present at rest?	Suggests inflammation, such as rheumatoid arthritis, or neuropathic pain
• Increased by motion? Activity?	Suggests abnormalities of the tendons or bursae Typical of overuse syndromes or athletic injuries
Is the pain in your leg (not related to a joint) induced or made worse	
• By sneezing? Coughing? Sitting or hyperextension of the back?	Lumbar nerve root pain
• Raising the leg up straight?	Lumbar spine lesion
• During stretching?	Inflamed tendons or bursae Sciatica
• By light touch?	Neuropathic pain, such as entrapment neuropathy
Does the pain occur	
• Climbing stairs or at night?	Trochanteric bursitis Piriformis syndrome
• After activity is over?	Tendinitis Quadriceps or hamstring strain
• After recent surgical procedure?	Coccydynia Entrapment neuropathies
Are you unable to bear weight?	Structural disorders of the hip joint such as fracture or aseptic necrosis of the femoral head
Are you unable to walk?	Related to pain rather than restricted motion Quadriceps muscle or hamstring strain
Are you unable to kick a ball?	Strain or inflammation of the muscles or tendons

(continued)

Modifying factors	Think about
Is the pain	
• *Greatest in the morning?*	*Rheumatoid arthritis (morning stiffness)*
• *Worse with prolonged use of the joint?*	*Osteoarthritis*
• *Better with use?*	*Hip adductor strain*
Do you have	
• *Fever or chills?*	*Septic arthritis or bursitis*
• *Numbness, tingling, or burning in the leg?*	*Neuropathic pain such as entrapment neuropathy*
	Sciatica
	LFCN syndrome
• *Swelling, redness, or dyspnea?*	*DVT with or without pulmonary thromboembolism*

DIAGNOSTIC APPROACH

- Characterize the pain: type, onset, associated complaints.
- Localize the pain: joints, tendons, soft tissues.
- Look for hints that the pain might be referred or neuropathic.
- Examine the functional anatomy of the pain: movements that cause, exacerbate, or relieve the pain.
- Identify potential causes: occupation, athletics, habits, and other musculoskeletal problems (eg, gait disorder, injury).

CAVEATS

While significant morbidity from musculoskeletal disorders of the lower extremity is rare, life- or limb-threatening disease may result from joint or soft tissue infection, DVT and its cardiopulmonary complications, or malignancy.

Neuropathic pain is the great mimicker. While investigation of the painful structure is necessary, do not ignore inflamed nerves, nerve roots, pain referred from other structures, or conditions that put the patient at risk for RSD/CRPS.

Descriptions are useful, but in an area such as the lower extremity that is easily accessible, there is no substitute for pointing to the area in question, performing the movement that causes the pain, or demonstrating the work-related or athletic activity that precipitates the pain.

PROGNOSIS

The vast majority of causes of lower extremity pain resolve spontaneously or with cessation of the inciting activity. Physical therapy helps many persons. Learning the importance of adequate warm up and stretching limits recurrences. Permanent disability is unusual. Systemic illnesses such as hypercoagulability or inflammatory disorders can radically change the prognosis of lower extremity conditions.

REFERENCES

1. Maigne JY, Doursounian L, Chatellier G. Causes and mechanisms of common coccydynia: role of body mass index and coccygeal trauma. *Spine.* 2000;25:3072–3079.
2. Hagen KB, Hilde G, Jamtvedt G, Winnem MF. The Cochran review of advice to stay active as a single treatment for low back pain and sciatica. *Spine.* 2002;27:1736–1741.
3. Kujala UM, Orava S, Jarvinen M. Hamstring injuries. Current trends in treatment and prevention. *Sports Med.* 1997;23:397–404.
4. Browning KH. Hip and pelvis injuries in runners careful evaluation and tailored management. *Phys Sportsmed.* 2001, 29.

5. Rich B, McKeag D. When sciatica is not disc disease: detecting piriformis syndrome in active patients. *Phys Sports Med.* 1992;20:104–115.

6. Reinders MF, Geertzen JH, Dijkstra PU. Complex regional pain syndrome type I: use of the International Association for the Study of Pain diagnostic criteria defined in 1994. *Clin J Pain.* 2002;18:207–215.

7. Grossman MG, Ducey SA, Nadler SS, Levy AS. Meralgia paresthetica: diagnosis and treatment. *J Am Acad Orthop Surg.* 2001;9:336–344.

8. Ryan JB, Wheeler JH, Hopkinson WJ, et al. Quadriceps contusions. West Point update. *Am J Sports Med.* 1991;19:299–304.

9. Holder-Powell HM, Rutherford OM. Unilateral lower limb injury: its long-term effects on quadriceps, hamstring, and plantar flexor muscle strength. *Arch Phys Med Rehab.* 1999;80:717–720.

10. Shbeeb MI, Matteson EL. Trochanteric bursitis (greater trochanter pain syndrome). *Mayo Clin Proceed.* 1996;71:565–569.

11. Biundo JJJ, Irwin RW, Umpierre E. Sports and other soft tissue injuries, tendinitis, bursitis, and occupation-related syndromes. *Curr Opin Rheumatol.* 2001;13:146–149.

12. Prather H. Pelvis and sacral dysfunction in sports and exercise. *Phys Med Rehab Clin N Am.* 2000;11:805–836.

13. Guerra JJ, Steinberg ME. Distinguishing transient osteoporosis from avascular necrosis of the hip. *J Bone Joint Surg.* 1995;77:616–624.

14. Gottlieb RH, Widjaja J. Clinical outcomes of untreated symptomatic patients with negative findings on sonography of the thigh for deep vein thrombosis: our experience and a review of the literature. *Am J Roentgenol.* 1999;172:1601–1604.

15. Avsar FM, Sahin M, Arikan BU, et al. The possibility of nervus ilioinguinalis and nervus iliohypogastricus injury in lower abdominal incisions and effects on hernia formation. *J Surg Res.* 2002;107:179–185.

16. Braithwaite RS, Col NF, Wong JB. Estimating hip fracture morbidity, mortality and costs. *J Am Geriatr Soc.* 2003;51:364–370.

17. Sowers M. Epidemiology of risk factors for osteoarthritis: systemic factors. *Curr Opin Rheumatol.* 2001;13:447–451.

18. Rasch EK, Hirsch R, Paulose-Ram R, Hochberg MC. Prevalence of rheumatoid arthritis in persons 60 years of age and older in the United States: effect of different methods of case classification. *Arthritis Rheum.* 2003;48:917–926.

SUGGESTED READING

Greene WB (editor). *Essentials of Musculoskeletal Care,* 2nd ed. American Academy of Orthopaedic Surgeons, American Academy of Pediatrics; 2001.

McCue FC III. *The Injured Athlete,* 2nd ed. JB Lippincott Co; 1992.

Knee and Calf Pain

52

Jane E. O'Rorke, MD

Ten to fifteen percent of adults report knee pain at some point in their lifetime. It accounts for 3–5% of visits to a physician, resulting in 33 million new visits per year.[1] Exact location of the initial pain is key to the diagnosis. A differential diagnosis can be formulated by the anatomic structures in the area. A thorough history combined with a meticulous examination should establish the etiology.

Very little is known about calf pain as an entity; some of the etiologies have been studied in depth, however. History taking in calf pain is the key to determining the diagnosis.

KEY TERMS

Buckling	*A complete collapse of the knee, often secondary to pain or muscle weakness of the quadriceps.[2]*
Effusion	*When fluid accumulates in the knee joint causing swelling.*
Giving way	*This occurs with normal walking but may be most prominent during pivoting movements, such as those that occur with quick changes in direction. One bony structure slides on another in an abnormal way. Usually associated with ligamentous injuries.[1]*
Intermittent claudication	*Pain, tension, and weakness in the legs with walking, which intensifies to produce lameness and is relieved by rest.*
Locking	*When the knee is stuck, usually in about 45 degrees of flexion, and patient is unable to unlock the knee without manipulating it in some fashion.[2]*
Positive predictive value	*Measures whether or not an individual has a disease if a given symptom is present.*
Pseudolocking	*This occurs with arthritis, when the adjacent rough surfaces stick momentarily as they glide over one another.[2]*

ETIOLOGY

Knee Pain

The etiology of knee pain depends on the anatomic location of the pain. Common causes include osteoarthritis (34%), meniscal injury (9%), collateral ligament injury (7%), cruciate ligament injury (4%), gout (2%), fracture (1.2%), sprains and strain (42%), rheumatoid arthritis (0.5%), infectious arthritis (0.3%), and pseudogout (0.2%).[6]

Differential Diagnosis	Possible Causes
Anatomic location of the pain	
Anterior knee	Patellofemoral syndrome
	Prepatellar bursitis
	Patellar fracture
	Patellar tendinitis
	Quadriceps femoris strain
	Osteoarthritis
Posterior knee	Hamstring strain
	Bursitis (semimembranous, popliteal, gastrocnemius)
	Baker cyst
	Deep venous thrombosis
	Popliteal aneurysm
Medial knee	Medial meniscal tear
	Medial collateral ligament sprain
	Anserine bursitis
	Hamstring (semimembranous) strain
	Patellofemoral syndrome
Lateral knee	Lateral meniscal tear
	Lateral collateral ligament tear
	Iliotibial band syndrome
	Biceps femoris strain
	Fibular head fracture/dislocation
Presenting symptoms	
Knee laxity (giving way not buckling)	Anterior cruciate ligament tear
	Posterior cruciate ligament tear
	Lateral collateral ligament tear
	Medial collateral ligament tear
Knee locking or clicking	Medial meniscal tear
	Lateral meniscal tear
Acute swelling (immediately following injury)	Anterior cruciate ligament tear
	Posterior cruciate ligament tear
	Patellar fracture
	Tibiofemoral dislocation
Delayed swelling (occurs hours after injury)	Medial meniscal tear
	Lateral meniscal tear

Calf Pain

There are no formal epidemiologic studies of calf pain. The incidence and prevalence of intermittent claudication ranges from 3% to 10%, with a sharp increase in patients aged 70 or older.[4] For patients with deep venous thrombosis, calf pain has a positive likelihood ratio of 1.1 and positive predictive value of only 10%.[5]

Differential Diagnosis

- *Intermittent claudication*
- *Deep venous thrombosis*
- *Popliteal artery entrapment syndrome (in younger individuals not yet at risk for atherosclerotic disease)*
- *Tear or contusion of the gastrocnemius or soleus muscle*
- *Distal dissection of a Baker cyst*
- *Soft tissue sarcoma*
- *Muscle hematoma*
- *Compartment syndrome*

GETTING STARTED

Open-ended questions	Tips for effective interviewing
Tell me about the problem with your knee or calf.	• *Let patients describe the problem in their own words.*
Describe the first time you felt this pain. What exactly were you doing at the time?	• *Push patients for exact details concerning initial episode of pain, and if recurrent, ask about the first episode.*
Describe position of knee and direction of force at time of injury or pain.	• *Be firm when asking patients to point with 1 finger. If entire area hurts, have them point to the spot where initial pain was felt.*
Point with 1 finger to the area that hurts the most.	

INTERVIEW FRAMEWORK

- Localize the pain into 1 of the 4 anatomic areas of the knee: anterior, posterior, medial, or lateral.
- Follow format for attributes of a symptom
  - Where does it hurt? (Determining location is key in narrowing your differential.)
  - What does the pain feel like? (eg, burning? sharp?)
  - How severe is the pain? Have the patient rate pain on a scale of 0–10. What is the pain like at different times during the day? Or with different activities?
  - Did the pain develop quickly over hours, or insidiously over weeks or months? Is it intermittent or constant?
  - What aggravates the pain?
  - What relieves pain? (Include over-the-counter medications, prescription medications, alternative and complementary medicines or therapies, positions.)
  - Do you have any associated symptoms such as swelling, stiffness, or fever?
- Occupational and sports history may give a clue to the etiology of pain.
  - What type of work do you do now? What work have you done in the past?
  - What sports do you play? What have you played in the past?
- Functional limitations are important in assessing severity of pain.
  - What can you not do now that you could do before you had the pain?
  - Are there any activities you have stopped due to the pain?
  - Are you able to do your activities of daily life? Dressing? Bathing? Shopping?

IDENTIFYING ALARM SYMPTOMS
Knee Pain

Serious Diagnoses **Prevalence**[a]

Septic joint

Ligamentous tear with joint give away

Meniscal tear with locking of the knee joint

Fracture of the tibia, fibula, or patella

[a]Prevalence is unknown when not indicated.

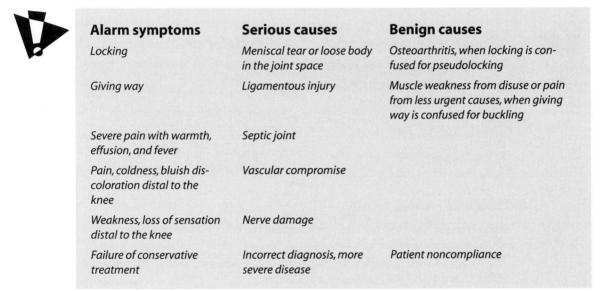

Alarm symptoms	Serious causes	Benign causes
Locking	*Meniscal tear or loose body in the joint space*	*Osteoarthritis, when locking is confused for pseudolocking*
Giving way	*Ligamentous injury*	*Muscle weakness from disuse or pain from less urgent causes, when giving way is confused for buckling*
Severe pain with warmth, effusion, and fever	*Septic joint*	
Pain, coldness, bluish discoloration distal to the knee	*Vascular compromise*	
Weakness, loss of sensation distal to the knee	*Nerve damage*	
Failure of conservative treatment	*Incorrect diagnosis, more severe disease*	*Patient noncompliance*

Calf Pain

Serious Diagnoses **Prevalence**[a]

Deep venous thrombosis

Intermittent claudication

Compartment syndrome

Soft tissue sarcoma

[a]Prevalence is unknown when not indicated.

Alarm symptoms	Serious causes	Likelihood ratio (LR+) [5]	Benign causes
Unilateral calf swelling	Deep venous thrombosis Cellulitis	1.5	Venous stasis
Calf pain	Deep venous thrombosis Cellulitis	1.1	Muscle strain Contusion
Redness	Deep venous thrombosis Cellulitis	0.6	Superficial skin irritation
Warmth	Deep venous thrombosis Cellulitis	1.4	

FOCUSED QUESTIONS FOR KNEE PAIN

If answered in the affirmative	Think about
Was there twisting of the knee? Was there a popping sensation? Does the knee give way (not buckle)? Was the knee in full extension? Was swelling immediate?	Ligamentous injury; history can support clinical suspicion but is probably of little value in distinguishing between ligamentous and meniscal injury or in pinpointing which ligament has sustained damage.[6]
Is there locking of the knee in a flexed position? Is there a click when you walk? Was there swelling over the next few hours or days?	Meniscal injury
Are you sexually active? (Especially in young patients without history of trauma and a warm, tender, swollen joint)	Gonococcal arthritis Reactive arthritis
Does stiffness of the knee last less than 15 minutes? Does pain worsen with activity?	Osteoarthritis
Was there trauma to the knee?	Fracture

Time course	Think about
Is the pain acute (less than 1 week)?	Fractures Contusions Ligamentous or meniscal tears Patellar subluxations Dislocations
Is the pain chronic?	Osteoarthritis Tumors Overuse syndromes (bursitis/tendinitis) Septic knee

FOCUSED QUESTIONS FOR CALF PAIN

If answered in the affirmative	Think about
Does the pain occur when walking?	Intermittent claudication
Does the pain occur at exactly the same distance each time?	Intermittent claudication
Is the pain relieved with rest?	Intermittent claudication
Have you been bedridden for more than 3 days in the past 4 weeks?	Deep venous thrombosis
Have you taken a long trip that required sitting still for hours?	Deep venous thrombosis
Have you had recent surgery?	Deep venous thrombosis
Is there a family history of blood clots?	Deep venous thrombosis
Do you take oral contraceptives?	Deep venous thrombosis
Do you take steroids or hormones for body building?[5]	Deep venous thrombosis
Did you have swelling behind your knee prior to the calf pain?	Dissecting Baker cyst
Have you had any trauma to the calf? Do you play sports? Were you doing an activity when the pain started?	Tear or contusion of the gastrocnemius or soleus muscle
Does the pain reoccur at the same distance every time?	Popliteal artery entrapment syndrome
Is the pain unilateral?	Popliteal artery entrapment syndrome
Do you have pain in the thighs, buttocks, or hips?[3]	Popliteal artery entrapment syndrome

CAVEATS

- Previous episodes may indicate an intermittent chronic process.
- When asking patients what medications they have used to treat the pain, determine exact dose and frequency. Patients may report a medication is not effective when a therapeutic dose was not being used or given adequate time to work.
- Sometimes patients will have unrecognized trauma to the knee, such as dancing. It is very important to ask exactly what the patient was doing at the time the pain started.
- Past and present occupational and sports history must be obtained.

PROGNOSIS

Most knee disorders can be diagnosed with a thorough history and physical. Although musculoskeletal problems often take weeks to months to resolve, many problems will resolve with conservative therapy.

Calf pain from deep venous thrombosis is potentially life-threatening and must be considered early in all patients presenting with calf pain. If the diagnosis is established early most complications will be averted. Pain due to intermittent claudication is likely to worsen with time, but progression can be slowed with intervention. In patients with intermittent claudication, disease of the coronary arteries and carotid arteries should also be considered. Disease in the latter can lead to considerable morbidity and mortality. Most other causes of calf pain have a good prognosis.

REFERENCES

1. Fernandez BB Jr. A rational approach to diagnosis and treatment of intermittent claudication. *Am J Med Sci.* 2002;323: 244–251.

2. Schmieder FA, Comerota AJ. Intermittent claudication: magnitude of the problem, patient evaluation, and therapeutic strategies. *Am J Cardiol.* 2001;87:3D–13D.

3. Solomon DH, Simel DL, Bates DW, et al. The rational clinical examination. Does this patient have a torn meniscus or ligament of the knee? Value of the physical examination. *JAMA.* 2001;286:1610–1620.

4. Wells PS, Anderson DR, Bormanis J, et al. Value of assessment of pretest probability of deep-vein thrombosis in clinical management. *Lancet.* 1997;350:1795–1798.

5. Scott S, Kelley M. Section Six: Knee and Lower Leg. In: Snider RK (editor). *Essentials of Musculoskeletal Care.* American Academy of Orthopaedic Surgeons; 1999.

6. Jackson JL, O'Malley PG, Kroenke K. Evaluation of acute knee pain in primary care. *Ann Intern Med.* 2003;139:575–588.

SUGGESTED READING

Anderson BC. *Office Orthopedics for Primary Care: Diagnosis and Treatment.* Philadelphia: WB Saunders Company; 1999.

Diagnostic Approach: Knee Pain

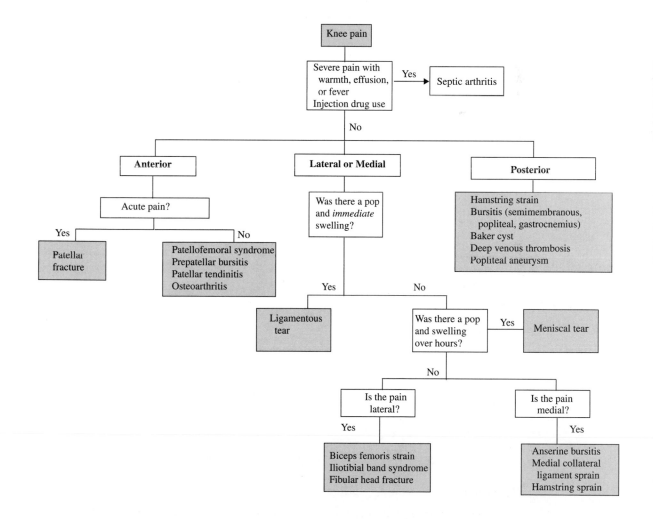

Diagnostic Approach: Calf Pain

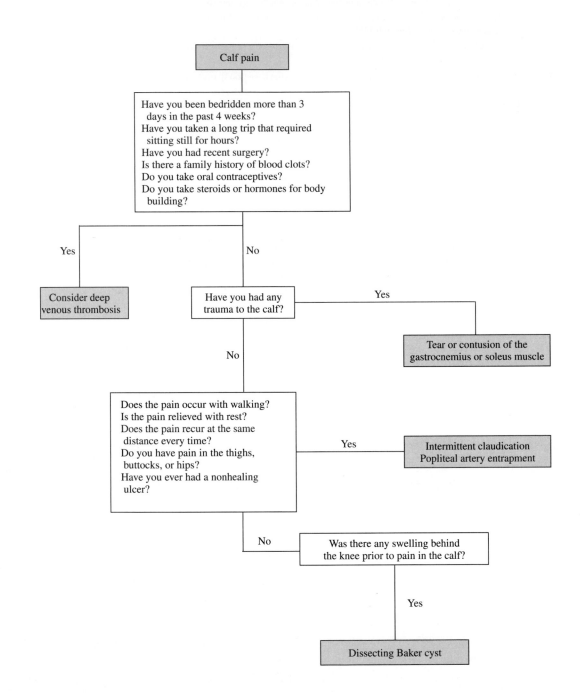

Ankle and Foot Pain

53

Jane E. O'Rorke, MD

More than 20% of musculoskeletal problems affect the foot and ankle.[1] Foot problems are rare among populations that do not wear shoes. Females are 9 times more likely than men to have foot problems. Chronic foot pain (lasting longer than 2 weeks) is more common than acute foot pain (less than 2 weeks duration).[2]

Between 5 and 10 million ankle injuries occur in the United States each year. Of these injuries, 85% are sprains. Adults, 21–30 years old, are at greatest risk.

KEY TERMS

Ankle sprain	*An injury to 1 or more ligaments of the ankle.*
Bunion	*The bony prominence and abnormal angle of the great toe.[3]*
Forefoot	*Includes toes and distal aspect of metatarsals.*
Hindfoot	*Includes the entire heel.*
Midfoot	*Area between distal metatarsals and beginning of calcaneus.*

ETIOLOGY

Foot Pain

In a study of 459 Italian persons, 21.8% had foot pain with standing and 9.6% had pain at rest. The most common physical findings included calluses/corns (64.8%), hypertrophic nails (29.6%), hallux deformities (21.2%) and absent arterial pulses (15.9%).[4] The Women's Health and Aging Study reported 316 (32%) of disabled women had moderate to severe foot pain. Obesity and osteoarthritis of the hands and feet were more common in these women.[5] Ultimately, determining the etiology of foot pain depends on the location and duration of pain.

Differential Diagnosis

Forefoot pain	*Midfoot pain*	*Hindfoot pain*
Bunions	*Osteoarthritis*	*Plantar fasciitis*
Hammer toes	*Midfoot plantar fasciitis*	*Posterior heel bursitis*
Claw toes	*Plantar fibromas*	*Achilles tendinitis*
Ingrown toenails	*Tarsal tunnel syndrome*	
Metatarsalgia		
Interdigital neuromas		
Hallux rigidus		

Ankle Pain

There are no studies addressing the etiology of ankle pain. Most ankle pain results from injury to the lateral ligaments of the ankle. Once again the location of the pain is the mainstay for determining the etiology.

Differential Diagnosis

Lateral ankle pain	**Medial ankle pain**	**Posterior ankle pain**
Sprain of the lateral ligaments	Sprain of the deltoid ligaments	Achilles tendinitis
Distal fibular fracture	Posterior tibial tendinitis	Achilles tendon rupture
Chronic ankle instability	Tarsal tunnel syndrome	**Chronic ankle pain**
Peroneal tendinitis	Distal tibial fracture	Arthritis
		Subtalar synovitis

GETTING STARTED

Open-ended questions

Tell me about the problem with your foot or ankle

Point with 1 finger to the area that is bothering you the most. Point to where you first felt the pain.

Describe the first time you felt this pain. What exactly were you doing at the time?

Have you ever had this pain before? If so, how was it treated?

Tips for effective interviewing

- Let patients describe the problem in their own words.
- Push patients for exact details concerning initial episode of pain and if recurrent, ask about the first episode.
- Be firm when asking patients to point with 1 finger. If entire area hurts have them point to the spot where initial pain was felt.

INTERVIEW FRAMEWORK

- Follow format for attributes of a symptom
  - Where does it hurt? (Determining location is key in narrowing your differential.)
  - What does the pain feel like? (ie, burning? sharp?)
  - How severe is the pain? Have the patient rate pain on a scale of 0–10. What is the pain like at different times during the day? Or with different activities?
  - Did the pain develop quickly over hours, or insidiously over weeks or months? Is it intermittent or constant?
  - What aggravates the pain?
  - What relieves the pain? (Include over-the-counter medications, prescription medications, alternative and complementary medicines or therapies, positions.)
  - Do you have any associated symptoms, such as swelling, stiffness, or fever?
- Occupational and sports history may give a clue to the etiology of pain.
  - What type of work do you do now? What work have you done in the past?
  - What sports do you play? What have you played in the past?
- Functional limitations are important in assessing severity of pain.
  - What can you not do now that you could do before you had the pain?
  - Are there any activities you have stopped due to the pain?
  - Are you able to do your activities of daily life? Dressing? Bathing? Shopping?

IDENTIFYING ALARM SYMPTOMS

Foot

Alarm symptoms	Serious causes	Benign causes
Fever, ulceration, or skin redness (warmth)	Cellulitis Septic arthritis	
History of trauma with inability to bear weight	Fracture	Bone contusion Sprain
Pain on weight bearing, swelling after a recent increase in activity	Stress fracture	Plantar fasciitis

Ankle

Alarm symptoms	Serious causes	Benign causes
Persistent rolling in or out of the foot	Ligamentous instability Posterior tibial dysfunction	Weakness of the muscles supporting the ankle Shoes with poor support
Pain on the medial aspect of the ankle anterior to the medial malleolus	Deltoid ligament sprain	Trauma without ankle instability
Pain in the lower anterior portion of the leg just above the ankle	High ankle (syndesmotic) sprain	Strain without ankle instability
Inability to walk 4 steps immediately after injury or during evaluation	Ankle fracture	Simple sprain
Numbness, weakness in the foot	Fracture with compromise of a nerve	
Feeling of being shot or kicked in the back of the ankle, sometimes with an audible pop	Achilles tendon rupture	Contusion of the Achilles tendon

FOCUSED QUESTIONS

Foot Pain

Questions	Think about
Are you having problems wearing your shoes?	Foot deformities, including ganglion cysts and plantar fibromas
Do your shoes rub on your big toe? Is there rubbing on any other toes?	Bunions Adventitial bursitis of the first metatarsophalangeal joint Hammer toes

(continued)

Questions	Think about
Does the weight of a sheet cause pain in your toe?	*Gout*
Are any of your toes numb? *Is there pain between your toes?* *Do tight shoes make your toes tingle?*	*Morton neuroma*
Do you have diabetes mellitus?	*Diabetic foot* *Charcot foot*
Do you have pain at night?	*Diabetic foot* *Charcot foot*
Do you have burning?	*Diabetic foot* *Charcot foot*
Do you have tingling?	*Diabetic foot* *Charcot foot*
Do you have progressive deformity?	*Diabetic foot* *Charcot foot*
Is the pain in your heel at its worst when you first step on it? *Does the pain improve with non–weight-bearing?*	*Plantar fasciitis*
Do you have tingling and burning along the bottom of your foot? *Does the arch of your foot cramp?*	*Tarsal tunnel syndrome*

Ankle Pain

Questions	Think about
Was there any twisting or rotation of the ankle? Did you land on the side of your foot?	*Ankle sprain* *Fracture*
Do have any lumps on the back of your heel?	*Pre-Achilles bursitis*
Does the back of your ankle hurt when climbing stairs?	*Retrocalcaneal bursitis*
Is there swelling around the back of your ankle? Are your shoes rubbing the inside of your ankle?	*Posterior tibialis tenosynovitis*
Have you played sports in your lifetime? Any history of dance?	*Ankle instability* *Osteoarthritis*
Have you had any past injuries to your ankle?	*Chronic ankle instability*

CAVEATS

- If a patient reports acute pain, ask about previous episodes because they may indicate a more chronic intermittent process.
- Get the patient to commit to the location of the pain with 1 finger.
- When asking patients about medications they have used to treat the pain, determine exact dose and frequency. Often, patients will report a medication is not effective when they were not taking a therapeutic dose or not allowing time for it to work.

- Sometimes patients will have trauma to the foot or ankle but they will not recognize it as trauma, such as dancing. It is very important to ask exactly what the patient was doing at the time the pain started.
- Do not skip occupational and sports history, past and present.

PROGNOSIS

Most foot and ankle disorders can be diagnosed with a thorough history and physical. Although musculoskeletal problems often take weeks to months to resolve, many problems will resolve with conservative therapy.

REFERENCES

1. Pfeffer GB. Foot and ankle. In: Snider RK (editor). *Essentials of Musculoskeletal Care.* American Academy of Orthopaedic Surgeons; 1997:366–489.

2. Balint GP. Foot and ankle disorders. In: *Best Practice & Research Clinical Rheumatology.* Elsevier Science Ltd; 2003:87–111.

3. Anderson BC. *Office Orthopedics for Primary Care: Diagnosis and Treatment,* 2nd ed. Philadelphia: WB Saunders Company; 1999:326.

4. Benvenuti F, Ferrucci L, Guralnik JM, et al. Foot pain and disability in older persons: an epidemiologic survey. *J Am Geriatr Soc.* 1995;43:479–484.

5. Leveille SG, Guralnik JM, Ferrucci L, et al. Foot pain and disability in older women. *Am J Epidemiol.* 1998;148:657–665.

Diagnostic Approach: Foot Pain

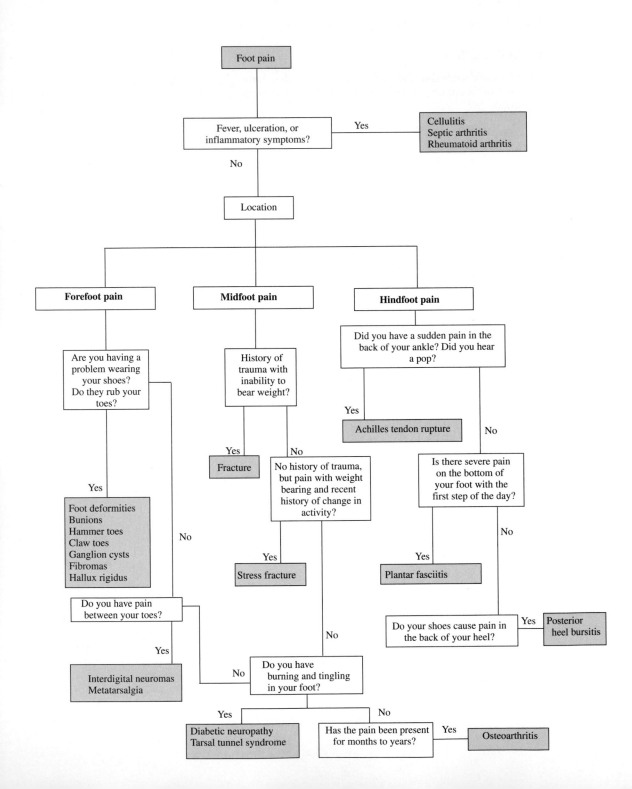

Diagnostic Approach: Ankle Pain

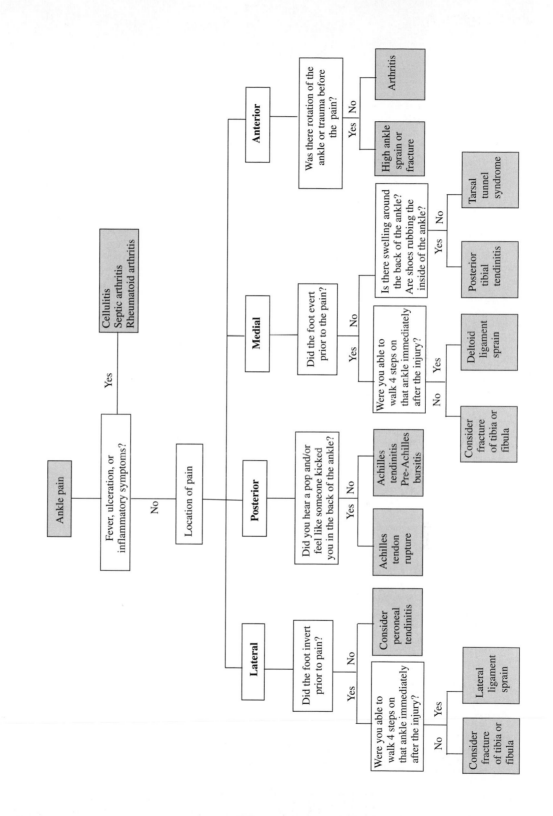

SECTION XI
Neurology

Confusion

Daniel Press, MD, & Michael Ronthal, MB, BCh

Confusion is the inability to maintain a coherent stream of thought or action. Altered level of consciousness is common in confusional states and can be the predecessor of stupor and coma if the underlying cause is not found and reversed. Delirium refers to a confusional state caused by a medical condition. Patients with delirium present a unique challenge in acquiring a history because the organ system required to report on symptoms, the central nervous system (CNS), is itself dysfunctional. For that reason, clinicians must obtain most of the historical information from caregivers and family members. Nonetheless, the history is crucial to determining the correct diagnosis. Often, delirium coexists with dementia.[1] Demented patients are particularly vulnerable to lapse into confusion, a state termed "beclouded dementia." Among patients who present to an emergency department with delirium, the diagnosis is overlooked in up to 40–60% of cases.[2] Regardless of cause, delirium confers a worse prognosis with higher hospital readmission rates and 30-day mortality, especially if untreated.[3] The causes of delirium differ greatly depending on the setting (ie, hospital versus nonhospital).

KEY TERMS

Alertness	*The level of arousal or responsiveness to external cues.*
Attention	*The ability to focus on specific stimuli and change from one stimulus to another when salient.*
Confusion	*Inability to maintain a coherent stream of thought.*
Delirium	*Acute impairment in attention with a fluctuating course and altered level of consciousness caused by a medical condition; also called acute confusional state and encephalopathy.*
Dementia	*Chronic degenerative condition affecting memory, behavior, and cognition.*

ETIOLOGY

The causes of delirium differ for persons in the community and those hospitalized for a medical illness. In the hospital setting, delirium generally occurs in patients with predisposing risk factors (see below).[4] While severe illnesses, large doses of CNS-active medications, and severe metabolic impairments can cause delirium even in low risk patients, a relatively mild insult can trigger it in patients with multiple risk factors. Causes of delirium in the community can be subdivided into 3 large categories: primary insults to the CNS (seizures, stroke, or meningitis), systemic metabolic conditions impairing CNS function (systemic infections, hypoxia, hypotension, renal failure, or hepatic failure), or the effect of medications (see Differential Diagnosis below).

Risk factors	Relative risk
Use of physical restraints	*4.4 (2.5–7.9)*
Malnutrition	*4.0 (2.2–7.4)*
> 3 medications added during hospital stay	*2.9 (1.6–5.4)*
Use of bladder catheter	*2.4 (1.2–4.7)*
Any iatrogenic event	*1.9 (1.1–3.2)*

Differential Diagnosis[a]	Prevalence[b]
Primary CNS causes	**35%**
Meningitis/encephalitis	
Stroke (primarily right hemisphere, either frontal, parietal, or occipital lobes)	
Seizures (postictal state or partial seizures)	
Head trauma	
Secondary CNS causes	**60%**
Infections, especially urinary tract infection (UTI), pneumonia, or sepsis	*5%*
Hypoxia	*25%*
Hypoperfusion (eg, congestive heart failure, shock)	*5%*
Hypoglycemia	*5%*
Renal failure	*5%*
Hepatic failure	
Toxins (carbon monoxide, heavy metals)	
Medications	**5%**
Alcohol (intoxication or withdrawal)	*3%*
Narcotic analgesics	
Opiates	
Amphetamines	
Anticholinergic drugs (especially diphenhydramine)	
Drug withdrawal syndromes	

[a]Causes of delirium among elderly patients presenting to emergency department.[2]
[b]Prevalence is unknown when not indicated.

GETTING STARTED

- The confused patient often cannot provide a coherent history. Ask focused questions regarding the presence of headache, recent drug use, and fevers.
- Confirm the history with a caregiver. Make every effort to contact a caregiver if no one is with the patient. This crucial task may require some detective work.

- Always determine the patient's current medications and whether any have changed. An accurate determination often requires calls to the patient's pharmacy or requests to have the family bring in all the medication bottles.
- In young patients, consider both the acute effects of drugs of abuse and withdrawal states.

INTERVIEW FRAMEWORK

- The goal is to determine the acute cause of the confusion and establish the presence of any baseline risk factors (eg, dementia, malnutrition).
- Inquire about timing of the episode
  - Previous episodes?
  - Suddenness of onset?
  - Any baseline confusion?
- Associated symptoms
  - Fever?
  - Shortness of breath?
  - Headache?
  - Abnormal motor activity?
- Drug usage
  - Any recent change in drug regimen?
  - Use of drugs of abuse or pain medications?
  - Recent drug withdrawal?

IDENTIFYING ALARM SYMPTOMS

Delirium itself usually reflects serious CNS dysfunction, especially if the onset has been acute. Delirium is a common presentation of life-threatening conditions, including subarachnoid hemorrhage, meningitis, and increased intracranial pressure due to a mass lesion. A number of investigations are often necessary to determine the cause; certain symptoms will suggest which tests should be done first.

Alarm symptoms	Serious causes	Benign causes
Fever or hypothermia	Meningitis Sepsis	UTI Upper respiratory tract infection (URI)
Abnormal motor activity or history of epilepsy	Seizures (status epilepticus) or postictal state	Myoclonus or asterixis from metabolic disturbance
Headache	Stroke Meningitis Mass lesion	Migraine and confusion due to excessive pain medication
Shortness of breath	Hypoxia (congestive heart failure, pneumonia)	URI
Diaphoresis, tremors	Hypoglycemia	Fever
Neglect (inattention to 1 side of space) or visual field loss	Stroke	Glaucoma Macular degeneration
Ataxia, nystagmus	Wernicke encephalopathy	Alcohol or drug intoxication

FOCUSED QUESTIONS[a]

Questions	Think about
Do you have	
• History of seizures?	Postictal state
	Nonconvulsive status epilepticus
• Pain on urination or recent urinary catheter?	UTI
	Urosepsis
• Shortness of breath?	Congestive heart failure
	Pneumonia
	Pulmonary embolism in postoperative patient
• History of insulin-requiring diabetes?	Hypoglycemia
• History of liver problems?	Hepatic encephalopathy
• Headache?	Meningitis
	Stroke
	Subarachnoid hemorrhage
Have you recently used sleep medications?	Anticholinergic or sedative toxicity
Have you fallen recently?	Unwitnessed head trauma
Have you experienced memory problems previously?	Underlying dementia

Quality	Think about
Is the confusion primarily a memory problem?	Dementia
Or does the patient have poor attention, especially with fluctuations?	Delirium

Time course	Think about
Is the onset	
• Sudden (over seconds)?	Seizure
	Stroke
	Subarachnoid hemorrhage
• Over minutes to hours?	Drug-induced
	Hypoxia
	Hypoglycemia
• Over hours to days?	Infection
	Renal failure
	Hepatic failure
• Gradual progression over months?	Dementia

Associated symptoms	Think about
Do you have	
• Altered level of consciousness?	Delirium of any cause
• Hypervigilence?	Drug or alcohol withdrawal
	Wernicke encephalopathy

• Shortness of breath?	*Congestive heart failure* *Myocardial infarction* *Pulmonary embolism*
• Headache?	*Subarachnoid hemorrhage* *Mass lesion* *Meningitis*
• Blurred vision? (monocular)	*Cavernous sinus disease* *Pituitary apoplexy*
• Blurred vision? (binocular)	*Parietal or occipital lobe stroke or mass lesion* *Hypertensive encephalopathy*
• Stiff neck?	*Meningitis (bacterial, viral, neoplastic, or aseptic)*
• Vertigo?	*Cerebellar or brainstem lesion*
• Jaundice?	*Hepatic encephalopathy*
• Dysuria or anuria?	*UTI* *Pyelonephritis* *Uremic encephalopathy*
Modifying factors	**Think about**
Are symptoms worse at nighttime?	*"Sundowning" (may be due to delirium or underlying dementia)*
Is there rapid improvement over seconds?	*Postsyncope (see Chapter 26)*
Is there improvement over minutes to hours?	*Postictal state*
Are symptoms worse when standing?	*Hypoperfusion*
History of seizures	*Nonconvulsive status epilepticus*

[a]Ask both patient and caregiver.

DIAGNOSTIC APPROACH

The diagnostic approach to confusion depends on 3 factors: the temporal course, the presence of focal neurologic signs, and the age of the patient. An acute onset over hours to days suggests delirium, while a gradual onset over months suggests underlying dementia. If the onset is acute, rapidly search for an underlying reversible cause that may be life-threatening without treatment. Focal symptoms (visual changes, headache, focal weakness or numbness) suggest a primary CNS process. The central causes include CNS infections (meningitis, abscess), strokes (ischemic or hemorrhagic), mass lesions (tumors), or seizures (with postictal state). If delirium develops without focal signs or symptoms, the patient's age may help determine the likely cause.

In younger patients without a focal CNS cause, drug use or withdrawal, unwitnessed head trauma, and unwitnessed seizure should be considered. When delirium develops in the elderly, likely causes include systemic infections (UTI, pneumonia), drugs (especially opiates and anticholinergic medications), hypoxia, hypoperfusion, and metabolic disturbances (renal failure, hepatic failure). In hospitalized patients, questions should focus both on the cause of the delirium and predisposing risk factors (see above).

A number of concomitant medical conditions bring up special concerns.

• **Epilepsy:** Confusion is most often due to a postictal state, but a sudden worsening in confusion or fluctuating course suggests ongoing seizures or nonconvulsive status epilepticus.

- **Diabetes:** Both hypoglycemia and hyperglycemia (with either acidosis or a hyperosmolar state) can present as confusion. In patients with diabetes, confusion can also develop from either cerebral ischemia (stroke) or coronary ischemia (myocardial infarction).
- **Hepatic cirrhosis:** Confusion can be a sign of worsening cirrhosis but may also herald upper gastrointestinal bleeding from varices (causing cerebral hypoperfusion or hepatic encephalopathy). Drug-induced delirium is also more common due to impaired hepatic metabolism.
- **Parkinson's disease:** In addition to the usual causes, anticholinergic drugs and dopamine agonists can cause confusion.
- **Cancer:** Cancer may cause confusion via direct cerebral mechanisms (metastases, carcinomatous meningitis), indirect mechanisms (drug effects, paraneoplastic states), and systemic mechanisms (hypercalcemia, hyponatremia, hepatic encephalopathy due to liver metastases, uremic encephalopathy due to obstructive uropathy).
- **HIV/AIDS:** HIV can predispose to confusion through CNS infections (toxoplasmosis, cryptococcal meningitis, progressive multifocal leukoencephalopathy) as well as directly (HIV dementia). Complicated treatment regimens with large numbers of medications can also predispose to confusion.
- **Postoperative patients:** If confusion is present immediately upon awakening from surgery, consider an intraoperative event (eg, global hypoxia/hypoperfusion or a focal stroke). In days 1–3 after surgery, hypoxia (from pneumonia or a pulmonary embolism) and drug withdrawal should be considered in addition to other causes of confusion in hospitalized patients.

CAVEATS

- The confused patient's ability to communicate and provide useful history can fluctuate markedly. Be sure to get ancillary information from other caregivers and, when in doubt, evaluate the patient at different times.
- Do not assume that confusion has been longstanding in a patient who appears "demented." Err on the side of assuming there is a treatable delirium present, even in patients with chronic cognitive deficits.
- Delirium and dementia often coexist. Determining whether an underlying dementia is present is nearly impossible in the setting of a delirium. Appropriate testing and interventions should be planned after the causes of the confusion have been treated.

PROGNOSIS

Some symptoms of delirium can persist for 6 months or longer in up to 80% of patients.[5] Those persons in whom delirium develops during a hospital stay are much more likely to require long-term institutional care; 43% reside in an institution at 6 months. The 1-month mortality for hospitalized patients with delirium is approximately 14% and is significantly higher than controls even when accounting for comorbid conditions.[6] Mortality for those with delirium is 39% at 1 year, roughly twice the likelihood compared with age-matched controls.[4] While delirium is frequently completely reversible, it is often the harbinger of more serious and chronic cognitive deficits.

REFERENCES

1. Rahkonen TR, Luukkainen-Markkula R, Paanila S, et al. Delirium episode as a sign of undetected dementia among community dwelling elderly subjects: a 2 year follow up study. *J Neurol Neurosurg Psychiatry.* 2000;69:519–521.
2. Lewis LM, Miller D, Morley JE, et al. Unrecognized delirium in ED geriatric patients. *Am J Emerg Med.* 1995;13:142–145.
3. Francis J, Kapoor WN. Prognosis after hospital discharge of older medical patients with delirium. *J Am Geriatr Soc.* 1992; 40:601–606.
4. Inouye SK, Charpentier PA. Precipitating factors for delirium in hospitalized elderly persons. Predictive model and interrelationship with baseline vulnerability. *JAMA.* 1996;275:852–857.
5. Francis J, Martin D, Kapoor WN. A prospective study of delirium in hospitalized elderly. *JAMA.* 1990;263:1097–1101.
6. Cole MG, Primeau FJ. Prognosis of delirium in elderly hospital patients. *CMAJ.* 1993;149:41–46.

SUGGESTED READING

American Psychiatric Association. Delirium: Practice Treatment Guideline: 1998. Available at http://www.psych.org/psych_pract/treatg/pg/pg_delirium_1.cfm

Brown TM, Boyle MF. Delirium. *BMJ.* 2002;325:644–647.

Francis J. Recognition and evaluation of delirium. 2003. UpToDate. B. Rose. Wellesley, MA. Available at http://www .uptodate.com

Diagnostic Approach: Confusion

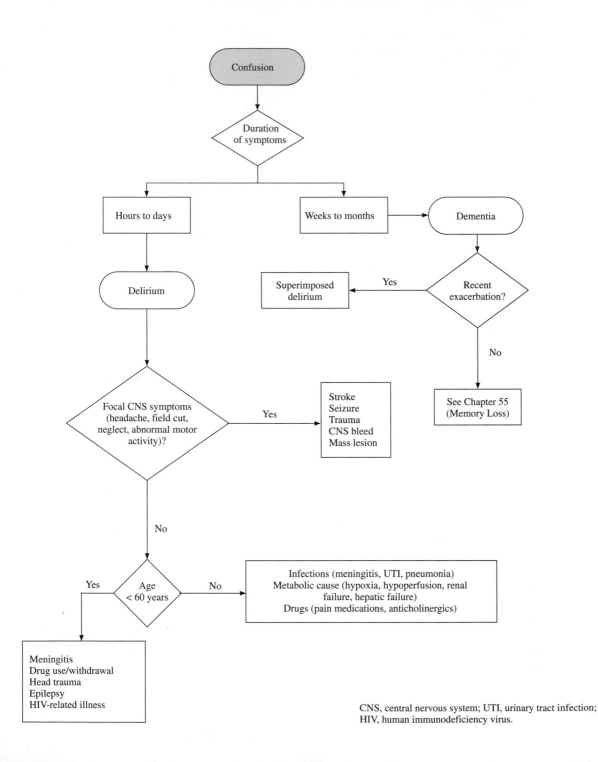

CNS, central nervous system; UTI, urinary tract infection;
HIV, human immunodeficiency virus.

Memory Loss

Calvin H. Hirsch, MD

Although recall and the speed of cognitive processing decline slightly with normal aging,[1] substantial memory loss is abnormal and reflects underlying pathology. While memory loss characteristically is the most prominent feature of early dementia, impairment in other domains of cognitive function, personality changes, or behavioral disturbances may be the earliest symptoms noted by observers. The prevalence of dementia doubles every 5 years after the age of 60, rising from 1% at age 60 to approximately 40% at age 85.[2] Nearly 67% of patients aged 75 and older with dementia have Alzheimer's disease.

KEY TERMS

Delirium
A state of global cognitive impairment with an acute onset, fluctuating course, short-term memory dysfunction, inattention, plus disorganized thinking or altered level of consciousness. Psychosis is common. Also called acute confusional state.

Dementia
A decline from a previous state of mental functioning that interferes with social or occupational activities. Dementia involves memory loss plus at least 1 of the following:
1. Aphasia (language impairment).
2. Impairment in executive function (eg, organizing, abstracting, judgment).
3. Apraxia (impaired ability to carry out familiar motor tasks despite intact motor function).
4. Agnosia (inability to identify familiar objects or substances despite intact sensation, such as failure to recognize the smell of coffee grounds).

ETIOLOGY

The accuracy and reliability of the diagnostic criteria for dementia vary, depending on the type of dementia. For Alzheimer's disease, the National Institute of Neurologic and Communicative Disorders and Stroke/Alzheimer's Disease and Related Disorders Association (NINCDS/ADRDA) criteria[3] enable expert clinicians to make an accurate diagnosis about 85% of the time. The several commonly used criteria for vascular dementia show accuracy in the range of 60% to 70%.

Major Causes of Memory Loss

Cause	Prevalence[a]	Definition
Mild cognitive impairment (MCI)	3%	Complaints and evidence of mild memory loss, with preservation of other cognitive abilities and daily functioning, in the absence of other explanations for the memory loss.[4] Approximately 8% per year of MCI cases progress to Alzheimer's disease.[5]
Alzheimer's disease	2.3–3.1%	Dementia that has an insidious onset and progresses steadily in the absence of focal neurologic signs or other identifiable causes. Autopsy reveals characteristic cortical degeneration with amyloid plaques and neurofibrillary tangles.
Vascular dementia	0.1–0.4%	Dementia temporally related to a stroke or due to chronic cerebral ischemia. Classically, the dementia progresses in a step-wise manner, but it may be steadily progressive. It may be difficult to distinguish from Alzheimer's disease. In the early stages, subcortical signs (eg, depression, subtle gait disturbances) and language difficulties often outweigh memory impairment, in contrast to early Alzheimer's disease, in which memory loss typically predominates.
Mixed dementia	0.2–0.7%	The coexistence of Alzheimer's disease and vascular dementia.
Diffuse Lewy body disease (DLBD)		The coexistence of dementia and Parkinsonism. Unlike Parkinson's disease, in which dementia begins years after the onset of extrapyramidal symptoms (EPS), the dementia of DLBD either precedes or occurs within 12 months of the onset of EPS. The cognitive impairment often fluctuates, and psychiatric symptoms—commonly, visual hallucinations—occur early in the course of the illness.
Frontotemporal dementia (FTD)		A progressive dementia in which personality changes (eg, apathy, self-neglect, perseveration, hyperorality) and speech impairment typically exceed memory loss during the early stages.[6]

[a]In persons over age 60; prevalence is not available when not indicated.

GETTING STARTED

Screening

Clinicians often fail to detect early dementia, in part because patients commonly deny having memory or other cognitive deficits, and in part because well-preserved social skills may conceal these deficits. In the absence of a complaint of memory loss, it is reasonable to screen patients for cognitive impairment approximately every 3 years from age 75 to 81, and then every other year thereafter. The most widely used screening instrument is the Folstein Mini-Mental State Examination (MMSE).[7] However, a sensitive alternative to the MMSE is the Mini-Cog,[8] which utilizes recall of 3 unrelated objects (eg, baseball, penny, chair) at 3 minutes and the drawing of a clock, involving inserting all the numbers and setting the hands to the requested time (Figure 55–1). Cognitive impairment is suggested if the patient fails to recall 2 of the 3 items or draws an abnormal clock. A failed screen should be followed by the full MMSE.

Family members or others who have frequent contact with the patient can be an invaluable source of information. An instrument like the Informant Questionnaire for Cognitive Decline in the Elderly (IQ-CODE)[9] gathers this information systematically and can improve diagnostic sensitivity for dementia.

Questions[a]	Comment
Do you sometimes have trouble remembering things or finding the right word?	• *If a family member or caregiver is present, discreetly interview them separately from the patient.*
Has there been a change in your ability to accomplish familiar tasks?	• *If a patient is suspicious or resentful of discussions behind his or her back, asking the nurse to obtain additional vital signs before the physical examination provides an excuse for you and the caregiver to leave the room.*
Can you give some recent examples?	• *Some patients and family members assume that memory loss is part of normal aging and discount its importance.*

[a]Consider asking these questions when there is a positive screen or a complaint of memory (or other type of cognitive) impairment.

INTERVIEW FRAMEWORK

A challenge in assessing memory loss is that other psychiatric and neurologic complaints may overshadow cognitive symptoms, which may go undetected unless specifically inquired about through directed questioning. The history should include the features and information presented below.

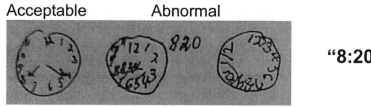

Figure 55–1. The Mini-Cog, which involves drawing a clock, inserting all the numbers, and setting the hands to the requested time, is a sensitive alternative to the Folstein Mini-Mental State Examination. Cognitive impairment is suggested if the patient draws an abnormal clock.

Feature	Specific information
Onset	Abrupt (onset can be dated to within days or weeks); if abrupt, ask about associated events (eg, fall, new medication) Insidious (exact onset impossible to pinpoint)
Duration	Days, weeks, months, or years
Overall course	Stable (no progression) Steadily progressive Step-wise decline (sudden worsening, period of stability, then sudden worsening)
Daily changes	Amount of fluctuation during the day and from 1 day to the next
Characteristics	Specific examples of memory problems
Associated cognitive problems	Language—word finding, fluency, naming Executive function—judgment, reasoning, planning, organization
Associated functional problems	Loss of ability to perform high-level intellectual tasks (recreational, occupational) Loss of ability to manage higher domains of functioning, such as driving, finances, shopping, meal preparation, housework Loss of ability to perform basic self-care, such as maintaining continence, hygiene, and appearance
Associated neurologic symptoms	Headache Focal neurologic symptoms Gait disorder
Concurrent medical conditions	Untreated or undertreated medical conditions, such as hyperthyroidism and hypothyroidism, B_{12} deficiency, chronic ethanol abuse, HIV infection
Prescribed and over-the-counter medications	Medications that can cause confusion, such as narcotics, benzodiazepines, major tranquilizers, and anticholinergic medications (eg, antihistamines)
Associated psychiatric symptoms	Personality changes Mood changes Behavioral problems (eg, aggression, agitation, psychosis, paranoia)

IDENTIFYING ALARM SYMPTOMS

Alarm symptoms can be classified into 2 types: (1) those reflecting the seriousness of the underlying cause of memory loss, and (2) those reflecting serious complications. Because persons with dementia residing in the community cannot survive without the close involvement of a caregiver, caregiver stress must be monitored as part of overall patient management.

Alarm symptoms	Consider
Abrupt onset	Delirium Vascular dementia Subdural hematoma
Dementia associated with urinary incontinence and wide-based gait	Normal-pressure hydrocephalus

Rapid progression over weeks	*Subdural hematoma* *Brain tumor*
Rapid progression over months	*Subacute spongiform encephalopathy* *Vascular dementia*
Dementia associated with depressed level of consciousness	*Delirium* *Chronic drug toxicity (eg, benzodiazepines)* *HIV with opportunistic central nervous system infection*
Disruptive behavior (agitation, aggressive or threatening behavior, purposeless behavior, wandering, inverted sleep-wake cycle, resistance to care)	*Common in the middle to late stages of dementias; assess caregiver well-being*
Psychosis, paranoia	*Common in middle to late dementia* *If visual hallucinations experienced early on, consider DLBD*
Inappropriate, involuntary movements of face or body	*Extrapyramidal side effects of neuroleptic medication* *Huntington's chorea*
Difficulty with gait, stiffness, postural instability	*AIDS dementia complex* *Subacute spongiform encephalopathy* *Parkinson's disease with dementia* *DLBD* *Vascular dementia* *Side-effects of neuroleptic medication* *Late Alzheimer's disease*
Seizures	*Mid to late stages of Alzheimer's disease* *Korsakoff syndrome with ethanol withdrawal* *Brain tumor* *Delirium from repeated seizures*
Signs or suspicion of abuse of patient by caregiver or abuse of caregiver by patient	*If present or strongly suspected, contact Adult Protective Services* *Risk of reciprocal abuse highest when demented patient physically aggressive and when premorbid relationship between patient and caregiver was poor*
Caregiver acts angry, short-tempered, depressed, or anxious; complains of not being able to cope	*Assess for caregiver stress, need for counseling, institutionalization of patient*

Serious Diagnoses

All dementias affect daily functioning and therefore are serious; most degenerative (progressive) dementias are irreversible. However, treatment of underlying conditions may halt the progression or even lead to partial or complete reversal of dementia. Some causes of memory loss or dementia can be life-threatening or produce substantial morbidity if not recognized. Although there is no known treatment for subacute spongiform encephalopathy, its potential for human-to-human transmission through organ transplantation or blood inoculation renders it a public health hazard if undiagnosed.[10]

Serious Diagnoses	Suggestive history	Differential diagnosis
Chronic subdural hematoma	Dementia of acute or subacute origin May progress History of falling or known fall Recent head trauma Focal neurologic symptoms may be present	Vascular dementia, "chronic" delirium (ie, lasting > 2 weeks)
Delirium	Short-term memory loss only part of syndrome Cardinal symptoms include acute onset with fluctuating course during the day, inattention, plus disorganized thinking, and/or altered level of consciousness (hyperalert, agitated versus somnolent, passive)	Ethanol or benzodiazepine withdrawal
AIDS dementia complex	An infrequent (< 2%) initial presentation of AIDS with features of a subcortical dementia Early on, there is psychomotor slowing and apathy, with later development of bradykinesia, altered posture, and parkinsonian gait disturbance Consider in a patient with HIV risk factors or who is HIV-positive	FTD Neurosyphilis Brain tumor Subacute spongiform encephalopathy Lewy-body dementia (in older patient)
Subacute spongiform encephalopathy (SSE)	The generic name given to prion-associated encephalopathies like Creutzfeldt-Jakob disease Rapidly progressive SSE should be considered when memory loss occurs at a young age Early stages dominated by psychiatric symptoms (dysphoria, withdrawal, irritability, apathy), with memory loss prominent in the middle stages[11]	Depression FTD Neurosyphilis AIDS dementia complex Vascular dementia Early-onset Alzheimer's disease (genetic – family history usually positive)
Late neurosyphilis	Memory loss often accompanied by delusions, paranoia, and emotional lability Signs of tabes dorsalis may be present (paresthesias, impaired proprioception, wide-based gait)[12]	AIDS dementia complex SSE Alzheimer's disease
Brain tumor	Complaints of memory loss usually associated with psychomotor retardation or apathy Patient or family members may also report headaches, altered level of consciousness, or focal neurologic changes	Depression FTD

Korsakoff syndrome	Memory loss due to thiamine deficiency Usually, history of alcohol abuse Patient typically unaware of deficit and confabulates	MCI Alzheimer's disease B_{12} deficiency
B_{12} deficiency	Symptoms of memory loss or mild dementia Complaints of ataxia, decreased lower extremity sensation (dorsal column disease) should increase suspicion Note: Neuropsychiatric symptoms may precede anemia	Early Alzheimer's disease MCI Korsakoff syndrome
Normal-pressure hydro-cephalus	Dementia associated with urinary incontinence and wide-based gait Low likelihood if complete triad not present[13]	B_{12} deficiency Late neurosyphilis
Hyperthyroidism	A rare but reversible cause of dementia in older persons Because older persons may not display the typical symptoms of hyperthyroidism (so-called "apathetic hyperthyroidism"), it should be ruled out in most cases of dementia	Alzheimer's disease B_{12} deficiency
Hypothyroidism	Hypothyroidism has been associated with dementia, but the incidence of complete reversibility of the dementia with thyroid replacement is low.	Alzheimer's disease Apathetic hyperthyroidism AIDS dementia complex B_{12} deficiency Depression
Pseudodementia	Defined as dementia-like symptoms due to depression Variable onset, usually traceable to within weeks Both subjective and objective evidence of memory loss Depressed mood and affect, apathy, weight loss support this diagnosis Patient may have variable somatic complaints. Note: Depression occurs in up to 50% of patients with Alzheimer's disease	Alzheimer's disease MCI FTD Hypothyroidism AIDS dementia complex

FOCUSED QUESTIONS

Use focused questions to determine the presence of associated and alarm symptoms. Questions about the order in which symptoms developed can help narrow the differential diagnosis. Screening tools like the MMSE only partially determine the severity of dementia, and systematic questioning about the impact of the memory loss or dementia on daily activities should comprise part of the evaluation.

Questions

What sort of activities or hobbies did you do 6 months ago? Have you had trouble with—or stopped doing—any of these in recent months? Why?

In the last few months, have you lost your way driving to a familiar destination?

Which came first—memory problems or stiffness and a shuffling gait?

(To the caregiver) What time of day does [specific disruptive behavior] occur or get worse? Are there any precipitating factors? What happens when the behavior occurs? How troublesome is this behavior to you? What do you do when it happens?

Think about

Impairment of daily activities due to cognitive problems suggests dementia rather than MCI or benign age-related changes
Depression also should be considered

Loss of visuospatial functioning suggests dementia

If memory first, think about DLBD or vascular dementia
If memory problems began more than a year after parkinsonian symptoms, consider Parkinson's disease with dementia

Think about ways to prevent disruptive behaviors, ways the caregiver can manage them without medications
If unsuccessful, consider a trial of a major tranquilizer

Quality

Involves only memory loss

Predominantly memory loss but other cognitive domains affected

Language affected more than memory

Age of onset under 65

Think about

MCI
Early dementia (impairment in other cognitive domains unrecognized)
Korsakoff syndrome
Depression/pseudodementia

Dementia, not otherwise specified

FTD

Early-onset Alzheimer's disease
FTD
SSE
AIDS dementia complex
Brain tumor

Time course

Acute onset

- *Fluctuating course throughout day*

- *Minimal diurnal variation or slow progression over days*

- *Minimal diurnal variation, stable over weeks to months or step-wise progression*

Insidious onset

- *Minimal diurnal variation, slow, steady progression over months*

Think about

Delirium

Subdural hematoma

Stroke (vascular dementia)

Alzheimer's disease
Vascular dementia
FTD
DLBD
SSE (relatively more rapid)
AIDS dementia complex (relatively more rapid)

• Step-wise progression over months	Vascular dementia
Associated symptoms	**Think about**
Apathy	Depression/pseudodementia
	FTD
	AIDS dementia complex
	SSE
	Hypothyroidism
Depression	Depression/pseudodementia
	Subcortical (vascular) dementia
	Alzheimer's disease
Psychosis	
• In early stages of dementia	DLBD
• In middle to late stages of dementia	Any progressive dementia
Disruptive behavior (eg, agitation, aggression, wandering, disrupted sleep-wake cycle)	Any moderate to advanced dementia
Extrapyramidal signs and symptoms (gait disturbance, stooped posture, decreased spontaneous movement)	Late Alzheimer's disease
	DLBD
	Dementia associated with Parkinson's disease
	Late SSE
	Vascular dementia
Incontinence	Any advanced dementia
• With wide-based gait	Normal-pressure hydrocephalus
Modifying factors	**Think about**
Acute illness	Superimposed delirium exacerbating memory loss or dementia
Chronic metabolic disorder (ie, hypothyroidism, hyperthyroidism, B_{12} deficiency)	May cause or exacerbate memory loss or dementia
Medications (major and minor tranquilizers, centrally acting antihypertensives, narcotics, anticonvulsants, nonsteroidal anti-inflammatory drugs, anticholinergic medications, others)	May cause or exacerbate memory loss or dementia

CAVEATS

- The clinician should not be lulled into assuming that every older patient with dementia has Alzheimer's disease. The diagnosis of the dementia type should follow a rigorous systematic process that includes a careful physical examination (emphasizing neurologic findings), followed, when indicated, by blood tests, cranial imaging, and (infrequently) lumbar puncture and electroencephalogram.
- The distinction between "benign" age-associated memory impairment (subjective without objective memory loss) and MCI (subjective plus objective memory loss) may be difficult without neuropsychological testing. An affective disorder (depression) should be ruled out for both entities.
- There is no such thing as acute Alzheimer's disease. A diagnosis of dementia cannot be made in the acutely ill patient, in whom delirium may cloud the picture.
- Given the prevalence of polypharmacy among older patients, the potential for adverse central nervous system effects, including chronic confusion mimicking dementia, is substantial.

PROGNOSIS

Currently, all dementias involving brain degeneration are irreversible, although acetylcholinesterase inhibitors may slow or delay progression slightly in Alzheimer's disease, DLBD, and (to a lesser extent) vascular and mixed dementia. Memantine has been shown to slow the progression of moderate to severe Alzheimer's disease. The prognosis for Alzheimer's disease varies according to the stage at which it was diagnosed, with a mean survival from diagnosis of approximately 8 years. Vascular dementia tends to follow a more rapid course than Alzheimer's disease. SSEs, which can be transmitted from animal to human (eg, "mad cow" disease), follow a rapid course measured in months and currently have no treatment available.

Because hypothyroidism, B$_{12}$ deficiency, and hyperthyroidism are common among older persons without dementia, treatment in persons with dementia will only infrequently lead to cognitive improvement. Patients who do improve generally have mild dementia; the improvement can take months following normalization of laboratory values.

REFERENCES

1. Christensen H. What cognitive changes can be expected with normal ageing? *Aust N Z J Psychiatry.* 2001;35:768–775.

2. von Strauss E, Viitanen M, De Ronchi D, et al. Aging and the occurrence of dementia: findings from a population-based cohort with a large sample of nonagenarians. *Arch Neurol.* 1999;56:587–592.

3. McKhann G, Drachman D, Folstein M, et al. Clinical diagnosis of Alzheimer's disease: report of the NINCDS-ADRDA Work Group under the auspices of Department of Health and Human Services Task Force on Alzheimer's Disease. *Neurology.* 1984;34:939–944.

4. Chertkow H. Mild cognitive impairment. *Curr Opin Neurol.* 2002;15:401–407.

5. Larrieu S, Letenneur L, Orgogozo JM, et al. Incidence and outcome of mild cognitive impairment in a population-based prospective cohort. *Neurology.* 2002;59:1594–1599.

6. Snowden JS, Neary D, Mann DM. Frontotemporal dementia. *Br J Psychiatry.* 2002;180:140–143.

7. Folstein MF, Folstein SE, McHugh PR. "Mini-mental state": a practical method for grading the cognitive state of patients for the clinician. *J Psychiatr Res.* 1975;12:189–198.

8. Borson S, Scanlan J, Brush M, Vitaliano P, Dokmak A. The mini-cog: a cognitive 'vital signs' measure for dementia screening in multi-lingual elderly. *Int J Geriatr Psychiatry.* 2000;15:1021–1027.

9. Jorm AF. A short form of the Informant Questionnaire on Cognitive Decline in the Elderly (IQCODE): development and cross-validation. *Psychol Med.* 1994;24:145–153.

10. Croes EA, van Duijn CM. Variant Creutzfeldt-Jakob disease. *Eur J Epidemiol.* 2003;18:473–477.

11. Spencer MD, Knight RS, Will RG. First hundred cases of variant Creutzfeldt-Jakob disease: retrospective case note review of early psychiatric and neurological features. *BMJ.* 2002;324:1479–1482.

12. Cintron R, Pachner AR. Spirochetal diseases of the nervous system. *Curr Opin Neurol.* 1994;7:217–222.

13. Dippel DW, Habbema JD. Probabilistic diagnosis of normal pressure hydrocephalus and other treatable cerebral lesions in dementia. *J Neurol Sci.* 1993;119:123–133.

SUGGESTED READING

Aguero-Torres H, Winblad B, Fratiglioni L. Epidemiology of vascular dementia: some results despite research limitations. *Alzheimer Dis Assoc Disord.* 1999;13 Suppl 3:S15–20.

Benecke R. Diffuse Lewy body disease—a clinical syndrome or a disease entity? *J Neurol.* 2003;250(Suppl 1):I39–42.

Croes EA, van Duijn CM. Variant Creutzfeldt-Jakob disease. *Eur J Epidemiol.* 2003;18:473–477.

Cummings JL, Cole G. Alzheimer disease. *JAMA.* 2002;287:2335–2338.

DeCarli C. Mild cognitive impairment: prevalence, prognosis, aetiology, and treatment. *Lancet Neurol.* 2003;2:15–21.

Packard RC. Delirium. *Neurology.* 2001;7:327–340.

Ritchie K, Lovestone S. The dementias. *Lancet.* 2002;360:1759–1766.

Zekry D, Hauw JJ, Gold G. Mixed dementia: epidemiology, diagnosis, and treatment. *J Am Geriatr Soc.* 2002;50:1431–1438.

Diagnostic Approach: Memory Loss

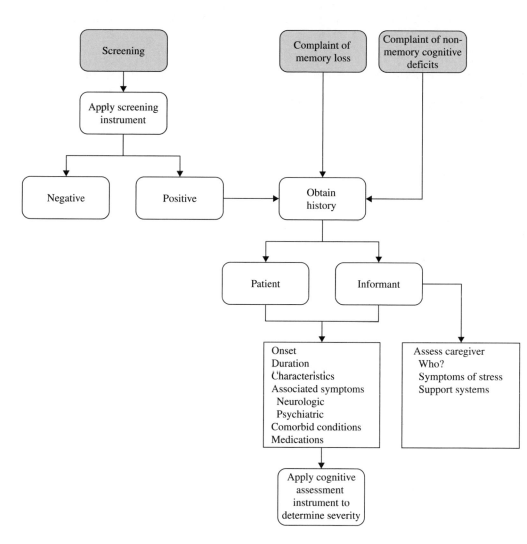

Diplopia

56

Jason J. S. Barton, MD, PhD, FRCPC

Diplopia is the condition of seeing more than a single image. In most cases, it is due to ocular misalignment (the eyes are not pointing at the same location in space). Thus, images of an object fall on different locations of the retinae of the eyes, giving the impression that there are 2 objects.

KEY TERMS

Abduction	Moving the eye away from the nose.
Adduction	Moving the eye toward the nose.
Binocular diplopia	Diplopia present only when both eyes are open.
Comitant diplopia	Diplopia that does not vary with gaze direction.
Depression	Moving the eye down.
Diplopia	Seeing a duplicate copy of an image, colloquially referred to as "double vision."
Elevation	Moving the eye up.
Esotropia	Crossed eyes, eyes pointing medially with respect to each other.
Exotropia	Eyes that are pointing laterally with respect to each other.
Hypertropia	One eye elevated with respect to the other.
Microvascular palsy	Palsies attributed to small vessel ischemia, often related to hypertension or diabetes.
Monocular diplopia	Diplopia with only 1 eye open.
Phoria	A tendency for the eyes to be misaligned when 1 eye is covered; with both eyes open the person's ocular motor control system can use vision to align the eyes so that there is no diplopia.
Polyopia	Seeing multiple copies of an image.

ETIOLOGY

Binocular diplopia stems from dysfunction of structures ranging from muscle, neuromuscular junction, and nerves in their course within and outside the brainstem, and prenuclear brainstem control problems. This anatomic division is a useful approach to evaluation and differential diagnosis.

Differential Diagnosis

Ocular myopathy	***Supranuclear (brainstem) disorders*[6]**
Graves ophthalmopathy[1]	*Stroke*
Neuromuscular junction	*Tumor*
Myasthenia gravis[2]	*Demyelination*
Botulism	*Infection*
***Cranial neuropathy (III, IV, VI)*[3–5]**	
Microvascular disease (diabetes)	
Tumor	
Infection	
Inflammation	
Cerebral aneurysm	

GETTING STARTED

Questions	**Remember**
Does double vision disappear when 1 eye is closed?	*If diplopia persists with 1 eye closed, the cause is a simple refractive problem, not an ocular motor problem.*
Does it hurt?	*Pain should raise considerations of more serious diseases, even though it can occur with benign microvascular palsies.*
How long have you had double vision? Is it getting worse?	*Progression is an ominous feature, suggesting a mass lesion.*

INTERVIEW FRAMEWORK

- Determine whether the problem is due to a refractive problem or ocular misalignment.
- For ocular misalignment, determine the pattern of diplopia in order to isolate the eye with weakness and determine which specific movement of that eye is weak.
- Determine the temporal evolution and probe for associated symptoms of serious disease.
- Identify risk factors from prior history, especially diabetes, or symptoms compatible with vasculitis.

IDENTIFYING ALARM SYMPTOMS

Diplopia can occasionally be a sign of ominous, even life-threatening disease. Fortunately this is unusual. Dangerous pathology is most often associated with lesions of the brainstem or peripheral nerve rather than muscle. The likelihood of serious causes depends on which nerve is involved, underscoring the importance of making an anatomic diagnosis first. The following data are from 4789 patients with cranial nerve palsies (III, IV and VI) who presented either to a hospital or ophthalmology clinic.[3–5] The distribution also differs by age; pediatric patients tend to have fewer microvascular palsies and more mass lesions.[7]

Serious Diagnosis	Prevalence[a]
Cerebral aneurysm	6%
Brain tumor	13%
Cavernous sinus mass lesion	
Increased intracranial pressure	
Infection	

[a]Among patients with cranial nerve palsies; prevalence is unknown when not indicated.

Alarm symptoms	Serious causes	Benign causes
Eye pain or headache	Cerebral aneurysm	Microvascular palsy
	Cavernous sinus mass lesion	Unrelated migraine
	Increased intracranial pressure	
	Meningitis	
Facial numbness	Cavernous sinus mass lesion	
Facial weakness	Brainstem lesion	
Limb weakness	Meningitis	
Limb numbness		
Imbalance		
Drowsiness		

FOCUSED QUESTIONS

Questions	Think about
Is double vision still present when you close 1 eye?	Refractive cause (ie, cataract)
Does double vision vary through the day?	Myasthenia gravis
Can you make vision single with concentration?	Congenital esophoria or exophoria, a latent tendency to benign ocular deviation that can emerge in later life with diplopia

Quality	*Think about*
Is diplopia vertical?	III nerve palsy
	IV nerve palsy
	Graves ophthalmopathy[1]
	Skew deviation[6]
Is diplopia horizontal?	VI nerve palsy
	Internuclear ophthalmoplegia
	Graves ophthalmopathy
Does it change with which way you look?	Nerve or muscle palsy

(continued)

Time course	Think about
Is the distance between the images about the same as when you first noticed diplopia?	Microvascular palsies Skew deviation from strokes
Is it increasing over time?	Tumor Meningeal infection
Does it vary from day to day?	Myasthenia gravis
Associated symptoms	**Think about**
Do you have eye, head, or facial pain?	Infection, tumor, or aneurysm (if pain is prolonged)
Has your eye changed in appearance?	Proptosis in Graves ophthalmopathy
Has your speech or swallowing changed?	Bulbar symptoms in myasthenia gravis
Do you have numbness anywhere in your face?	Cavernous sinus lesion
Do you have weakness or numbness of 1 side of your body?	Brainstem lesion
Is your balance affected?	Brainstem or cerebellar lesion
Modifying symptoms	**Think about**
Does the double vision increase with certain visual activities like driving or reading?	Myasthenia gravis

DIAGNOSTIC APPROACH

See Figure, Diagnostic Approach: Diplopia. First, determine if diplopia is monocular or binocular (Does each eye alone see single?).

Monocular Diplopia

If 1 eye sees double while the other is covered, this is a refractive problem. Among elderly patients, this is most commonly a cataract.

Binocular Diplopia

If diplopia only occurs with both eyes open, the problem is a misalignment between the 2 eyes. Next, determine whether the diplopia is horizontal or vertical (see Figure, Diagnostic Approach: Vertical Diplopia).

Horizontal Diplopia

In evaluating horizontal diplopia, the following 3 questions are necessary:

- Which eye sees the right-most image?
- Is diplopia worse (separation between the images increases) in left or right gaze?
- Is diplopia worse for near or far vision?

Because of the optics, the eye that sees the right-most image is pointing left of the other eye. For example, if the left eye sees the right image, it is pointing left of where the right eye is looking. Hence the eyes are diverged, or exotropic, usually indicating a weakness of adduction. If the left eye sees the left image, the eyes are crossed, or esotropic, from abduction weakness (Figure 56–1). This does not yet establish which eye is the weak eye. It just tells the relative position of the 2 eyes.

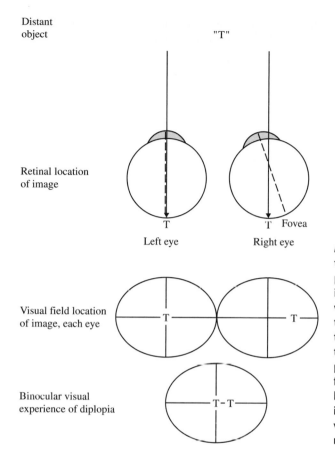

Distant object   "T"

Retinal location of image

T   T Fovea

Left eye   Right eye

Visual field location of image, each eye

T   T

Binocular visual experience of diplopia

T–T

Figure 56–1. Image pattern in esotropia. The position of the eyes in a patient with a right VI nerve palsy is shown, as the patient fixates on the letter "T" in the distance. Because the right eye is deviated towards the nose, the image of the "T" in this eye falls to the left of the fovea, whereas in the good left eye the "T" is projected onto the fovea (see 'retinal location of image'). Because of the inversion of images projected onto the retina, a retinal image left of the fovea is perceived as right of center (see 'visual field location of image'). Thus the "T" seen by the right eye is right of the "T" seen by the left eye (see 'binocular visual experience'). This is an "uncrossed diplopia", meaning that the right eye sees the right image

Diplopia worsens when you make the weak nerve or muscle work. For example, if diplopia gets worse in left gaze, this implies a problem with either abducting the left eye or adducting the right eye. If diplopia is worse looking close, adduction is the problem (because we cross our eyes to look close). If it is worse at far, abduction is the problem. Thus, a left VI nerve palsy, which causes weakness of the lateral rectus that abducts the left eye, will cause a horizontal diplopia worse at far and in left gaze.

Vertical Diplopia

The 3 questions for vertical diplopia are similar to the 3 for horizontal diplopia:

- Which eye sees the lower image?
- Is the diplopia worse in left or right gaze?
- Is the diplopia worse in up or down gaze?

The higher eye sees the lower image. Diplopia may be due to weakness of the depressor muscles (inferior rectus or superior oblique) of the higher eye, or the elevator muscles (superior rectus or inferior oblique) of the lower eye.

The 3 questions above can isolate a weakness of any single oblique or vertical rectus muscle. However, in practical terms, the main differential of vertical diplopia is between 5 items (see Figure, Diagnostic Approach: Vertical Diplopia):

1. Graves ophthalmopathy[1]: Look for associated signs of proptosis, conjunctival injection, and lid lag or retraction. Patients may have other signs of hyperthyroidism or hypothyroidism, but also consider euthyroid Graves disease.

2. Myasthenia gravis[2]: This disorder can mimic any palsy. The hallmark is variability, with diplopia changing throughout the day, sometimes worse with visually demanding tasks like driving or reading. Often the findings vary with different examiners or visits.

3. IV nerve palsy: The 3 questions will suggest that the affected eye is higher, and this separation is worse when looking in the direction of the lower (normal) eye or when looking down.

4. III nerve palsy: Various combinations of weakness of adduction, elevation and depression, ptosis, and/or a larger pupil in the affected eye.

5. Skew deviation[6]: This results from disruption of brainstem vestibular pathways. The above 4 conditions should be excluded. A neurologic examination may reveal damage to sensory or motor tracts to the limbs (as they passed through the brainstem) or cerebellar signs.

CAVEATS

- Binocular diplopia is most often due to a weakness of a muscle or nerve; however, it may infrequently be due to restriction. That is, an eye fails to move because the muscle that moves it in the opposite direction is tethered and unable to stretch. The 2 main causes of this are muscle inflammation (eg, Graves ophthalmopathy), and orbital fractures from facial trauma. Suspect these entities if there is proptosis, conjunctival redness, a history of thyroid disease, or recent facial trauma.

- If you suspect myasthenia, ask about generalized symptoms of limb weakness, dyspnea, or dysphagia. These patients may be at risk for respiratory failure or aspiration.

- If painful diplopia is present, always obtain neuroimaging to screen for the possibility of a parasellar mass, infection, or cerebral aneurysm. Obtain a magnetic resonance imaging (MRI) scan of the pituitary (cavernous sinus) region, not a standard brain MRI.

- If a patient has mild ocular motor weakness that causes diplopia only in 1 or a few directions of gaze, he or she may report that the diplopia is intermittent. However, if the diplopia is always present when looking in a given direction, the problem is not really intermittent but persistent.

- The history of onset is not useful in trying to determine whether the problem is an acute or chronically progressive one. Diplopia is either present or it is not. It is more useful to determine whether the *distance* between the images has been gradually increasing with time.

- The "Pupil Rule": The III nerve innervates the lid, the pupil dilator, and all extraocular muscles except the lateral rectus and superior oblique. If a patient appears to have a complete III nerve palsy except for completely normal pupil function (ie, same size as other pupil in both light and dark), it is very unlikely due to a cerebral aneurysm pressing on the III nerve.[8] This is because the location of the pupil fibers in the III nerve make them prone to compression by an adjacent aneurysm.

PROGNOSIS

Prognosis depends on the cause of diplopia. Patients with ocular myopathy such as Graves ophthalmopathy generally have a very slowly progressive diplopia. Occasionally, this disease leads to more rapid orbital mass effect with risk of corneal exposure and compressive optic neuropathy.

Ocular myasthenia will progress to generalized myasthenia in 50% of patients (80% of these doing so within 2 years of diagnosis).[9] Therefore, these patients must be monitored carefully.

Cranial neuropathies most often result from microvascular disease, and most patients recover spontaneously within 12–14 weeks. Cerebral aneurysms must be identified and treated promptly because of a high risk of subarachnoid hemorrhage and death.

REFERENCES

1. Bartley G, Gorman C. Diagnostic criteria for Graves' ophthalmopathy. *Am J Ophthalmol.* 1995;119:792–795.

2. Barton JJS, Fouladvand M. Ocular aspects of myasthenia gravis. *Semin Neurol.* 2000;20:7–20.

3. Berlit P. Isolated and combined pareses of cranial nerves III, IV and VI. A retrospective review of 412 patients. *J Neurol Sci.* 1991;103:10–15.

4. Green W, Hackett E, Schlezinger N. Neuro-ophthalmologic evaluation of oculomotor nerve paralysis. *Arch Ophthalmol.* 1964;72:154–167.

5. Richards BW, Jones FR, Younge BR. Causes and prognosis in 4278 cases of paralysis of the oculomotor, trochlear, and abducens cranial nerves. *Am J Ophthalmol.* 1992;113:489–496.

6. Keane J. Ocular skew deviation. Analysis of 100 cases. *Arch Neurol.* 1975;32:185–190.

7. Kodsi SR, Younge BR. Acquired oculomotor, trochlear and abducent cranial nerve palsies in pediatric patients. *Am J Ophthalmol.* 1992;114:568–574.

8. Nadeau S, Trobe J. Pupil sparing in oculomotor palsy: a brief review. *Ann Neurol,* 1983;13:143–148.

9. Bever CJ, Aquino A, Penn A, et al. Prognosis of ocular myasthenia. *Ann Neurol.* 1983;14:516–519.

SUGGESTED READING

Acierno M. Vertical diplopia. *Semin Neurol.* 2000;20:21–30.

Barton JJS. Infranuclear and nuclear ocular motor palsies. In: Rosen ES, Eustace P, Thompson HS, Cumming WJK (editors). *Neuro-ophthalmology.* Mosby; 1998:15.1–15.13.

Barton JJS. Neuroophthalmology III: Eye movements. In: Joynt R, Griggs R (editors). *Baker's Clinical Neurology on CD-ROM.* Lippincott Williams & Wilkins; 2002.

Leigh RJ, Zee DS. The diagnosis of peripheral ocular motor palsies and strabismus. In: *The Neurology of Eye Movements,* 3rd ed. Oxford University Press; 1999:321–404.

Diagnostic Approach: Diplopia

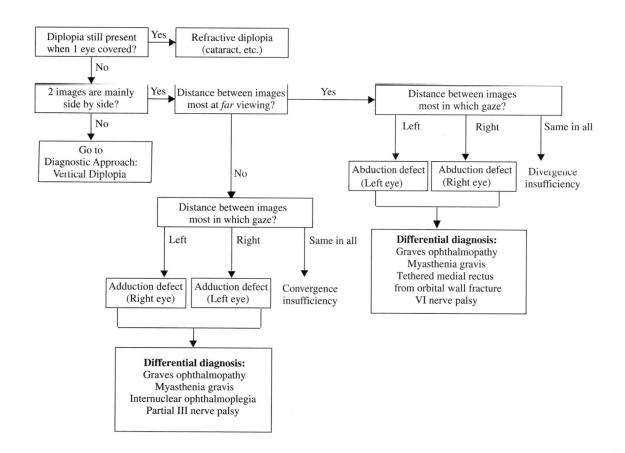

Diagnostic Approach: Vertical Diplopia

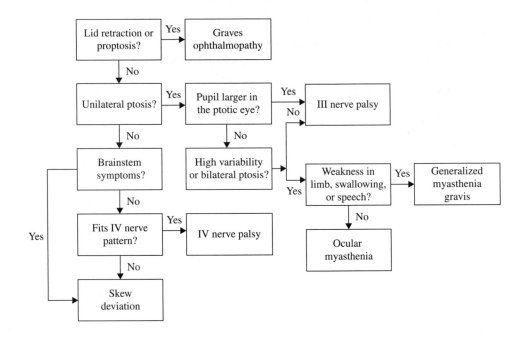

Gait Abnormalities

Jeff Wiese, MD

Ambulation (gait) is an exercise in controlled falling. The upright body falls forward and the outstretched foot and leg must prevent the body from falling by supporting the body's weight and rotating the weight over the limb. Gait abnormalities result from 1 of 5 disorders:

1. Inadequate muscle strength to flex the hip (to raise the knee), flex the knee (to lift the foot), or dorsiflex the ankle (to keep the foot from dragging on the ground).
2. Inadequate sensation in the foot (or excess sensation with neuropathies) to tell the brain when the foot has planted and is ready for the body to rotate over the limb.
3. Inadequate muscle strength in the leg to maintain extension of the leg (knee) to support the body's weight.
4. Inability to relax the muscles of the leg as the body moves over the extended leg and transfers weight to the opposite leg (in preparation for extending the leg for the next step).
5. Disorders of the cerebellum, which normally receives sensory input and coordinates muscle contraction (the stepping limb) and relaxation (the opposite limb).

KEY TERMS

Ataxia	Unbalanced or uncoordinated ambulation.
Cerebellar ataxia	Ataxia due to impaired cerebellar function.
Normal-pressure hydrocephalus	A triad of dementia, ataxia, and incontinence that results from obstruction of the arachnoid granulations that drain cerebrospinal fluid. The fluid accumulation compresses the brain causing the symptoms.
Peripheral neuropathy	Abnormal sensory or motor nerve function leading to weakness, altered sensory perception, or both.
Sensory ataxia	Ataxia due to impaired proprioceptive or sensory feedback from the lower extremities.
Spastic paraplegia	Tonic muscular contraction leading to an inability to relax the muscles. The increased tone is due to damage of the inhibitory neurons in the spinal cord or brain.

ETIOLOGY

Gait disorders result from disease of muscles, nerves, bones and joints, or the cerebellum.

GETTING STARTED

- Review the patient's past medical history. Most gait abnormalities are due to chronic or congenital diseases.
- Assess the time course of the symptoms. Acute changes in gait suggest an injury or stroke. A gradual, protracted onset suggests a systemic disease, peripheral neuropathy, or cerebellar disease.
- Avoid leading questions. It may be necessary to follow-up with a close-ended questions directed at the most likely disorder.

INTERVIEW FRAMEWORK

- Assess for alarm symptoms.
- Ask about conditions that make the gait abnormality worse (ie, walking in darkness or walking up stairs).
- Ask about weakness involving other parts of the body (ie, the arms, neck).
- Ask about sensory abnormalities involving other parts of the body.
- Ask about alcohol and drug use.
- Take a thorough dietary history.
- Determine the temporal pattern and duration of symptoms, accompanying symptoms, and precipitating factors.

IDENTIFYING ALARM SYMPTOMS

Outside of spinal cord impingement and stroke, gait abnormalities are rarely a life-threatening condition. For all cases of gait abnormalities, a sudden onset of the abnormality is alarming; the less serious etiologies, such as degenerative joint disease, are insidious in onset. Chronic neurologic degenerative diseases, such as parkinsonism and cerebellar degeneration, are also insidious.

Serious Diagnoses

- Spinal cord impingement
- Stroke
- Normal-pressure hydrocephalus
- Aortic dissection causing spinal cord ischemia

Alarm symptoms	Consider
Use of injection drugs Recent bacterial infection Fever	Spinal cord impingement from an epidural or spinal abscess
History of cancer Incontinence Numbness in your buttocks and groin area (saddle anesthesia)	Spinal cord impingement from a metastatic malignancy
Atrial fibrillation Hypertension History of stroke Lost vision Arm weakness	Stroke
Incontinence Decline in thinking ability (ask family members)	Normal-pressure hydrocephalus

| Chest pain | Aortic dissection causing spinal cord ischemia |
| Hypertension | |

FOCUSED QUESTIONS

Causes of Muscle Weakness

See Chapter 13 for causes of muscle weakness. It is important to distinguish whether the weakness is isolated to 1 muscle (traumatic injury, radiculopathy), 1 limb (stroke), or both limbs (systemic disease or spinal cord disease).

Questions	**Think about**
When you walk, do you waddle like a duck? Are other parts of your body weak?	***Gluteal or quadriceps weakness:*** *To begin walking, the body must lift the leg to keep it from dragging on the ground. To do this, the hip must be raised by contraction of the gluteal (buttocks) and quadriceps muscles. If either is weak, the patient swings the leg laterally to keep it from dragging, creating a gait that looks like the waddle of a duck.*
When you walk, do you feel as if you are walking up steps?	***Damage to the peroneal nerve:*** *Weakness of dorsiflexion due to peroneal nerve damage prevents the patient from lifting the toes as he or she moves forward. The patient will compensate by lifting the knee higher than normal to lift the foot so that the toes clear the ground. This has the appearance of the patient walking up steps.*
Have you had recent surgery? Have you had trauma to the lower extremity?	***Damage to the peroneal nerve:*** *Occurs commonly following trauma to the lower extremity or surgery during which the patient's leg has become pinned against the bed-rail, paralyzing the peroneal nerve.*
Are you unable to stand prior to initiating gait?	***Systemic weakness*** *(see Chapter 13)*

Sensory Abnormalities

Questions	**Think about**
Do you slap your feet down as you walk? Do you walk with a wider stance than normal? Describe your diet. Are you a strict (vegan) vegetarian? (B_{12} deficiency) Have you had unprotected sex or a history of sexually transmitted diseases? (syphilis) Do you have a history of diabetes? Do you consume excessive amounts of alcohol?	***Sensory abnormality:*** *Normal gait requires adequate position sense, which is accomplished by proprioceptive input from the leg muscles. Disease of the dorsal columns (eg, B_{12} deficiency, syphilis, or diabetes mellitus) impairs proprioception, causing the patient to fall. To increase stability, the patient widens the distance between the legs as he walks. The patient may also slap the feet down as he walks to increase sensory input.*

(continued)

Questions	Think about
Is your gait worse with the eyes closed?	**Dorsal column disease:** Visual input compensates for lack of proprioceptive sensory input
Is your gait equally bad with eyes open or closed?	**Cerebellar dysfunction**
Do your feet hurt or burn as you walk?	**Hyperasthetic gait (due to a sensory neuropathy):** With hyperasthesia, the patient walks as if on hot coals; similar to walking on a foot after it has fallen asleep (pins and needles).

Inability to Relax Muscles

All causes of spastic paraparesis are due to upper motor neuron disease (from the cerebral cortex to the anterior horn.

Questions	Think about
Do you have trouble getting yourself going forward when you try to walk? (festination) Do you have trouble stopping yourself once you begin walking? (propulsion) Do you walk in small steps?	**Parkinsonism:** Motor output to legs is chronically hyperstimulated. The muscles are tonically contracted, making it difficult to relax and allow the leg to be lifted as the patient tries to extend it forward during gait. To compensate, the patient takes small, short steps like a wind-up robot (march a petite pas).
Where there any complications associated with your birth? Do you have a history of multiple sclerosis?	**Spastic paraplegia:** The legs are locked in spastic contraction. The patient takes short steps with toes never leaving the floor. The knees cross and rub against each other as the patient moves forward, like the blades of a scissors (scissors gait). The most common causes of this gait are cerebral palsy and multiple sclerosis.
Have you experienced a decline in the sharpness of your thinking ability? Have you had difficulty holding your urine? When you walk, do you feel like your feet are magnetically "stuck" to the floor?	**Normal-pressure hydrocephalus:** A disease of older patients characterized by dementia, urinary incontinence, and ataxia. The characteristic gait is a magnetic gait.

Cerebellar Disorders

Questions	Think about
Have you noticed difficulty keeping your balance? Do you consume alcohol on a regular basis?	**Cerebellar disease:** The midline cerebellum (vermis) processes proprioceptive input from the legs and adjusts motor input to the legs accordingly. When damaged or impaired (by alcohol), the patient cannot make fine motor adjustments to keep moving forward.

When you walk, do you stumble from side to side as you try to move forward?	*Acute intoxication or chronic alcohol abuse (both lobes of the cerebellum involved)*
When you walk, do you consistently deviate or 'fall' toward one side?	*Unilateral cerebellar disease (eg, tumor, abscess)*

CAVEATS

- The observed pattern of gait abnormalities can be a helpful clue to the etiology.
- Hysterical gait is characterized by wide swings from left to right, hitting the walls of the hall as the patient moves forward.
- Unless intoxicated, patients with cerebellar damage will consistently deviate to one side of the hall (the side of the lesion).
- The malingering patient will lurch from the hips (maintaining enough control to avoid falling until he means to) while the patient with cerebellar disease will lurch from the knees.
- Do not assume that the cerebellum is healthy because the patient can successfully perform finger-to-nose and heel-shin testing. All patients should have their ambulation observed if cerebellar disease is suspected.

PROGNOSIS

The prognosis of gait abnormalities depends on the underlying disease.

SUGGESTED READING

Jackson GR, Owsley C. Visual dysfunction, neurodegenerative diseases, and aging. *Neurol Clin.* 2003;21:709–728.

Mayer M. Neurophysiological and kinesiological aspects of spastic gait: the need for a functional approach. *Funct Neurol.* 2002; 17:11–17.

Mayeux R. Epidemiology of neurodegeneration. *Annu Rev Neurosci.* 2003;26:81–104.

Nielsen JB, Sinkjaer T. Afferent feedback in the control of human gait. *J Electromyogr Kinesiol.* 2002;12:213–217.

Patrick JH. Case for gait analysis as part of the management of incomplete spinal cord injury. *Spinal Cord.* 2003;41:479–482.

Rietman JS, Postema K, Geertzen JH. Gait analysis in prosthetics: opinions, ideas and conclusions. *Prosthet Orthot Int.* 2002; 26:50–57.

Rodda J, Graham HK. Classification of gait patterns in spastic hemiplegia and spastic diplegia: a basis for a management algorithm. *Eur J Neurol.* 2001;8 (Suppl 5):98–108.

Wilder RP, Wind TC, Jones EV, Crider BE, Edlich RF. Functional electrical stimulation for a dropped foot. *J Long Term Eff Med Implants.* 2002;12:149–159.

Diagnostic Approach: Gait Abnormalities

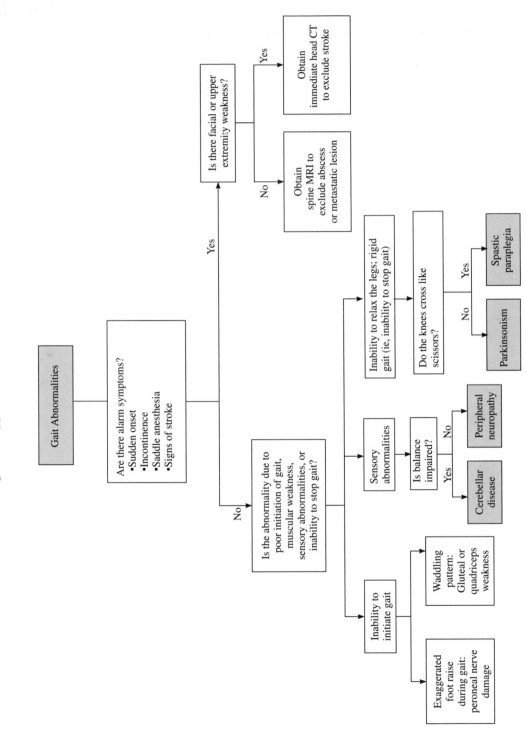

MRI, magnetic resonance imaging; CT, computed tomography.

Tremor

Raymond Kevin Ryan, MD, & Daniel Tarsy, MD

Tremor is rarely a chief complaint. Tremor is of general interest because nearly every person experiences a tremor at some point in his or her life.[1] People may not attribute tremor to underlying disease and so often do not seek medical attention. When evaluating tremor, determine whether the tremor is truly a new symptom and whether it interferes with a patient's activities or causes social dysfunction. Typically, the most common concern among patients is whether or not they have Parkinson's disease.[2] However, essential tremor is the most common type of organic tremor.

Tremor can be subdivided into 3 major types: resting, action, and postural. Resting tremor is typical of parkinsonian tremor. Action tremor is more often the result of essential tremor, cerebellar disease, or intoxication. Pathologic postural tremors can be due to many causes. In terms of alarm symptoms, tremor is rarely an urgent chief complaint. The evaluation of tremor usually occurs in the outpatient setting.

KEY TERMS

Tremor	The rhythmic oscillation of antagonist groups of muscles, in either an alternating or synchronous fashion.
Action tremor	An oscillation that occurs or increases with voluntary movement, generally of mid range frequency (6–8 Hz). Also called kinetic tremor.
Postural tremor	An oscillation that occurs with maintaining a fixed posture against gravity or during a fixed posture (clenched fist, standing), generally of an upper mid to higher range frequency (8–14 Hz).
Essential tremor	Isolated postural or action tremor involving the hands and sometimes the head and voice without other neurologic findings. Genetically determined with a positive family history ("familial tremor") in approximately 50% of cases.
Intention tremor	A type of action tremor in which an oscillation occurs orthogonal to the direction of movement and increases in amplitude as the target is approached. Usually denotes cerebellar disease.
Physiologic tremor	Irregular oscillations of 8–10 Hz occurring during maintenance of a posture, which disappear when the eyes are closed or a gravity load is placed on the muscles. By definition, physiologic tremor of varying intensity is a normal finding and common in the general population.

(continued)

KEY TERMS

Enhanced physiologic tremor	*Physiologic tremor increases in amplitude during times of fatigue, sleep deprivation, treatment with certain drugs, caffeine use, or stress.*
Rest tremor	*Usually a low frequency (3–6 Hz) oscillation that occurs with no action (voluntary contraction of muscles) and without resisting gravity.*
Task-specific tremor	*A tremor elicited by a specific task, such as speaking or writing.*

ETIOLOGY

It is necessary to distinguish primary neurologic tremors (eg, due to Parkinson's disease, essential tremor, multiple system atrophy) from secondary tremors resulting from a non-neurologic etiology (eg, medication effects, intoxication, metabolic derangement). The clinician should also address what functional impairment results from the tremor to help differentiate between rest, action, or postural tremor. Many diseases result in 1 or more tremor types.

Differential Diagnosis	Prevalence[a]
Primary tremors	
Essential tremor	*0.4–4%[3]*
Parkinson's disease (PD)	*0.057–0.37%[3,4]*
Parkinsonian syndromes	
• Multiple system atrophy (MSA)	*.002–.006%[5]*
• Progressive supranuclear palsy (PSP)	*.004%[5,6]*
Peripheral neuropathy	
Psychogenic tremor	
Wilson's disease	*.003%[3,7]*
Cerebellar dysfunction	
Midbrain tremor (rubral)	
Secondary tremors	
Adrenergic agents (eg, amphetamines, bronchodilators, β-adrenergic agonists, peripheral vasoconstrictors, tricyclic and serotonin reuptake inhibitor antidepressants)	
Miscellaneous drugs (eg, lithium, corticosteroids, antipsychotics, caffeine, cyclosporine, valproic acid, and amiodarone)	
Fatigue, anxiety, fear	

[a]In the general population; prevalence data are unavailable when not indicated.

GETTING STARTED

As with any history, try to let the patient tell as much as possible in his or her own words. Ask the patient to tell a story. This will prevent the patient from simply showing you a shaking hand.

Questions	Remember
Chief complaint	
Why did you come to the office? *What about the tremor made you come in today?* *Has something about your tremor changed?*	*Establishes tremor as the complaint, and delineates activities affected, progression, and acuity while encouraging the patient to tell his or her own story.*
Onset	
Who first noticed the tremor?	*Often people seek medical help because a spouse or coworker has noticed an abnormal movement.*
When did you first notice the tremor? When and how did it first interfere with your life?	*These questions encourage the patient to tell the full story.*
Did it start in one hand/side, or both?	*Strictly unilateral tremor suggests PD as opposed to essential tremor.*
Quality	
When do you notice the tremor the most? At rest, while holding an object, or while moving the affected body part?	*This question translates rest, postural, and action tremors into layman's terms.*
Does it interfere with sitting still?	*A feature of rest tremor*
Does it interfere with writing, eating, drinking, or any other action?	*If yes, consider action, task-specific, or intention tremors. If the answer is no, consider a rest tremor. If someone complains of being unable to hold a camera or read a newspaper, consider a postural tremor.*
Progression	
How has the tremor changed over time?	*Reemphasizes the need to think of the history as a story. A long time course suggests a slower neurodegenerative disease or essential tremor.*

INTERVIEW FRAMEWORK

Use the following checklist to establish acuity and tremor type:

- Reasons for seeing the doctor (helps establish tremor type).
- Onset (duration).
- How has it changed over time (progression)?
- Who noticed the tremor: the patient or someone else?
- What part of the body is affected?
- Is it focal, unilateral, or bilateral?
- Does it occur at rest, during action, or during a fixed position?

The next items are the associated factors that allow a differential diagnosis to be developed from the history.

- Precipitating and alleviating factors.
- Associated problems with movements and gait.

- Family history.
- Exposure to medications.
- Exposure to intoxicants or poisons.
- Other medical or psychiatric conditions.
- Continuous versus paroxysmal?

IDENTIFYING ALARM SYMPTOMS

The following features suggest that a serious diagnosis should be considered:

1. Recent, sudden onset (within hours to days).
2. Rapid progression (over hours to days).
3. Exposure to new medications, controlled substances, intoxicants, or toxins.
4. Associated sudden alteration of mental status.
5. Underlying disease (eg, cancer or immunodeficiency) and acute onset tremor.

In an emergency situation, the chief complaint will most likely not be tremor, but another symptom. Psychogenic tremor is an exception.

Serious Diagnoses: Acute tremor[a]

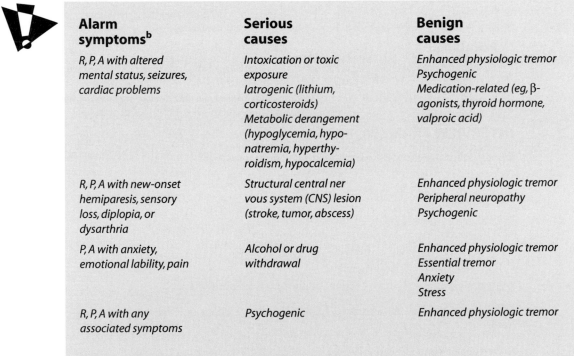

Alarm symptoms[b]	Serious causes	Benign causes
R, P, A with altered mental status, seizures, cardiac problems	Intoxication or toxic exposure Iatrogenic (lithium, corticosteroids) Metabolic derangement (hypoglycemia, hyponatremia, hyperthyroidism, hypocalcemia)	Enhanced physiologic tremor Psychogenic Medication-related (eg, β-agonists, thyroid hormone, valproic acid)
R, P, A with new-onset hemiparesis, sensory loss, diplopia, or dysarthria	Structural central nervous system (CNS) lesion (stroke, tumor, abscess)	Enhanced physiologic tremor Peripheral neuropathy Psychogenic
P, A with anxiety, emotional lability, pain	Alcohol or drug withdrawal	Enhanced physiologic tremor Essential tremor Anxiety Stress
R, P, A with any associated symptoms	Psychogenic	Enhanced physiologic tremor

[a]See reference 10 (pages 426–427) for an expanded list.
[b]Tremor type with associated symptoms; R, resting; A, action; P, postural.

Serious Diagnoses: Nonacute tremor[a]

Symptoms[b]	Serious causes	Positive likelihood ratio (LR+)[c]	Benign causes
R, P with rigidity, bradykinesia, gait instability, hypophonia, incontinence, orthostasis	PD (70–100% have resting tremor, often as the initial presentation[8]) PSP or MSA[d]	1.3–1.5[9]	Neuroleptic-induced tremor
P, A with gait instability and a definite family history	Wilson's disease		Essential tremor Enhanced physiologic tremor Multiple sclerosis Anxiety Stress Psychogenic

[a]See reference 10 (pages 426–427) for an expanded list.
[b]Tremor type with associated symptoms; R, resting; A, action; P, postural.
[c]Data on likelihood ratios are unavailable when not indicated.
[d]Tremor occurs in 17% of patients with PSP, and up to 29% of patients with MSA. In contrast, other parkinsonian features occur more commonly than tremor in PSP and MSA.

FOCUSED QUESTIONS

Questions	Think about
Does anyone in your family have tremor? (Ask separately about hands, voice, and head.)	Essential or familial tremor Familial PD, Wilson's disease
Was your tremor originally on 1 or both sides of your body?	PD often begins as a unilateral tremor Essential tremor and atypical parkinsonism will often be bilateral Structural lesions may cause unilateral tremor
Do you have any other problems with movement • Standing up from a couch or deep chair? (movement initiation) • Brushing your teeth or turning doorknobs? (bradykinesia) • Any recent falls? (gait instability or ataxia)	Focal weakness may indicate a structural lesion. Ataxia results from cerebellar dysfunction, CNS lesions, intoxications, or essential tremor. Gait instability, bradykinesia, movement initiation problems, and rigidity are all parkinsonian symptoms.
Do you have any problems with urinary incontinence, lightheadedness when you stand, sexual dysfunction, changes in bowel or bladder habits, uncontrolled sweating for no specific reason, or difficulty swallowing?	Suggest autonomic dysfunction, as can be seen in MSA. Urinary incontinence is also a feature of normal-pressure hydrocephalus (NPH). NPH can rarely manifest with parkinsonian features and a resting tremor.

(continued)

Quality

Does the tremor occur when you are sitting still and your hands are resting?

Does the tremor occur when you are trying to do something, such as drinking, writing, eating, or picking up something?

Is your tremor most noticeable when you are trying to hold something up or maintain a pose?
Do you have problems reading a newspaper or using a camera?

Think about

Resting tremor suggests parkinsonian (from PD, MSA, PSP, or neuroleptics), essential tremor, multiple sclerosis, or infectious diseases.

Action tremor.
End-point tremor suggests essential tremor, multiple sclerosis, structural lesions, neuropathies, cerebellar pathology, or toxins.
Task-specific tremor (writing, speaking) suggests essential tremor or dystonic tremor.

Postural tremor suggests neuropathies, parkinsonian syndromes, essential tremor, metabolic derangements, or structural lesions.

Time course

Did the tremor start suddenly?

How long have you had this tremor?

Has this been getting worse over time?
Have there been any recent changes in your tremor?

Think about

Acute tremor suggests intoxication, toxic exposure, structural lesion, or psychogenic.
Ask about exposure to pesticides (organophosphates), heavy metals (mercury, lead), or other chemicals (manganese, arsenic, carbon monoxide, cyanide, alcohol).

Chronic tremor suggests PD, essential tremor, parkinsonian syndromes, dystonia, multiple sclerosis, chronic ethanol abuse, or neuropathy.

Acute progression (over hours to days or over weeks to months) suggests acute toxic exposure, anoxic event, or psychogenic etiology.
Chronic progression (over weeks to months or over years) suggests long-term toxic exposure; multiple sclerosis; an atypical or "parkinson plus" syndrome like PSP or MSA, PD, or essential tremor.

Associated symptoms

Have you had recent falls?
Has anyone commented on changes in how you walk?
Have you had the feeling that you were falling?

Have you had urinary or bowel incontinence?
Have you had fainting spells or felt light-headed when you stood up?
Have you had sexual dysfunction?

Think about

Bradykinesia, rigidity, falls, and gait instability suggest PD, an atypical parkinsonian syndrome, or tremor secondary to neuroleptic medication.

Autonomic symptoms suggest MSA.

Medications and drugs

What medications do you take?
Do you smoke?
Do you drink a lot of coffee, tea, or sodas?

Think about

Many medications and drugs have an adrenergic enhancing effect. Such adrenergic effects cause postural tremors, especially the first 3 medications on the following list:

Do you have any medical problems, and if so, what medications do you take?	*Theophylline and caffeine*
	β-agonist inhalers (for asthma)
	Nicotine
	Valproic acid
	Lithium (considered a peripheral tremor, not of CNS origin)
	Amiodarone (may be related to peripheral and CNS damage)
	Methylphenidate, amphetamines
	Corticosteroids
	Tricyclic antidepressants
	Serotonin reuptake inhibitors
	Calcium channel antagonists
	Ethanol
Have you ever taken medication for hallucinations, psychotic episodes, depression, or mood swings?	*Neuroleptic medications (eg, haloperidol, chlorpromazine) may cause any type of tremor: resting, postural, and action.*
Modifying symptoms	**Think about**
Do stress, anxiety, or fatigue worsen the tremor?	*Can occur in all tremor types, so differentiation must be made by ascertaining what functions are worsening (action or sitting still)*
Does alcohol improve the tremor?	*About 65–70% of patients with essential tremor report this.*

DIAGNOSTIC APPROACH

First, establish acuity of the tremor and then establish the tremor type. The goal is to distinguish between primary neurologic tremors (eg, Parkinson's disease, essential tremor, MSA) and secondary tremors from non-neurologic etiologies (eg, medication effects, intoxication, metabolic derangement). If the medical history and exposure history are negative, then a primary neurologic tremor is most likely.

1. Establish the acuity of onset.
2. Establish the tremor type.
3. Consider causes of primary versus secondary tremor.
4. Ask about associated symptoms.

CAVEATS

- The patient will describe his or her tremor in functional terms. The interviewer should break down activities step by step to understand if the tremor occurs at rest, while holding a posture, or during activity.
- Clinicians may not easily distinguish PD from related atypical parkinsonian syndromes except at postmortem examination; differentiation often only takes place over time.
- The patient may not want or need treatment so much as the comfort or reassurance of a specific diagnosis.
- A patient with essential tremor may report a unilateral onset because the patient first noticed that the dominant hand was affected.
- The history should establish a baseline for future monitoring of the tremor and its treatment.
- Stress, common stimulants (eg, caffeine, nicotine), and fatigue commonly cause tremor. Ask about coffee consumption, sleep habits, and stressors if the patient describes an enhanced physiologic

tremor. Anything that increases adrenergic effect (eg, fatigue, stress, caffeine, and certain medications) can lead to enhanced physiologic tremor.

- Primary tremors due to a primary neurologic disorder are likely to progress.
- Many patients and families have access to a variety of information, especially from the Internet. If the patient describes the tremor as "resting" or "postural," do not be misled. For diagnostic purposes, do not assume the informant is using those terms correctly.
- Other involuntary movements that may be confused with tremor include:

  Myoclonus: Isolated or serial, high-velocity muscle contractions. Myoclonic jerks are a descriptive term, not associated with a specific diagnosis.

  Asterixis: Sudden, transient, repetitive loss of muscle tone when holding a posture. This is sometimes called "negative myoclonus." Associated with decompensated liver disease.

  Dystonia: Fixed contraction of a muscle or group of muscles causing abnormal posturing, and possibly a rhythmic tremor if antagonist muscles synchronously contract.

  Tic: Isolated, generally arrhythmic, focal muscle contractions. Associated with a premonitory urge and temporary, subjective relief.

  Athetosis: An arrhythmic, twisting movement.

  Chorea: Another hyperkinetic, involuntary movement of arrhythmic jerks, non-patterned, and with unpredictable timing and distribution, more rapid than athetosis. These movements are often incorporated into voluntary movements.

- History alone cannot distinguish between tremor, myoclonus, asterixis, chorea, and other movement disorders. This distinction must be made by the physical examination, laboratory findings, and electrophysiologic studies.

PROGNOSIS

Acute tremor usually results from more serious pathology, which ultimately determines prognosis. In primary tremors, prognosis varies. Essential tremor, although sometimes called "benign" tremor, can be progressive and debilitating; however, it is not typically associated with the disability of PD and other parkinsonian syndromes. Idiopathic PD has a mean age of onset ranging from 55 to 65 years. PSP and MSA have faster progression and a shorter life expectancy.[5,6,10] At this time, there are no abortive or regenerative therapies for PD to halt or reverse disease progression. Wilson's disease has a poor prognosis if left untreated but is potentially reversible, and so should be considered in any patient with unexplained tremor.

REFERENCES

1. Tarsy D. Movement Disorders. In: Samuels M, Feske SK (editors). *Office Practice of Neurology.* 2003.
2. Pullman SL, Yim JHC. Essential insights on essential tremor. *Pract Neurol.* 2002:42–46.
3. Louis ED. Essential tremor. *N Engl J Med.* 2001;345:887–891.
4. Parkinson's Disease: Etiology Diagnosis, and Management. Movement Disorders Virtual University. 2002. Available at http://www.wemove.org
5. Schrag B, Ben-Schlomo Y, Quinn NP. Prevalence of progressive supranuclear palsy and multiple system atrophy: a cross-sectional study. *Lancet.* 1999;354:1771–1775.
6. Golbe LI. The epidemiology of PSP. *J Neural Transm.* 1994;(Suppl.)42:263–273.
7. Reilly M, Daly L, Hutchinson M. An epidemiological study of Wilson's disease in the Republic of Ireland. *J Neurol Neurosurg Psychiatry.* 1993;56:298–300.
8. Hughes AJ, Daniel SE, Kilford L, Lees AJ. Accuracy of clinical diagnosis of idiopathic Parkinson's disease: a clinico-pathological study of 100 cases. *J Neurol Neurosurg Psychiatry.* 1992;55:181–184.
9. Rao G, Fisch L, Srinivasan S, et al. Does this patient have Parkinson's disease? *JAMA.* 2003;289:347–353.
10. Jankovic J, Tolosa E (editors). *Parkinson's Disease and Movement Disorders,* 3rd ed. Lippincott Williams & Wilkins; 1998.

Diagnostic Approach: Tremor

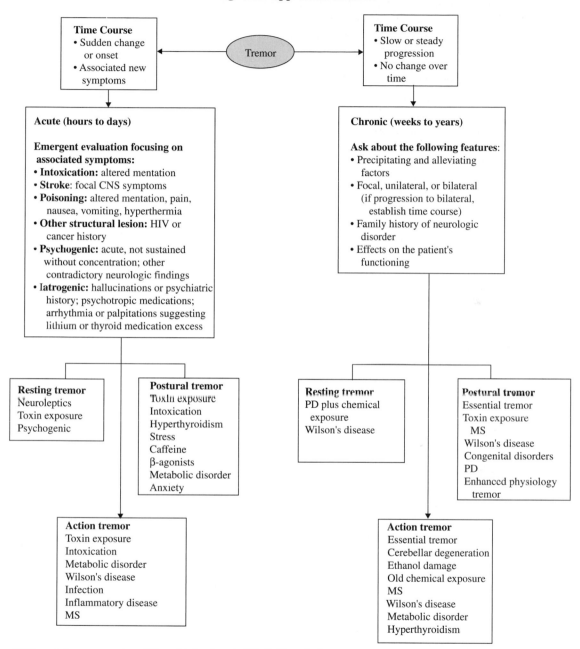

CNS, central nervous system; MS, multiple sclerosis; PD, Parkinson's disease.

SECTION XII
Psychiatry

Anxiety

Michael H. Zaroukian, MD, PhD

Anxiety can be a normal and adaptive short-term, fear-based response to perceived threats of physical or psychological harm. An anxiety disorder exists when recurrent or persistent episodes of anxiety are so intense, frequent, or situationally inappropriate that they cause significant distress or impair normal functioning, activities, or relationships. Anxiety disorders are common but are underrecognized both by patients and providers.

Diagnosing anxiety disorders depends heavily on history taking, since physical examination and laboratory testing add little to the evaluation. An important starting point is to keep anxiety disorders in mind, particularly in patients who have a history of unexplained medical symptoms, high utilization of health care resources, major life stresses, prior physical or psychological trauma, depression or substance abuse, or disruptions in social or occupational functioning. Once recognized, anxiety disorders can be classified into 1 of the major categories listed below.

KEY TERMS[1]

Agoraphobia	*Anxiety about being confined without easy egress or escape, causing avoidance or endurance with marked distress.*
Anxiety	*Apprehension, uneasiness, or fear in response to a real or perceived threat.*
Anxiety disorder	*Excessive anxiety and worry, recurring more days than not, for at least 6 months.*
Anxiety due to drugs, medications, and medical illness	*Anxiety primarily resulting from the effects of drugs (cocaine, amphetamines, caffeine), drug withdrawal (alcohol, narcotics, sedatives, nicotine, caffeine); medications (decongestants, β-agonists, fluoxetine); or medical conditions (see Alarm Symptoms).*
Generalized anxiety disorder (GAD)	*Excessive anxiety, recurring more days than not for at least 6 months, associated with various objects, circumstances, or events.*
Obsessive-compulsive disorder (OCD)	*Recurrent, persistent, and intrusive thoughts, impulses, or images causing marked anxiety and distress, with an irresistible need to perform repetitive, time-consuming behaviors.*
Panic attacks	*Rapidly peaking (10 min), intense fear or alarm and at least 4 of the following 13 symptoms: abnormal heart beat, chest discomfort, sweating, shakiness, dyspnea or choking, smothering sensation, abdominal symptoms, dizziness or faintness, sense of unreality, fear of going crazy or losing control, fear of dying, numbness or tingling, hot flashes or chills.*

(continued)

KEY TERMS[1]

Panic disorder	*Recurrent, unexpected panic attacks, followed by at least 1 month of persistent concern about additional attacks, worry about implications or consequences, or a significant change in behavior in relation to the attacks.*
Phobia	*Persistent, irrational, intense anxiety and worry in response to specific external objects, activities, or situations.*
Posttraumatic stress disorder (PTSD)	*Persistent reexperience of a traumatic event involving the threat of death or serious injury to self or others, resulting in intense fear, helplessness, or horror.*
Social phobia	*Marked and persistent fear of social activities or performances involving possible scrutiny or evaluation by others, resulting in avoidance or endurance with intense anxiety or stress. Recognized as excessive or unreasonable.*
Specific phobia	*Marked and persistent fear precipitated immediately and consistently by the presence or anticipation of a specific object or situation, resulting in avoidance or endurance with intense anxiety or stress. Recognized as excessive or unreasonable.*

ETIOLOGY

Environmental factors, rather than specific genetic abnormalities, play a much more important role in the anxiety disorders. Studies have identified various alterations in neurotransmitters, regional brain activity, and hypothalamic-pituitary axis function, but no unifying theory has emerged. Among environmental factors, childhood adversity, traumatic experiences and major stress were associated with anxiety disorders in adulthood.[2]

Differential Diagnosis	Lifetime prevalence in US adults[a]
GAD	3–5%[3]
Panic attacks	7.3%[3]
Panic disorder	2–5%[3]
PTSD	9–12%[4]
Anxiety due to drugs, medications, and medical illness	
OCD	2–3%[5]
Agoraphobia	3.5–7%[3]
Social phobia	13.3%[3]
Specific phobias	15.7%[3]

[a]Prevalence estimate is unavailable when not indicated.

GETTING STARTED

• Before the visit, review the patient's problems; medications; past, family, social, and occupational history for relevant clues.

- Conduct the interview in an environment that is quiet, comfortable, private, and calming.
- Remind the patient that you will protect his or her confidentiality.
- Avoid distractions.
- Don't rush the patient's story.
- Use open-ended questioning, empathic listening, validation, and affirmation.
- After you have listened to the patient's story, proceed to focused, non-leading questions.
- Consider the NURS (naming, understanding, respecting, and supporting) framework for handling emotions and relationship-building.[6]
- Remember that many patients are not consciously aware of their anxiety or the relationship between anxiety and their symptoms.
- Screen for predisposing or aggravating factors, including comorbid mental disorders, stresses, substance abuse, and past abuse or neglect.
- Use decision-support tools and reminder systems as needed, including questionnaires and interview tools. Some useful online resources include the following:

Resource	Web site address
Anxiety Disorders Association of America	http://www.adaa.org/index.cfm
National Institute of Mental Health	http://www.nimh.nih.gov/anxiety/anxietymenu.cfm
Patient Health Questionnaire	http://www.depression-primarycare.org/clinicians/toolkits/materials/forms/phq9/questionnaire/
Hamilton Anxiety Scale	http://www.anxietyhelp.org/information/hama.html
Liebowitz Social Anxiety Scale	http://www.anxietyhelp.org/information/leibowitz.html

Open-ended questions

Tell me about your worries, fears, concerns and stresses, and how they affect you.

Can you identify anyone or anything that tends to bring on or worsen your feelings of worry, fear, concern, or stress?

When you feel worried, fearful, concerned or stressed, what helps you feel better?

Tips for effective interviewing

- *Establish a setting of comfort and trust*
- *Listen actively and empathically*
- *Be supportive and nonjudgmental*
- *Handle emotions effectively (NURS)*
- *Avoid distractions, leading questions*
- *Involve family members as appropriate*

INTERVIEW FRAMEWORK

- Assess for alarm symptoms.
- Classify the anxiety disorder: generalized, phobic, obsessive-compulsive, posttraumatic, panic, drugs.
- Identify important comorbidities and risk factors.

IDENTIFYING ALARM SYMPTOMS

Anxiety can be serious or even life-threatening when it aggravates a serious underlying medical condition (eg, angina, heart failure, asthma), or when it precipitates a reaction that is maladaptive (substance abuse) or actively self-destructive (suicide).

Serious Diagnoses	Lifetime prevalence by condition[a]
Major depression	*60–90% of patients have GAD, social phobia, or panic disorder*
Alcoholism	*Social phobia: 16%*[7]
Suicide	
Medical illnesses	
Dementia	
Eating disorders	
Somatization disorder	
Personality disorders	

[a]Prevalence estimate is unavailable when not indicated.

Alarm symptoms	Consider
Cognitive impairment	*Dementia*
Confusion or agitation	*Substance abuse or withdrawal*
	Medications
	Hypoxia
	Infection
	Head injury
	Hypoglycemia
Syncope	*Temporal lobe epilepsy*
	Cardiac arrhythmia
Severe or changing headache	*Head injury*
	Brain infection
	Central nervous system tumor or hemorrhage
	Temporal arteritis
Dyspnea	*Panic disorder*
	Asthma
	Pneumothorax
	Pulmonary embolism
	Heart failure
	Hypoxia
Exertional chest pain	*Angina pectoris*
Thyroid enlargement	*Hyperthyroidism*
	Hypothyroidism
Rash, arthralgia, hematuria	*Vasculitis*
	Rheumatoid arthritis
	Systemic lupus erythematosus
Jaundice	*Infectious mononucleosis*
	Viral hepatitis

FOCUSED QUESTIONS

After listening to the patient's worries, fears, concerns, stresses, precipitating factors and coping responses, proceed to focused questions to determine the specific anxiety disorder.[8] Remember that multiple disorders may be present.

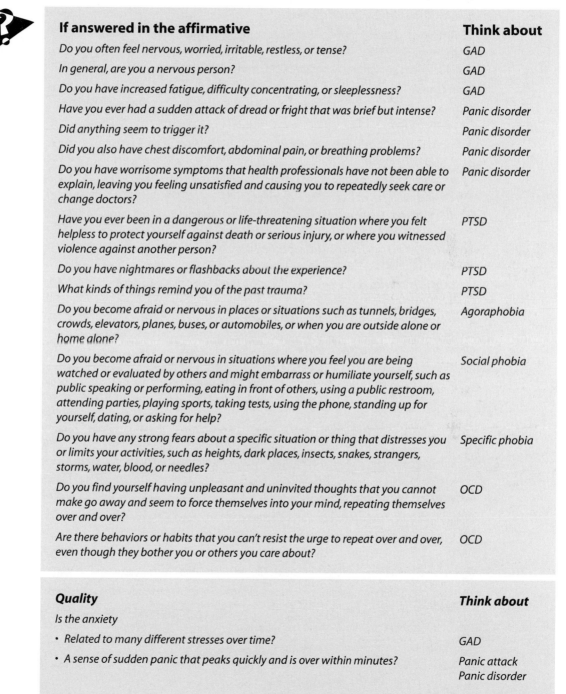

If answered in the affirmative	Think about
Do you often feel nervous, worried, irritable, restless, or tense?	GAD
In general, are you a nervous person?	GAD
Do you have increased fatigue, difficulty concentrating, or sleeplessness?	GAD
Have you ever had a sudden attack of dread or fright that was brief but intense?	Panic disorder
Did anything seem to trigger it?	Panic disorder
Did you also have chest discomfort, abdominal pain, or breathing problems?	Panic disorder
Do you have worrisome symptoms that health professionals have not been able to explain, leaving you feeling unsatisfied and causing you to repeatedly seek care or change doctors?	Panic disorder
Have you ever been in a dangerous or life-threatening situation where you felt helpless to protect yourself against death or serious injury, or where you witnessed violence against another person?	PTSD
Do you have nightmares or flashbacks about the experience?	PTSD
What kinds of things remind you of the past trauma?	PTSD
Do you become afraid or nervous in places or situations such as tunnels, bridges, crowds, elevators, planes, buses, or automobiles, or when you are outside alone or home alone?	Agoraphobia
Do you become afraid or nervous in situations where you feel you are being watched or evaluated by others and might embarrass or humiliate yourself, such as public speaking or performing, eating in front of others, using a public restroom, attending parties, playing sports, taking tests, using the phone, standing up for yourself, dating, or asking for help?	Social phobia
Do you have any strong fears about a specific situation or thing that distresses you or limits your activities, such as heights, dark places, insects, snakes, strangers, storms, water, blood, or needles?	Specific phobia
Do you find yourself having unpleasant and uninvited thoughts that you cannot make go away and seem to force themselves into your mind, repeating themselves over and over?	OCD
Are there behaviors or habits that you can't resist the urge to repeat over and over, even though they bother you or others you care about?	OCD

Quality	*Think about*
Is the anxiety	
• *Related to many different stresses over time?*	GAD
• *A sense of sudden panic that peaks quickly and is over within minutes?*	Panic attack Panic disorder

(continued)

Quality	*Think about*
• *Related to situations in which you would have trouble escaping if trapped?*	Agoraphobia
• *Characterized by a fear of embarrassment and humiliation?*	Social phobia
• *Limited to a specific situation or object?*	Specific phobia
• *Described as a repetitive series of intrusive, irrational thoughts and irresistible urges to do something?*	OCD
• *Characterized by nightmares or flashbacks of traumatic experiences?*	PTSD

Time course	*Think about*
Describe a typical episode of worry, fear, or anxiety. What triggers it and how long does it usually last?	
It comes on in a rush, gets very bad very fast, but goes away fast.	Panic attack Panic disorder
It starts when I have to do something in front of a group, but it goes away soon afterwards.	Social phobia
It starts when I have to be in a crowded room far from the door, and goes away when I get out or get close to the door.	Agoraphobia
It comes on when I start climbing a ladder, and doesn't go away until my feet are back on the ground.	Specific phobia
Lots of different things can bring it on and I'm not sure it ever goes away completely. I'm just a worrier.	GAD
It comes on whenever I get thoughts about being responsible for my family getting hurt and it doesn't go away until I've checked to make sure the stove is off and the doors are locked, 12 times!	OCD
I seem to get it more if I drink less, and I feel better if I have a beer or take a sleeping pill. It seems to be worse since my thyroid medication was increased.	Anxiety due to medications, sedative-hypnotic withdrawal, or alcohol withdrawal
It happens if I get short of breath after I fall asleep, or if I get chest pain when I walk.	Anxiety due to medical illness

Associated symptoms	*Think about*
When your worry, fear, or anxiety is bad, do you notice any other symptoms?	
My face turns red, my heart beats fast, and my hands get clammy	Social phobia Specific phobia
I get really fatigued, my muscles tighten up, I forget things, and I can't sleep.	GAD
My head, chest, and stomach hurt; my heart beats fast; I feel faint; and my hands go numb.	Panic attack Panic disorder
I "fly off the handle," ache just about everywhere, or just feel numb all over.	PTSD
I get a bad rash on my hands or bald spots.	OCD

Modifying symptoms	Think about
Does anything in particular tend to trigger an episode of fear, worry, or distress?	
It seems like it can be almost anything, depending on what's going on in my life.	GAD
Anytime I have to perform a solo on my instrument at a band concert.	Social phobia
Whenever I have to clean out the garage, where there might be a spider.	Specific phobia
I get it every time I'm in a crowded room where I can't see a way to get out easily.	Agoraphobia
I get it whenever the thought of germs pops into my head.	OCD
It happens whenever a car engine backfires suddenly.	PTSD
I had it right after my mother died, and again after my car slid across the highway in a snowstorm and I barely missed getting hit by a cement truck.	Panic disorder
Every time my asthma gets bad, and I have to go to the emergency department.	Anxiety due to medical illness

DIAGNOSTIC APPROACH

The first step in diagnosing anxiety disorders is to determine whether a serious underlying medical condition or a separate primary mental health disorder is causing the patient's anxiety. In addition, anxiety due to drugs should be excluded.

Questioning should then focus on whether anxiety comes on as a sudden attack without warning as is characteristic of panic disorder, or is more predictably associated with known triggering objects, events, or circumstances. When anxiety triggers are diverse and persistent, general anxiety disorder is the likely diagnosis. When they are specific and known, phobias, OCD, or PTSD is likely.

CAVEATS

- Somatic symptoms of severe anxiety can cause affected people to worry that they have a serious undiagnosed medical illness. Such patients are at risk for potentially harmful tests and treatments as well as distress when a diagnosis that explains their symptoms is not forthcoming. The approach to such patients includes careful assessment for underlying medical conditions and patient education about the relationship between anxiety and somatic symptoms.

- Remember that a patient's beliefs about the causes of their symptoms can significantly affect the diagnosis made by their provider. Patients who "explain away" (normalize) their anxiety-associated symptoms ("I'm tired because I don't have time to exercise") are much less likely to be diagnosed with anxiety than patients who use psychological terms ("I'm emotionally worn-out").[10]

- Patients with anxiety are often ashamed or embarrassed, or concerned that they will be judged by their provider. Establishing a positive relationship with anxious patients may encourage them to reveal, acknowledge, and undergo treatment for the disorder.

PROGNOSIS

Without treatment, anxiety disorders generally persist and cause significant hardship to patients and their families. Since most patients benefit considerably from therapy, accurate and timely diagnosis helps them get the care needed to enhance their functioning and happiness.

GAD	*Treated patients generally have a reduction in symptoms but typically relapse if therapy is discontinued.*
Agoraphobia	*Some untreated patients abuse sedatives and alcohol to allay anxiety. Nearly all agoraphobic patients respond well to therapy.*
Social phobia and specific phobia	*With treatment, the great majority of patients show at least moderate improvement.*
Obsessive-compulsive disorder	*With the advent of potent serotonin reuptake inhibitors, the great majority of treated patients improve but few go into remission. Continued therapy is required to prevent relapse.*
PTSD	*With prompt intervention, most patients with early PTSD respond rapidly and well. Chronic PTSD is more difficult to treat and more likely to be associated with ongoing and variable disability.*

REFERENCES

1. American Psychiatric Association. *Diagnostic and Statistical Manual of Mental Disorders.* 4th ed. American Psychiatric Association; 1994.

2. Molnar BE, Buka SL, Kessler RC. Child sexual abuse and subsequent psychopathology: results from the National Comorbidity Survey. *Am J Public Health.* 2001;91:753–760.

3. Kessler RC, McGonagle KA, Zhao S, et al. Lifetime and 12-month prevalence of DSM-III-R psychiatric disorders in the United States. Results from the National Comorbidity Survey. *Arch Gen Psychiatry.* 1994;51:8–19.

4. Breslau N, Davis GC, Andreski P, Peterson E. Traumatic events and posttraumatic stress disorder in an urban population of young adults. *Arch Gen Psychiatry.* 1991;48:216–222.

5. Karno M, Golding JM, Sorenson SB, Burnam MA. The epidemiology of obsessive-compulsive disorder in five US communities. *Arch Gen Psychiatry.* 1988;45:1094–1099.

6. Smith RC. *The Patient's Story: Intergrated Patient-Doctor Interviewing.* 1st ed. Little, Brown and Company; 1996.

7. Schneier F, Martin L, Liebowitz M, et al. Alcohol abuse in social phobia. *J Anx Disord.* 1989;3:15.

8. Zimmerman M. *Diagnosing DSM-IV Psychiatric Disorders in Primary Care Settings: An Interview Guide for the Nonpsychiatrist Physician.* East Greenwich: Psych Products Press; 1994.

9. Feldman M. Managing psychiatric disorders in primary care: 2. Anxiety. *Hosp Pract.* 2000;35:77–84.

10. Kessler D, Lloyd K, Lewis G, Gray DP. Cross sectional study of symptom attribution and recognition of depression and anxiety in primary care. *BMJ.* 1999;318:436–439.

SUGGESTED READING

Levinson W, Engel C. Anxiety. In: Feldman M, Christensen J, editors. *Behavioral Medicine in Primary Care: A Practical Guide.* Appleton & Lange; 1997:193-211.

Moses S. Anxiety. In: Moses S, editor. *Family Practice Notebook.* Family Practice Notebook, LLC: Lino Lakes. Electronic text. 2003.

Diagnostic Approach: Anxiety

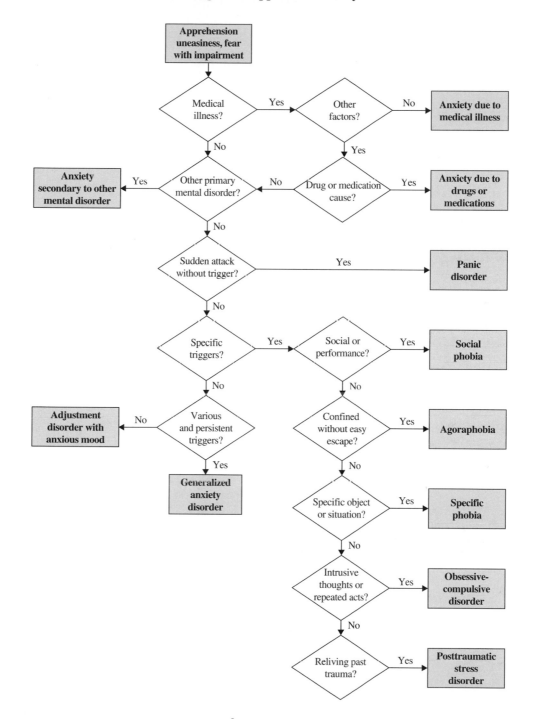

(Adapted , with permission, from Feldman M.[9])

Depressed Mood

John W. Williams Jr., MD, MHSc, & Linda Harpole, MD, MPH

Clinical depression is a syndrome characterized by the following cardinal symptoms: depressed mood or anhedonia, additional psychological (eg, decreased concentration) or somatic symptoms (eg, insomnia), and impaired functioning. In settings where primary care patients are screened systematically for clinical depression, 10–30% report depressed mood. The US Preventive Services Task Force recommends a brief 2-item screen in settings organized to offer high quality depression care.[1] Although depressed mood is a cardinal feature of depression, most patients present with physical complaints. If systematic screening is not implemented, clinicians should consider clinical depression in patients who present with a "red flag" for clinical depression such as insomnia, fatigue, chronic pain, recent life changes or stressors, fair or poor self-rated health, and unexplained physical symptoms.[2]

KEY TERMS[3]

Anhedonia	*Markedly diminished interest or pleasure in almost all activities most of the day, nearly every day.*
Appetite or weight change	*Substantial change in appetite nearly every day or unintentional weight loss or gain (eg, ≥ 5% of body weight in 1 month).*
Decreased concentration	*Diminished ability to think or concentrate, or indecisiveness nearly every day.*
Decreased energy	*Fatigue or loss of energy nearly every day.*
Depressed mood	*Depressed mood most of the day, nearly every day.*
Guilt or feelings of worthlessness	*Feelings of worthlessness or excessive guilt nearly every day.*
Increased or decreased psychomotor activity	*Psychomotor agitation or retardation nearly every day.*
Sleep disturbance	*Insomnia or hypersomnia nearly every day.*
Suicidal ideation	*Recurrent thoughts of death or suicide.*

ETIOLOGY[4]

Female gender, prior depression, chronic medical illness, and depression in a first-degree relative are risk factors for clinical depression. Among patients with depressed mood or a positive depression screen, the prevalence of clinically significant depressive disorders varies depending on the clinical setting and patient characteristics. In primary care settings, approximately 25–50% of such patients will have transient dysphoria (eg, feeling down because their sports team lost the big game) or more persistent but mild symptoms that do not impair function and do not meet formal criteria for a psychiatric diagnosis.

Among the remaining patients, approximately 25% will have major depression, 25% will have dysthymic disorder or depression not otherwise specified (NOS), and a small proportion will have bipolar disorder or general medical causes for the depressive symptoms.

Major depressive disorder is characterized by ≥ 5 of 9 depressive symptoms, including depressed mood or anhedonia, which impair function and last ≥ 2 weeks. Dysthymic disorder is a chronic but milder depressive disorder, characterized by depressed mood that is present more days than not for 2 or more years, in addition to other depressive symptoms. Depressive disorder NOS is a milder depressive disorder that does not meet criteria for major depression or dysthymia. It is characterized by 2 to 4 depressive symptoms, including depressed mood or anhedonia, which impair function and last ≥ 2 weeks. Depressive disorders commonly co-occur with other psychiatric disorders.

Differential Diagnosis[5–8]	Prevalence[a]	Prevalence in unselected primary care patients
Bipolar disorder	2–10%	0.5–2%
Major depressive disorder	20–30%	4.8–8.6%
Dysthymic disorder	5–15%	2.1–3.7%
Depression NOS	10–15%	4.4–5.4%
Adjustment disorder		Approximately 4%
Bereavement		1–2%
Mood disorder due to a general medical condition	Uncertain but < 5%	Uncertain but very low
Premenstrual dysphoric disorder		2–9% of women of reproductive age
Other psychiatric illness, such as alcohol or anxiety disorders	10–50% (may co-occur with depressive disorder)	Alcohol use disorder 5.2–9% Anxiety disorder 7.3–11.8%
Transient dysphoria or mild symptoms not meeting criteria for a psychiatric diagnosis	25–50%	5–30%

[a]Among persons with depressed mood or a positive depression screen; prevalence is unknown when not indicated.

GETTING STARTED

- It may be useful to begin with a general question such as "How are things at home or work?" or "How are you doing emotionally?"
- Since clinically significant depression requires 1 of 2 cardinal symptoms, an efficient strategy is to ask specifically about depressed mood and anhedonia. Since different age groups use differing terms for depression, it is best to use several synonyms. The screen is considered positive if patients endorse depressed mood or anhedonia; the likelihood ratio for a positive screen (LR+) = 2.7 and likelihood ratio for a negative screen (LR−) = 0.14.[9]

Questions	Remember
Over the past month, have you been feeling down, depressed, or hopeless?	Depressed patients may make the interviewer feel sad. Use your emotional response as a diagnostic clue.

Over the past month, have you been bothered by little interest or pleasure in doing things?	*This symptom is often more prominent than depressed mood in older adults.*

INTERVIEW FRAMEWORK

- If depressed mood or anhedonia is present, inquire about additional depressive symptoms by clinical interview or administer a depression questionnaire such as the "Patient Health Questionnaire."[10]
- Ask about impact on daily functioning, since impaired function at home, work, or in interpersonal relationships is required to diagnose clinical depression.
- Assess for alarm symptoms of suicidality.
- Consider secondary causes such as medications, hypothyroidism, malignancy, autoimmune or central nervous system disorders.
- Consider symptom pattern, duration, and associated symptoms to make a specific diagnosis.

Medications Associated with Clinical Depression

Definite causal relationship	**Possible causal relationship**
• *High-dose reserpine*	• *Oral contraceptives*
• *High-dose glucocorticoids*	• *Carbamazepine*
• *Anabolic steroids*	• *Phenobarbital*
• *Cocaine or amphetamine withdrawal*	
• *Interferon*	

IDENTIFYING ALARM SYMPTOMS

Since patients rarely volunteer thoughts of suicide, it is important to ask directly. The topic may be introduced by asking "Have you been feeling that life is not worth living or that you would be better off dead?" Another approach is to ask "Sometimes when a person feels down or depressed they might think about dying. Have you been having any thoughts like that?" If patients have suicidal ideation, ask more detailed questions to distinguish passive from active suicidal ideation and to assess risk for suicide. Physical symptoms that are inconsistent with the overall severity of depression, such as marked weight loss with otherwise mild depression, suggest alternative diagnoses such as underlying malignancy.

Alarm symptoms	**Comment**
Suicide[10,11]	
Have you had any thoughts of hurting yourself in some way?"	*A response of "not at all" puts the patient at very low risk.*
Have you made any plans or considered a method that you might use to harm yourself?	*If yes, ask for details.*
Have you ever attempted to harm yourself?"	*Past attempts are a risk factor for future attempts.[11]*

(continued)

Suicide[10,11]	Comment
There's a big difference between having a thought and acting on a thought. Do you think you might actually make an attempt to hurt yourself in the near future?	A positive response puts the patient at very high risk for suicide.
Serious general medical conditions	**Think about**
Have you lost weight despite having a normal or near normal appetite?	Malignancy
Have you felt cold when everyone else felt comfortable? Have you noticed dry skin or constipation?	Hypothyroidism
Have you noticed a rash, dry eyes or mouth, difficulty swallowing food, or pain/swelling in the hands or feet?	Autoimmune disorders (eg, Sjögren syndrome)
Have you noticed a tremor or a change in gait? Have you had episodes of weakness on 1 side of the body?	Central nervous system disorders (Parkinson disease or recurrent strokes)

FOCUSED QUESTIONS

Assessing DSM Symptoms[3,9,12]

- To assess the effects of depressive symptoms on function, ask "How difficult has the (fill in the pertinent symptoms) made it for you to do your work, take care of things at home, or get along with other people?"

Questions	Think about
How has your mood been lately? Have you been feeling down, depressed, or hopeless? How often does that happen? How long does it last?	Depressed mood
Have you lost interest in your usual activities? Do you get less pleasure in things you used to enjoy?	Anhedonia
How have you been sleeping? How does that compare to your normal sleep?	Sleep disturbance
Has there been any change in your appetite or weight?	Appetite or weight change
Have you noticed a decrease in your energy level?	Decreased energy
Have you been feeling fidgety or had problems sitting still? Have you felt slowed down, like you were moving in slow motion or stuck in mud?	Increased or decreased psychomotor activity
Have you been having trouble concentrating? Is it harder to make decisions than before?	Decreased concentration
Are you feeling guilty or blaming yourself for things? How would you describe yourself to someone who had never met you before?	Guilt or feelings of worthlessness

Have you felt that life is not worth living or that you would be better off dead?	*Suicidal ideation*
Sometimes when a person feels down or depressed, they might think about dying. Have you been having any thoughts like that?	

Quality

Think about

At least 5 DSM symptoms including depressed mood or anhedonia	*Major depressive disorder*
Milder severity including depressed mood or anhedonia	*Dysthymia* *Depressive disorder NOS* *Adjustment disorder*
Mild symptoms that do not impair function	*Transient dysphoria*

Time course

Think about

Did these symptoms begin after the death of a loved one?	*Bereavement*
Did these symptoms begin during a time of stress?	*Adjustment disorder with depressed mood*
Have you ever seen or experienced a traumatic event in which you or someone else's life was in danger? How about threat of serious injury?	*Posttraumatic stress disorder*
Have these symptoms been present on most days for at least 2 years?	*Dysthymia or chronic major depressive disorder*
Do these episodes occur at a particular time of the year?	*Seasonal affective disorder*
Do your symptoms begin during the week prior to menses and remit within a few days of menses?	*Premenstrual dysphoric disorder*

Associated symptoms

Think about

Have you ever had periods where your mood was very good, or too good, for no reason?	*Bipolar disorder*
Were these periods accompanied by racing thoughts, reduced need for sleep, or increased energy?	*Bipolar disorder*
Did it get you into trouble, for instance spending too much money, impulsively traveling, or taking on too many projects?	*Bipolar disorder*
Have you ever had visions or seen things that other people could not see? Have you heard things that other people could not hear, such as noises, or the voices of people whispering or talking?	*Depressive disorder with psychotic features* *Psychotic disorders such as schizophrenia or schizoaffective disorder*
Have you ever had a panic attack, where out of the blue, you experienced intense anxiety, fear, or discomfort for no apparent reason?	*Panic disorder*
Have you felt nervous, anxious, or on edge on more than half the days in the last month?	*Generalized anxiety disorder (see Chapter 59)*

(continued)

Associated symptoms	Think about
Do you drink alcohol? Tell me about your drinking habits.	
• Was there ever a time when you drank too much?	Alcohol disorder Substance-induced mood disorder
• Has drinking alcohol ever caused problems such as missing work, legal problems, driving while intoxicated?	Alcohol disorder Substance-induced mood disorder
Modifying symptoms	**Think about**
Some people find their mood changes frequently—as if they spend every day on an emotional roller coaster. Does this sound like you? Some people prefer to be the center of attention, while others are content to remain on the edge of things. How would you describe yourself?	Personality disorder is suggested by frequent mood swings or need to be the center of attention (particularly if bothered by others being in the spotlight)

DIAGNOSTIC APPROACH

Once a clinical depression is diagnosed, additional history should be elicited about factors that may affect treatment. First, explore the patient's understanding and acceptance of the diagnosis. Stigmatizing beliefs about depression or outright rejection of the diagnosis may interfere with treatment adherence. Second, ask about prior episodes and response to treatment. The risk of relapse, and hence the need for longer-term treatment, increases with the number of prior episodes. Treatments that have been effective for past episodes are likely to be effective for the current episode. See Diagnostic Approach: Depressed Mood.

CAVEATS

- Men and adolescents may describe excessive irritability rather than depressed mood.
- Because the psychological and physical symptoms of depression may overlap with other physical illness, diagnosing depression in patients with severe or multiple chronic medical illnesses can be especially challenging. The DSM criteria suggest counting symptoms toward a clinical depression diagnosis unless the symptom is "clearly and fully accounted for by a general medical condition."
- Distinguishing early dementia from depression may be difficult; in many instances the conditions co-occur. If the depressive symptoms are at least as prominent as those suggesting dementia, diagnose and treat for depression. If the patient does not respond to depression treatment, further evaluation is needed.
- Although depressive disorders are common globally, symptom descriptions (eg, "nervios") and illness attributions (eg, susto, Hwa-byung) may vary across cultures.[13]

PROGNOSIS

Major depression is a relapsing illness for many patients; the probability of recurrence is 50% after a single episode, increasing to 90% after 3 episodes. Antidepressant medication and depression specific psychological therapies improve symptoms significantly for about 70% of individuals completing a course of therapy. Chronic major depression (lasting ≥ 2 years) is more treatment resistant and combined antidepressant and psychotherapy is more effective. For patients with depressive symptoms only, major depression will develop in approximately 25% within 2 years.

REFERENCES

1. US Preventive Services Task Force. Screening for depression: recommendations and rationale. *Ann Intern Med.* 2002;136: 760–764.

2. Jackson JL, O'Malley PG, Kroenke K. Clinical predictors of mental disorders among medical outpatients. Validation of the "S4" model. *Psychosomatics.* 1998;39:431–436.

3. American Psychiatric Association. *Diagnostic and Statistical Manual of Mental Disorders: DSM-IV.* Washington, DC; American Psychiatric Association, 1994.

4. Depression Guideline Panel. Depression in Primary Care: Volume 1. Detection and Diagnosis. Clinical Practice Guideline, Number 5. ed. Rockville, MD: US Department of Health and Human Services, Public Health Service, Agency for Health Care Policy and Research, AHCPR Publication No. 93-0550; 1993.

5. Coyne JC, Fechner-Gates S, Schwenk TL. Prevalence, nature, and comorbidity of depressive disorders in primary care. *Gen Hosp Psychiatry.* 1994;16:267–276.

6. Piver A, Yatham LN, Lam RW. Bipolar spectrum disorders: new perspectives. *Can Fam Physician.* 2002;48:896–904.

7. Narrow WE, Rae DS, Robbins LN, Regier DA. Revised prevalence estimates of mental disorders in the United States. *Arch Gen Psychiatry.* 2002;59:115–123.

8. Sherbourne CD, Jackson CA, Meredith LS, Camp P, Wells KB. Prevalence of comorbid anxiety disorders in primary care outpatients. *Arch Fam Med.* 1996;5:27–34.

9. Williams JW Jr, Noel PH, Cordes JA, Ramirez G, Pignone M. Is this patient clinically depressed? *JAMA.* 2002;287:1160–1170.

10. Depression Management Tool Kit, Macarthur Initiative on depression in primary care at Dartmouth and Duke. 2003 Trustees of Dartmouth College. Appendix II. http://www.depression-primarycare.org/clinicians. Accessed 8/21/03.

11. Mann JJ. A current perspective of suicide and attempted suicide. *Ann Intern Med.* 2002;136:302–311.

12. Zimmerman M. Diagnosing DSM-IV psychiatric disorders in primary care settings. An interview guide for the nonpsychiatrist physician. East Greenwich, RI: Psych Products Press; 1994.

13. Kirmayer LJ . Cultural variations in the clinical presentation of depression and anxiety: implications for diagnosis and treatment. *J Clin Psychiatry.* 2001;62:22–28.

Diagnostic Approach: Depressed Mood

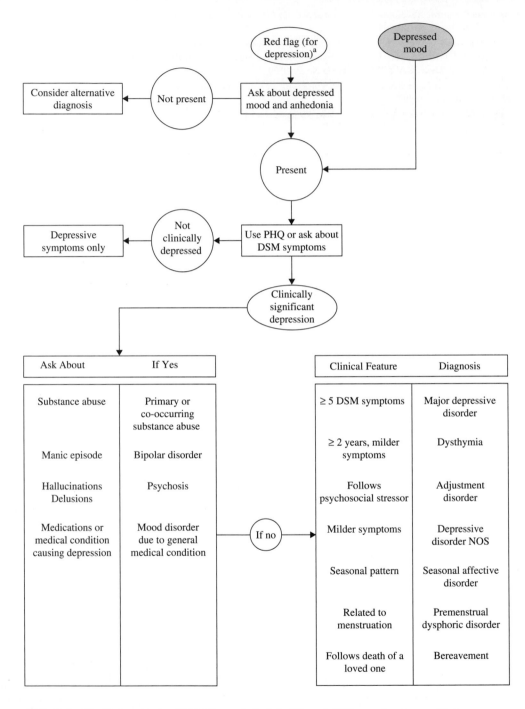

PHQ, Patient Health Questionaire; DSM, Diagnostic Statistical Manual; NOS, not otherwise specified.

aRed flags for clinical depression include: insomnia, fatigue, chronic pain, recent life changes or stressors, fair or poor self-rated health, and unexplained physical symptoms.

SECTION XIII
Communicating the History

The Case Presentation

Lawrence M. Tierney, Jr., MD

The spoken case presentation is the concise summary of the history and physical examination. Unlike the written version in a patient's chart, the oral presentation is dynamic and ranges from a brief summary given by phone to a consultant to a more formal presentation to a large medical audience at an academic session. Succinctness and organization are especially important, as the presenter has neither the luxury of omitting important details nor time for repetition. Brevity is of paramount importance; simply reading from the chart defeats the purpose of the exercise. Highlighted in this chapter are the essential components of the presentation: the chief complaint, the history of present illness (HPI), the past medical history, the family and social history, the review of systems and, finally, the physical examination findings.

The chief complaint should be as brief as possible, in essence articulating the principal subject under consideration. Invariably, there is one overriding problem in the majority of patients, and a listener is helped enormously by recognizing what it is at the start. Indeed, from the first words of a presentation, a listener is formulating possible diagnoses. A lengthy chief complaint that includes details of past history serves only to confuse the listener, and lengthen the presentation—a cardinal sin. The patient's own words need be mentioned only if they illuminate the problem under consideration. The source is always assumed to be the patient, and its content accurate; if considered otherwise by the presenter, this qualification must be made clear. The patient is best identified as a man or woman, which are more respectful designations than male or female. Mentioning the patient's occupation is often helpful.

The HPI is the most important part of the exercise. If the problem is not understood by the conclusion of a properly presented HPI, it is unlikely to be understood after extensive evaluation. Instead of calendar dates, the duration of time prior to the episode of care should be specified. Calendar dates require a listener to remember the current date and subtract backwards to determine the length of the problem, an unnecessary distraction.

The initial step in organizing the HPI is identifying the logical parts of the present illness. For example, *beginning* the HPI with a history of hypercholesterolemia is sensible in a middle-aged man with chest pain. Thereafter, events should be given chronologically, up to the present moment. Many presentations are confusing because they include recent information first, followed by previous but relevant data. Instead, the HPI should be related like a story, with a beginning and an end.

What about the inclusion of pertinent negative historical information? Presenting negative data is often unnecessary when positive data tell the story. However, negative data become extremely significant in narrowing the differential diagnosis when the positive data leave the listener uncertain. For example, a 27-year-old woman with crushing substernal chest pain that radiates to both arms and is associated with a sense of impending doom sparks the interest of the listener; the differential diagnosis includes psychiatric, cardiovascular, gastrointestinal, or drug-induced causes. In this case, presenting the absence of symptoms helps the listener focus his or her differential diagnosis.

The past medical history, while a crucial component of the patient's written record, adds little to the presentation. If a historical fact is deemed important, it likely belongs in the HPI, and some past history may be eliminated entirely in the interest of time. The same is true for the family history; a lengthy pedigree often serves no function.

Presenting the social history is always important, and is a humanizing endeavor. Statements such as "the social history was noncontributory" diminish the practice of medicine by rendering patients pathophysiologic specimens rather than human beings. In addition, such knowledge may facilitate the doctor–patient interaction. Although medications and habits are often included at this point, such items may be more relevant in the HPI.

The review of systems should be as brief as possible, containing only those symptoms felt to be significant enough to merit further investigation. Including numerous positive responses by well-meaning patients only dilutes the significance of truly important symptoms.

It is of utmost importance that in the spoken presentation information not be repeated. The presenter decides where a fact best belongs, and its repetition would only consume precious time.

Though the physical examination is beyond the scope of this book, a few words are in order. It is best delivered in simple declarative sentences. Qualifiers such as remarkable and unremarkable, though widespread in medical parlance, are clichés that do not assist the listener. A complete examination can be presented in less than 1 minute, and a brief mention of each system tells the listener that they all have been examined. For instance, "the chest was clear" is an entirely appropriate elucidation of the pulmonary exam in a patient whose symptoms do not suggest lung disease. All positive findings, expected or not, are given, while negative data focus on signs logically expected by a listener. "There were no spider angiomata" in the patient with liver disease tells the listener that the examiner sought them. Announcing the *system* being presented (for example, "*chest*—he had no wheezes, rales, or rhonchi") is unnecessary because the listener will know what part of the body is being described.

Although laboratory or other diagnostic tests, problem lists, and the assessment are not the focus of this book, a few points are pertinent. The specific laboratory data presented depend on the setting, such as a hospital or clinic, and the nature of the patient's symptoms or clinical problem. Some listeners prefer that the presentation be concluded with a brief case synthesis, but a lengthy assessment and plan is better placed in the written record. Once again, the issue is time, and it is well known that the captive audience attention span rarely exceeds 7 minutes.

In summary, the best oral presentation resembles a narrative, given chronologically and delivered in language similar to routine conversation. The ability to articulate a crisp, clear presentation requires practice and skill. It is a lost art, but not one that cannot be retrieved.

Index

Note: Page numbers followed by *f* and *t* indicate figures and tables, respectively.